Moderate and Deep Sedation in Clinical Practice

Moderate and Deep Sedation in Clinical Practice

Third Edition

Edited by

Richard D. Urman, MD, MBA, FASA
Jay J. Jacoby Professor and Chair
Department of Anesthesiology
Anesthesiologist-In-Chief
The Ohio State University Health System
Columbus, Ohio, USA

Alan David Kaye, MD, PhD, DABA, DABPM, DABIPP, CCSM, FASA
Immediate Former Vice Chancellor of Academic Affairs, Chief Academic Officer, and Provost
Interventional Pain Program Fellowship Director
Vice Chairman of Research, Department of Anesthesiology
Professor, Department of Anesthesiology and Pharmacology, Toxicology, and Neurosciences
Louisiana State University School of Medicine
Shreveport, Louisiana, USA

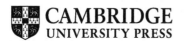

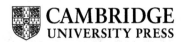

Shaftesbury Road, Cambridge CB2 8EA, United Kingdom

One Liberty Plaza, 20th Floor, New York, NY 10006, USA

477 Williamstown Road, Port Melbourne, VIC 3207, Australia

314–321, 3rd Floor, Plot 3, Splendor Forum, Jasola District Centre,
New Delhi – 110025, India

103 Penang Road, #05–06/07, Visioncrest Commercial, Singapore 238467

Cambridge University Press is part of Cambridge University Press &
Assessment, a department of the University of Cambridge.

We share the University's mission to contribute to society through the
pursuit of education, learning and research at the highest international levels
of excellence.

www.cambridge.org
Information on this title: www.cambridge.org/9781009233316

DOI: 10.1017/9781009233293

When citing this work, please include a reference to the
DOI 10.1017/9781009233293

First published 2012
Second edition 2017
Third edition 2025

A catalogue record for this publication is available from the British Library

*A Cataloging-in-Publication data record for this book is available from the
Library of Congress*

ISBN 978-1-009-23331-6 Paperback

Cambridge University Press & Assessment has no responsibility for the
persistence or accuracy of URLs for external or third-party internet websites
referred to in this publication and does not guarantee that any content on
such websites is, or will remain, accurate or appropriate.

....

Every effort has been made in preparing this book to provide accurate and
up-to-date information that is in accord with accepted standards and practice
at the time of publication. Although case histories are drawn from actual
cases, every effort has been made to disguise the identities of the individuals
involved. Nevertheless, the authors, editors, and publishers can make no
warranties that the information contained herein is totally free from error,
not least because clinical standards are constantly changing through research
and regulation. The authors, editors, and publishers therefore disclaim all
liability for direct or consequential damages resulting from the use of
material contained in this book. Readers are strongly advised to pay careful
attention to information provided by the manufacturer of any drugs or
equipment that they plan to use.

To my wife Dr. Kim Kaye for being the best
spouse a man could ask for in his life.
To my mother Florence Feldman who while
enduring a lifetime of pain and suffering with
seven back surgeries, taught me tremendous things
about pain, to accomplish tasks with the highest
of quality, and to reach my dreams and goals.
To my brother Dr. Adam M. Kaye, Pharm D,
for his loving support and help over the past
50 plus years.
To all my teachers and colleagues at the University
of Arizona in Tucson, Ochsner Clinic in New
Orleans, Massachusetts General Hospital/Harvard
School of Medicine in Boston, Tulane School of
Medicine in New Orleans, Texas Tech Health
Sciences Center in Lubbock, LSU School of
Medicine in New Orleans, and LSU School of
Medicine in Shreveport.

Alan David Kaye, MD, PhD

To my patients who inspired me to write this book
to help other practitioners improve their care
To my mentors for their encouragement and
support
To my students and trainees so that they can
use this guide to better understand the needs
of these patients
To my family: my wife Dr. Zina Matlyuk, MD,
my daughters Abigail and Isabelle who make it
all possible and worth it, every day.
And finally, to my parents, Tanya and Dennis
Urman.

Richard D. Urman, MD, MBA

Contents

Contributors

Mary Antonelli PhD, RN, MPH
Tan Chingfen Graduate School of
Nursing, University of Massachusetts
Chan Medical School Worcester, MA,
USA

Nicholas M. Bacher, MD
David Gefen School of Medicine at UCLA,
Los Angeles, CA, USA

Ezra Burch, MD
Brigham and Women's Hospital, Boston,
MA, USA and Harvard School of
Medicine, Boston, MA, USA

Elyse M. Cornett Bradley, PhD, RYT
Louisiana State University Health Sciences
Center, Shreveport, Shreveport, LA, USA

Katherine S. Cox, MD
Tulane University Medical Center, New
Orleans, LA, USA

**Laurie Demeule, MSN, RN, CNL,
CVRN-BC**
Brigham and Women's Hospital, Boston,
MA, USA

Karen B. Domino, MD
University of Washington, Seattle, WA,
USA

Chelsi J. Flanagan, DO, MPH
Ochsner Clinic Foundation, New Orleans,
LA, USA

Charles J. Fox III, MD
Louisiana State University Health
Shreveport, School of Medicine,
Shreveport, LA, USA

**John P. Gaillard, MD FACC, FACEP,
FCCM, FCCP**
Wake Forest Baptist Medical Center,
Winston Salem, NC, USA

Iaswarya Ganapathiraju, DO
Wake Forest Baptist Medical Center,
Winston Salem, NC, USA

Julie A. Gayle, MD
Louisiana State University Health Sciences
Center, School of Medicine, New Orleans,
LA, USA

G. E. Ghali, DDS, MD, FACS, FRCS(Ed)
Louisiana State University Health
Shreveport, School of Medicine,
Shreveport, LA, USA

Emily Goldenberg, MD
University of California – Irvine, CA, USA

Lisa Govoni, MSN RN CNL CCRN
Brigham and Women's Hospital, Boston,
MA, USA

Deniz Gungor
Louisiana State University Health Sciences
Center, Shreveport, LA, USA

Paul B. Hankey, BS
Kansas City University, Kansas City, MO,
USA

Eugenie S. Heitmiller, MD, FAAP
Division of Anesthesiology, Pain and
Perioperative Medicine, Children's
National Hospital, Washington, DC and
George Washington University School of
Medicine and Health Sciences,
Washington, DC, USA

K. Elliott Higgins III, MD
David Geffen School of Medicine,
University of California – Los Angeles,
CA, USA

Christopher Hoffman, DO
Sidney Kimmel Medical College, Thomas
Jefferson University, Philadelphia, PA,
USA

Eric Hsu, MD
David Gefen School of Medicine at UCLA,
Los Angeles, CA, USA

Liang Huang, MD, PhD
Langone Medical Center, New York, NY,
USA

**Jennifer Kales, MS, APRN, BC,
ACHPN, PhD**
Beth Israel Lahey Health, Boston, MA,
USA

Aaron J. Kaye, MD
Wake Anesthesia, Raleigh, NC, USA

Adam M. Kaye, PharmD, FASCP, FCPhA
Thomas J. Long School of Pharmacy,
Pharmacy Practice, University of the
Pacific, Stockton, CA, USA

Alan D. Kaye
Louisiana State University Health Sciences
Center, Shreveport, LA, USA

**Ashish K. Khanna, MD, MS, FCCP,
FCCM, FASA**
Wake Forest University School of
Medicine, Atrium Health Wake Forest
Baptist Medical Center, Winston Salem,
NC, USA

Vesela Kovacheva, MD, PhD
Brigham and Women's Hospital, Boston,
MA, USA

Lyubov Kozmenko, BSN, RN
Independent International Healthcare
Simulation Consultant

Valeriy Kozmenko, MD
University of South Dakota, Sioux Falls,
SD, USA

Lisa Lee, MD MS
David Geffen School of Medicine
University of California – Los Angeles,
CA, USA

Stacy Lee
Louisiana State University Health Sciences
Center, Shreveport, Shreveport, LA, USA

Henry Liu, MD
Perelman School of Medicine, University
of Pennsylvania Philadelphia, PA, USA

Bryan Lynn, MD
Tulane University Medical Center, New
Orleans, LA, USA

Saninuj Nini Malayaman, MD
University of Pennsylvania, PA, USA

Laxmaiah Manchikanti, MD
Pain Management Center of Paducah,
Paducah, KY, USA and University of
Louisville, KY, USA

Julia Metzner, MD
University of Washington, Seattle, WA,
USA

Renata M. Miketic, MD
Nationwide Children's Hospital, Ohio
State University Wexne Medical Center,
Columbus, OH, USA

**James D. Morris, MD, FACG, FACP,
AGAF, FASGE**
Louisiana State University Health
Shreveport, Shreveport, LA, USA

Debra E. Morrison, MD
University of California – Irvine, CA, USA

Maryam Mubashir, MD
Louisiana State University Health
Shreveport, Shreveport, LA, USA

Heikki E. Nikkanen MD
Harvard Medical School, Boston, MA, USA and Mount Auburn Hospital, Cambridge, MA, USA

Eshel A. Nir
Rambam Health Care Campus, Haifa, Israel and Rappaport Faculty of Medicine, Technion – Israel Institute of Technology, Haifa, Israel

Fredrik Olsen, MD, PhD
Sahlgrenska University Hospital, Gothenburg, Sweden

Shilpa Patil, MD
Louisiana State University Health Sciences Center, Shreveport, LA, USA

Andrea Poon, MD
David Gefen School of Medicine at UCLA, Los Angeles, CA, USA

Ryan Reichert
University of Illinois Chicago Medical School, Chicago, IL, USA

Anish P. Saikumar, DO
Texas Institute for Graduate Medical Education and Research, San Antonio, TX, USA

Benjamin A. Sanofsky, MD, MS Ed
Stanford University School of Medicine, Stanford Children's Health, Lucile Packard Children's Hospital, Stanford, CA, USA

David E. Seaver, RPh, JD
Brigham and Women's Hospital, Boston, MA, USA

Patricia M. Sequeira, MD
NYU Grossman School of Medicine, New York City, NY, USA and NYU Langone Health, New York City, NY, USA

Allie Shea, PA
Brigham and Women's Hospital, Boston, MA, USA

Harish Siddaiah, MD, FASA
Louisiana State University Health Sciences Center, Shreveport, LA, USA

Joel Stockman, MD
David Geffen School of Medicine, University of California – Los Angeles, CA, USA

Heather Trafton
Evergreen Nephrology, Nashville, TN, USA

Richard D. Urman
Department of Anesthesiology, Ohio State University, Columbus, OH, USA

Dev Vyas, MD
Tulane University Medical Center, New Orleans, LA, USA

Jue Teresa Wang, MD
Boston Children's Hospital, Boston, MA, USA and Harvard Medical School, Boston, MA, USA

Emmett E. Whitaker, MD, FAAP
University of Vermont Larner College of Medicine, Burlington, VT, USA and University of Vermont Medical Center, Burlington, VT, USA

Melissa Wibowo, MD
Stanford University School of Medicine, Fontana, CA, USA

Jennifer E. Woerner, DMD, MD, FACS
Health Sciences Center, Louisiana State University, Shreveport, LA, USA

Jennifer S. Xiong
Brigham and Women's Hospital, Boston, MA, USA

Micaela Zywicki, MD
UCLA Health, University of California – Los Angeles, CA, USA

Preface

A significant number of procedures performed under sedation are administered by non-anesthesia providers. As the number of medical and surgical procedures performed under moderate and deep sedation continues to grow, it is essential for all physicians, nurses, physician assistants, and other healthcare providers and administrators to develop appropriate policies and educational programs to provide safe patient care. Since guidelines and regulations put forth by many professional societies, the Joint Commission, and the Centers for Medicare and Medicaid Services are constantly evolving, it is important to stay current and well informed so that we can provide the best possible care for our patients.

Interventional procedures performed under moderate and deep sedation are increasing in complexity and duration, and patients may present with significant preexisting medical problems. A vast majority of these procedures are performed outside of the operating room in both inpatient and outpatient settings. Consequently, non-anesthesia providers are becoming more involved in the supervision and administration of moderate and deep sedation.

In this significantly updated third edition, our intention was again to compile a practical, comprehensive, up-to-date guide that can be used to set up and maintain a safe moderate and/or deep sedation program in your healthcare facility. There are a number of additional chapters reflecting emerging fields that require sedation. We cover all essential topics such as definitions of sedation levels, patient evaluation and recovery, pharmacology, monitoring and equipment, legal and patient safety issues, controversies, and emergency resuscitation. We discuss specific clinical and administrative aspects for the nursing and physician assistant staff. The handbook describes special considerations for unique patient populations such as pediatrics, the elderly, and patients with significant medical problems. Finally, we cover topics related to the procedures performed in the endoscopy, cardiology, and radiology suites, the intensive care unit, the emergency department, the dental practice, and the infertility clinic. Our chapter contributors constitute many national experts in their respective fields.

We hope that you find the third edition of this handbook an invaluable resource, whether you are a clinician or an administrator. Our goal is the safest possible administration of sedation with appropriate monitoring, medications, and personnel. Enjoy our book!

Introduction to Moderate and Deep Sedation

Benjamin A. Sanofsky, Renata M. Miketic,
Eugenie S. Heitmiller, and Emmett E. Whitaker

Background and History

The development of sedation and analgesia may be one of the preeminent advances in both medical science and human technology. The ability to alter human consciousness and perception of pain has opened the door to extraordinary possibilities for medical practice. However, the origins of these advances are ancient, likely reaching beyond the limits of written history. Ancient Greeks recognized that naturally occurring substances such as mandrake root and alcohol could alter consciousness and be used during surgical manipulations[1, 2]. Incan shamans used coca leaves to assist in trephination operations, in which burr holes drilled into the skull in an attempt to cure illnesses[1]. Surgeons in the Middle Ages used ice and so-called refrigeration anesthesia to dull pain sensation prior to incision [2, 3]. The development of procedural techniques and use of exogenous substances to alleviate suffering is one example of human ingenuity that is integral to our existence, and is ubiquitous across time and place.

Today's use of sedation derives primarily from more recent developments in medical science that emerged during the Industrial Revolution, and its origins are widely attributed to the public acceptance of the analgesic properties of ether. On October 16, 1846, this agent was used to facilitate the surgical removal of a vascular tumor from a patient's neck in front of an audience of physicians at Massachusetts General Hospital in Boston [4, 5, 6]. The procedure was well tolerated by the patient who endorsed feeling nothing more than a "scratch," and news of the successful demonstration quickly reached medical communities around the world [4, 5, 6]. The amphitheater hosting this landmark display later became known as the Ether Dome, and is credited with playing a key role in propelling exploration into the medical utility of mind-altering inhalational agents, laying the foundation for modern anesthetic practice.

Since then, continued pharmacologic advances have bestowed a variety of oral, intravenous, and inhalational medications capable of reliably inducing a range of desired sedative effects with increased specificity, predictability, and safety. Early sedatives generally had a slower onset and longer duration of action than many modern drugs, as well as many undesirable side effects. Over time, new agents with fewer side effects have been developed. Midazolam, for example, is one of the most widely used sedative medications today, and is popular for its quick onset, short duration of action, and overall safety profile [7]. Although lacking analgesic properties, its amnestic effects are especially helpful in facilitating procedures that are not especially painful but might be unpleasant for the patient. Propofol is another commonly used medication that provides little analgesia but is frequently utilized for its hypnotic effects, with rapid onset/offset and titratability [7]. Propofol also possesses antiemetic properties that are particularly beneficial in the ambulatory setting, where mitigation of post-procedural nausea helps improve recovery room efficiency and patient satisfaction with perioperative care [8]. Currently, the opioid chosen by many practitioners for procedural analgesia is fentanyl. Again, this popularity is likely related to its potency, short duration of action, and overall safety when administered by an experienced practitioner [7].

Improvements in physiologic monitoring have also drastically enhanced sedation safety. Equipment designed to quantitatively measure a patient's oxygenation, ventilation, blood circulation, and body temperature helps providers quickly recognize and attend to physiologic changes associated with varying levels of sedation. One of the most significant advances in monitoring was the development of pulse oximetry during World War II [9]. Using optics to monitor hemoglobin oxygen saturation, pulse oximetry offers a wealth of information pertaining to a patient's respiratory and hemodynamic status with a level of fidelity that, even to the trained and vigilant eye, cannot be achieved with clinical assessment alone.

As monitoring equipment and medications have improved, so has our ability to provide varying levels of sedation to precisely fit the needs of the patient. Rather than a one-size-fits-all approach, sedation is now viewed on a continuum, with "mild sedation" on one end of the spectrum and "general anesthesia" on the other [10]. Surgical techniques have also evolved to become less invasive and shorter in duration, allowing many procedures to transition out of the operating room and into a variety of clinical settings. This has increased the need for a tailored approach to sedation based on the type of procedure and the patient's anticipated sedative/analgesic requirements. From a provider standpoint, sedation is often preferred to general anesthesia when possible, as it allows for procedures to take place in a broader range of locations, is more cost effective, and may result in better patient satisfaction.[7, 11] Patients also tend to feel more comfortable with sedation when given the choice, as the complete loss of consciousness with general anesthesia is a common source of preoperative anxiety [12].

One of the central questions surrounding the practice of sedation relates to who should administer it. The growth of the healthcare system has created a diverse clinical milieu, with a need for sedation across a wide array of medical settings. Furthermore, the types of providers administering sedatives to patients have diversified in tandem. It should be recognized that practitioners of early dental and oral maxillofacial surgery were at the forefront of developing the practice of sedation, and by the 1980s most sedatives were administered by a registered nurse (RN) under supervision by a physician [13]. Today, procedural sedation is delivered by many different types of medical professionals including nurses (RNs), physician assistants

(PAs), certified registered nurse anesthetists (CRNAs), certified anesthesiologist assistants (CAAs), anesthesiologists, non-anesthesiologist physicians, dentists, and even computer-assisted devices.[14, 15]. As healthcare has evolved, the demand for such providers has outpaced the supply, and groups including the American Society of Anesthesiologists (ASA) have been called upon to develop guidelines for the administration of sedation and analgesia by non-anesthesiologists. Regardless of title, those providing sedation must be trained in the administration of sedative/hypnotic drugs, airway management, and patient resuscitation. Perhaps most importantly, those administering sedation must be prepared and able to care for a patient who inadvertently surpasses the planned plane of sedation.

The Continuum of Sedation

In 1995, a task force supported by the American Society of Anesthesiologists (ASA) put together practice guidelines for non-anesthesiologists administering sedation and analgesia [7]. These guidelines addressed pre-sedation preparation, personnel training and competency, recommended equipment, and considerations for post-sedation recovery. The original guidelines have been updated over the years to address the needs of our growing healthcare system, defining varying levels of depth on a continuum, and with a focus on providing recommendations on the administration of "moderate" and "deep" sedation in particular [10]. Levels of sedation are categorized according to the degree of impact on patient responsiveness, airway, ventilation, and cardiovascular function (shown in Table 1.1), each of which are described as follows:[10]

Minimal sedation (anxiolysis) is a drug-induced state during which patients respond normally to verbal commands. Although cognitive function and physical coordination

Table 1.1 Continuum of depth of sedation, definition of general anesthesia, and levels of sedation/ analgesia [10]

	Minimal sedation (anxiolysis)	Moderate sedation/ analgesia (conscious sedation)	Deep sedation/ analgesia	General anesthesia
Responsiveness	Normal response to verbal stimulation	Purposeful* response to verbal or tactile stimulation	Purposeful* response following repeated or painful stimulation	Unarousable even with painful stimulus
Airway	Unaffected	No intervention required	Intervention may be required	Intervention often required
Spontaneous ventilation	Unaffected	Adequate	May be inadequate	Frequently inadequate
Cardiovascular function	Unaffected	Usually maintained	Usually maintained	May be impaired

*A reflexive withdrawal from a painful stimulus is not considered purposeful response.

may be impaired, airway reflexes, and ventilatory and cardiovascular functions are unaffected.

Moderate sedation/analgesia ("conscious sedation") is a drug-induced depression of consciousness during which patients respond purposefully to verbal commands, either alone or accompanied by light tactile stimulation. No interventions are required to maintain a patent airway, and spontaneous ventilation is adequate. Cardiovascular function is usually maintained.

Deep sedation/analgesia is a drug-induced depression of consciousness during which patients cannot be easily aroused but respond purposefully following repeated or painful stimulation. The ability to independently maintain ventilatory function may be impaired. Patients may require assistance in maintaining a patent airway, and spontaneous ventilation may be inadequate. Cardiovascular function is usually maintained.

General anesthesia is a drug-induced loss of consciousness during which patients are not arousable, even by painful stimulation. The ability to independently maintain ventilatory function is often impaired. Patients often require assistance in maintaining a patent airway, and positive pressure ventilation may be required because of depressed spontaneous ventilation or drug-induced depression of neuromuscular function. Cardiovascular function may be impaired.

The ASA further states that practitioners aiming to produce a given level of sedation should be proficient in airway management and advanced life support and should be able to rescue patients whose level of sedation becomes deeper than initially intended. For example, individuals who administer moderate sedation/analgesia should be able to rescue patients who enter a state of deep sedation/analgesia, and those administering deep sedation/analgesia should be able to rescue patients who enter a state of general anesthesia.

Guidelines for Sedation and Analgesia by Non-Anesthesiologists

With the tremendous growth in the number and complexity of procedures, sedation needs have expanded considerably, with many different types of healthcare professionals providing sedation in a range of practice settings. Currently, there is little in terms of federal regulation for who may provide sedation. Instead, state and institutional policies, guided by recommendations from a number of professional organizations, are largely responsible for setting the framework within which clinicians practice. The American Society of Anesthesiologists (ASA), Association of Perioperative Registered Nurses (AORN), and American Association of Nurse Anesthesiology (AANA) are just a few of the leading associations providing these recommendations, each with their own sets of practice guidelines but with a common aim to improve safety, efficacy, and access to medical care for patients in need of procedural sedation.

Across these organizations, it is widely felt that *mild sedation* generally entails minimal risk to the patient, and that deeper levels of sedation require a higher level of care to ensure patient safety. For *moderate sedation*, the ASA provides guidelines pertaining to periprocedural considerations and the administration of sedatives (Table 1.2). These guidelines are designed to be applicable to procedures performed by practitioners who are not specialists in anesthesiology but who are qualified and licensed to provide sedation in a variety of settings. During moderate sedation, a single provider

Table 1.2 Guidelines for the administration of moderate sedation

Periprocedural focus	Recommendations
Patient evaluation	• Review previous medical records and interview the patient or family to identify: abnormalities of the major organ systems or airway, adverse experiences with sedation/analgesia, current medications, substance use, or frequent exposure to sedation/analgesic agents. • Conduct focused physical exam. • Review available laboratory test results and order additional tests as needed. • When possible, perform the pre-procedure evaluation far enough in advance to allow for optimal patient preparation, and reevaluate the patient immediately before the procedure.
Pre-procedure preparation	• Inform patients of the benefits, risks, and limitations associated with this sedation, as well as possible alternatives. • Consult with a medical specialist for patients with significant underlying conditions when appropriate, before administration of sedation. If it is likely that sedation to the point of unresponsiveness will be necessary to obtain adequate conditions, a physician anesthesiologist should be consulted. • Inform patients or legal guardians before the day of the procedure that they should not drink fluids or eat solid foods for a sufficient period of time to allow for gastric emptying before the procedure[a]. • On the day of the procedure, assess the time and nature of last oral intake in order to determine the target level of sedation and whether the procedure should be delayed. • In urgent or emergent situations where complete gastric emptying is not possible, moderate sedation should not be delayed based on fasting time alone.
Monitoring	• *Level of consciousness*: Periodically monitor a patient's response to verbal commands. During procedures where a verbal response is not possible (e.g., oral surgery, restorative dentistry, upper endoscopy), check the patient's ability to give a "thumbs up" or other indication of consciousness in response to verbal or tactile (light tap) stimulation. • *Ventilatory function and oxygenation*: Continually monitor ventilatory function by observation of qualitative clinical signs and with capnography unless precluded or invalidated by the nature of the patient, procedure, or equipment. For uncooperative patients, institute capnography after moderate sedation has been achieved. Continuously monitor all patients by pulse oximetry with appropriate alarms[b]. • *Hemodynamics:* Continually monitor blood pressure and heart rate during the procedure unless such monitoring interferes with the procedure (e.g., MRI where stimulation from the blood pressure cuff could arouse an appropriately sedated patient). Use electrocardiographic monitoring in patients with clinically significant cardiovascular disease or those who are undergoing procedures where dysrhythmias are anticipated.

Table 1.2 (cont.)

Periprocedural focus	Recommendations
Contemporaneous recording of monitored parameters	• Level of consciousness, respiratory function, and hemodynamics should be recorded at a frequency that is appropriate for the procedure and the patient's condition. At a minimum, this should be: (1) before the beginning of the procedure, (2) after administration of sedative/analgesic agents, (3) at regular intervals during the procedure, (4) during initial recovery, and (5) just before discharge. • Set device alarms to alert the care team to critical changes in patient status.
Availability of an individual responsible for monitoring	• Ensure that a designated individual other than the proceduralist is present to monitor the patient during the procedure. This individual should not be a member of the procedural team but may assist with minor, interruptible tasks once the patient's level of sedation/analgesia and vital signs have stabilized, provided that adequate monitoring is maintained.
Supplemental oxygen	• Use supplemental oxygen unless specifically contraindicated for a particular patient or procedure.
Emergency support	• Ensure that emergency medications and equipment are immediately available, and that an individual is present who is proficient in effectively using them. • Suction, advanced airway equipment, and resuscitation medications should be immediately available and in good working order. • A functional defibrillator should be immediately available, and an individual with advanced life support skills should be present or immediately available.
Sedative or analgesic medications *not* intended for general anesthesia	• Combinations of sedatives and analgesic agents may be administered as appropriate for the procedure and the condition of the patient. The propensity for combinations of sedative and analgesic agents to cause respiratory depression and airway obstruction emphasizes the need to appropriately reduce the dose of each component as well as the need to continually monitor respiratory function. • Ensure that vascular access is be maintained (for all patients receiving medications intravenously, and on a case-by-case basis for those receiving medications by non-intravenous routes).
Sedative or analgesic medications intended for general anesthesia	• In addition to recommendations above, provide care consistent with that required for general anesthesia. • Ensure that those administering sedation are able to reliably identify and rescue patients from unintended deep sedation or general anesthesia.
Reversal agents	• Ensure that specific antagonist medications are available whenever opioid analgesics or benzodiazepines are administered. • Prior to or concomitantly with pharmacologic reversal, patients who become hypoxemic or apneic during sedation/analgesia should: (1) be encouraged or stimulated to breathe deeply; (2) receive

Table 1.2 (cont.)

Periprocedural focus	Recommendations
	supplemental oxygen; and (3) receive positive pressure ventilation if spontaneous ventilation is inadequate.
	• Following pharmacologic reversal, patients should be observed long enough to ensure that sedation and cardiorespiratory depression does not recur once the effect of the antagonist dissipates.
	• The use of sedation regimens that include routine reversal of sedative or analgesic agents is discouraged.
Recovery care	• Observe patient in an appropriately staffed and equipped area until they are near their baseline level of consciousness and no longer at risk for cardiopulmonary depression prior to discharge.
	• Discharge criteria should be designed to minimize the risk of central nervous system or cardiorespiratory depression following discharge from observation by trained personnel.
Implementation of patient safety processes	• Create and implement a quality improvement process based on established national, regional, or institutional reporting protocols, and update them periodically in light of new technologies, equipment, or other advances in procedural sedation.
	• Create an emergency response plan.

Adapted from "Practice guidelines for moderate procedural sedation and analgesia 2018" [10].
[a] Refer to the American Society of Anesthesiologists' "Practice guidelines for preoperative fasting and the use of pharmacologic agents to reduce the risk of pulmonary aspiration: application to healthy patients undergoing elective procedures – an updated report" [16].
[b] The term continual is defined by the ASA as "repeated regularly and frequently in steady rapid succession," whereas continuous means "prolonged without any interruption at any time" [17]

typically assumes the dual role of performing the procedure and supervising the sedation, and may at times have their attention diverted to their primary focus, the procedure [18] For this reason, the ASA recommends that another individual take the primary role of continually monitoring the patient [19]. In recent years, an emphasis has been placed on improving the safety of *deep sedation*, and it is currently felt that the participation of a physician anesthesiologist should be involved when this level of sedation is needed [20]. While older guidelines have incorporated both moderate and deep sedation into one set of recommendations, a new set of guidelines specific to the administration of deep sedation is currently in development by the ASA [10]. Similar guidelines have not been created for the administration of *general anesthesia*, as this level of sedation requires direct supervision by a licensed provider credentialed specifically in the practice of anesthesia.

Apart from sedation's continuum, the ASA describes another category of sedation known as *monitored anesthesia care* (*MAC*). During MAC, an independent provider separate from the proceduralist takes primary responsibility for the sedation, focusing exclusively on the patient for any airway, hemodynamic, or physiologic derangements. MAC is often employed in settings where procedural needs or patient response to sedative medications are less predictable, making it more difficult for a non-anesthesia provider to safely induce and maintain the intended level of sedation. Additionally, according to the ASA, those delivering MAC must be licensed anesthesia providers qualified and prepared to convert to general anesthesia if needed [18].

The Anesthesia Care Team and the Role of Nurses in the Provision of Sedation and Analgesia

The scope of practice for non-physician healthcare professionals in anesthesia has grown to support an anesthesia care team (ACT) model, inclusive of anesthesiologists, CRNAs, and CAAs, in addition to a multitude of other medical personnel involved in providing perioperative patient care. The ACT developed in order to more efficiently provide patients with access to the full spectrum of anesthetic care while maintaining patient safety. At the time of this publication, the ASA states that while selected tasks may be delegated to qualified members of the ACT, overall responsibility for the team's actions and patient safety ultimately rests with the physician anesthesiologist [21]. The World Health Organization–World Federation of Societies of Anesthesiologists also recommends this model to ensure that one standard of safety is maintained among all provider groups [22]. Nurses are vital to this system, and over time, the responsibilities of each member of the ACT have grown in a consistent effort to improve medical efficiency. This became particularly relevant during height of the coronavirus pandemic, when the infrastructure for medical services struggled to support the demands of the population [23].

As the field advances with new techniques, safer practice methods, and targeted training programs, the degree of autonomy granted to non-physician providers is continually being evaluated to better fulfill growing healthcare needs. With this growth has come a wide range of patients requiring more complex care, necessitating a nuanced approach to risk stratification and the assessment of sedation needs for each patient. Distinguishing sedation from MAC has enabled a broader workforce to take part in safely administering sedation and analgesia for patients who do not require the full spectrum of anesthesia care. As with the ACT, nurses also play an integral role in this setting.

Comprising the largest component of the healthcare workforce and with a range of differentiated and advanced training pathways, the collective breadth and scope of practice for nurses is broad [24]. The desire to lend safety to the practice of sedation by non-anesthesia-trained nurses has led to the development of practice guidelines such as those provided by the ASA (Table 1.2). A number of nurse-led organizations including the AORN, AANA, the Society for Gastrointestinal Nurses and Associates, the American Society of PeriAnesthesia Nurses, the Emergency Nurses Association, and the American Association of Critical Care Nurses have also put forth position statements on sedation practice specific to their respective groups. Position statements are continually developed and, in the absence of clinical evidence, are based largely on expert opinion. Practice guidelines are then systematically refined to assist the practitioner in making clinical decisions on a day-to-day basis. These recommended practices are frequently used in concert with state law to create institutional sedation protocols and to regulate practice through legislation. The Joint Commission also surveys all healthcare organizations to ensure that professional standards are maintained and protocols are followed. These steps help ensure patient safety, and with a thoughtful approach to delegating the provision of sedation needs throughout a diverse workforce, patients benefit from improved access to care.

Summary

The practice of sedation has evolved significantly over the past century. Once mainly the task of anesthesiology personnel, the demand for sedation services has exceeded the supply. The result has been the expansion of the scope of practice of other professionals. With continued attention to a high standard of safety, many different healthcare providers are able to offer sedation services to those patients who need them.

References

1. Sabatowski R, Schäfer D, Kasper SM, Brunsch H, Radbruch L. Pain treatment: a historical overview. *Curr Pharm Des.* 2004;10(7):701–16. doi:10.2174/1381612043452974

2. Houghton IT. Some observations on early military anaesthesia. *Anaesth Intensive Care.* 2006;34(Suppl 1):6–15. doi:10.1177/0310057X0603401S01

3. Furnas DW. Topical refrigeration and frost anesthesia. *Anesthesiology.* 1965;26(3):344-7. doi:10.1097/00000542-196505000-00012

4. Finder RL. The art and science of office-based anesthesia in dentistry: a 150-year history. *Int Anesthesiol Clin.* 2003;41(3):1–12. doi:10.1097/00004311-200341030-00003

5. López-Valverde A, Montero J, Albaladejo A, Gómez de Diego R. The discovery of surgical anesthesia: discrepancies regarding its authorship. *J Dent Res.* 2011;90(1):31-4. doi:10.1177/0022034510385239

6. Desai SP, Desai MS, Pandav CS. The discovery of modern anaesthesia: contributions of Davy, Clarke, Long, Wells and Morton. *Indian J Anaesth.* 2007;51(6):472–8.

7. Watson DS, Odom-Forren J. *Practical Guide to Moderate Sedation/Analgesia,* 2nd ed. New York, NY: Mosby, 2005.

8. Kim EG, Park HJ, Kang H, Choi J, Lee HJ. Antiemetic effect of propofol administered at the end of surgery in laparoscopic assisted vaginal hysterectomy. *Korean J Anesthesiol.* 2014;66(3):210–15. doi:10.4097/kjae.2014.66.3.210

9. Severinghaus JW, Astrup PB. History of blood gas analysis. VI. Oximetry. *J Clin Monit.* 1986;2(4):270–88. doi:10.1007/BF02851177

10. Practice guidelines for moderate procedural sedation and analgesia 2018. *Anesthesiology.* 2018;128(3):437–79. doi:10.1097/ALN.0000000000002043

11. Meredith JR, O'Keefe KP, Galwankar S. Pediatric procedural sedation and analgesia. *J Emerg Trauma Shock.* 2008;1(2):88–96. doi:10.4103/0974-2700.43189

12. Eberhart L, Aust H, Schuster M, et al. Preoperative anxiety in adults: a cross-sectional study on specific fears and risk factors. *BMC Psychiatry.* 2020;20(1):140. doi:10.1186/s12888-020-02552-w

13. Ash HL. Anesthesia's dental heritage (William Thomas Green Morton). *Anesth Prog.* 1985;32(1):25–9.

14. ASGE Technology Committee, Banerjee S, Desilets D, et al. Computer-assisted personalized sedation. *Gastrointest Endosc.* 2011;73(3):423–7. doi:10.1016/j.gie.2010.10.035

15. Pambianco DJ, Whitten CJ, Moerman A, Struys MM, Martin JF. An assessment of computer-assisted personalized sedation: a sedation delivery system to administer propofol for gastrointestinal endoscopy. *Gastrointest Endosc.* 2008;68(3):542–7. doi:10.1016/j.gie.2008.02.011

16. Practice guidelines for preoperative fasting and the use of pharmacologic agents to reduce the risk of pulmonary aspiration: application to healthy patients undergoing elective procedures. An updated report by the American Society of Anesthesiologists Task Force on Preoperative Fasting and the use of

pharmacologic agents to reduce the risk of pulmonary aspiration. *Anesthesiology.* 2017;126(3):376–93. doi:10.1097/ALN.0000000000001452

17. American Society of Anesthesiologists. Standards for basic anesthetic monitoring. www.asahq.org/standards-and-guidelines/standards-for-basic-anesthetic-monitoring (accessed March 26, 2022)

18. American Society of Anesthesiologists. Distinguishing monitored anesthesia care ("MAC") from moderate sedation/analgesia (conscious sedation). www.asahq.org/standards-and-practice-parameters/statement-on-distinguishing-monitored-anesthesia-care-from-moderate-sedation-analgesia (accessed March 16, 2022)

19. American Society of Anesthesiologists. Statement of granting privileges for administration of moderate sedation to practitioners. www.asahq.org/standards-and-guidelines/statement-of-granting-privileges-for-administration-of-moderate-sedation-to-practitioners (accessed March 16, 2022)

20. American Society of Anesthesiologists. Advisory on granting privileges for deep sedation to non-anesthesiologist physicians. www.asahq.org/standards-and-guidelines (accessed March 16, 2022)

21. American Society of Anesthesiologists. Statement on the anesthesia care team. www.asahq.org/standards-and-guidelines/statement-on-the-anesthesia-care-team (accessed March 16, 2022)

22. Gelb AW, Morriss WW, Johnson W, et al. World Health Organization–World Federation of Societies of Anaesthesiologists (WHO–WFSA) International Standards for a Safe Practice of Anesthesia. *Anesth Analg.* 2018;126(6):2047–55. doi:10.1213/ANE.0000000000002927

23. Callan V, Eshkevari L, Finder S, et al. Impact of COVID-19 pandemic on certified registered nurse anesthetist practice. *AANA J.* 2021;89(4):334–40.

24. American Association of Colleges of Nursing. Nursing workforce fact sheet. www.aacnnursing.org/news-Information/fact-sheets/nursing-fact-sheet (accessed March 16, 2022)

Pharmacology Principles in Sedation

Aaron J. Kaye, Alan D. Kaye, Julie A. Gayle,
Richard D. Urman, and Adam M. Kaye

Introduction

Today, there are an increasing number of procedures requiring moderate and deep sedation being performed outside the surgical suite. As a result, qualified non-anesthesia providers are administering varying levels of sedation to patients for a variety of diagnostic, therapeutic, and/or surgical procedures. Practitioners should provide patients with the benefits of sedation and/or analgesia while minimizing the associated risks. To do so, providers should understand the pharmacology of the agents being administered as well as the role of pharmacologic antagonists for opioids and benzodiazepines. Today's practitioners are equipped with an abundance of versatile sedative agents that can be used alone and in combination. Furthermore, combinations of sedative and analgesics should be administered as appropriate for the procedure being performed and the condition of the patient. Policies and standards regarding administration of sedation and analgesia by non-anesthesia providers are addressed elsewhere in the book. This chapter focuses on the pharmacology of the drugs most used to provide moderate and deep sedation and their available reversal agents.

Pharmacology Basics

A drug that activates a receptor by binding to that receptor is called an *agonist*. An *antagonist* is a drug that binds to the receptor without activating the receptor and simultaneously prevents the agonist from stimulating the receptor. *Synergism* is when the effect of two drugs exceeds their algebraic summation. Often, this is seen with benzodiazepines and opioids when they are used in combination. *Pharmacokinetic*

Table 2.1 Causes of variability of individual responses to a drug

1. Drug interactions	
2. Pharmacokinetics	Age
	Renal function
	Hepatic function
	Cardiac function
	Bioavailability
	Body composition
3. Pharmacodynamics	Genetic differences
	Enzyme activity

properties of a drug determine its onset of action and duration of drug effect. More specifically, pharmacokinetics describes the absorption, distribution, metabolism, and excretion of a drug (i.e., what the body does to the drug.) *Pharmacodynamics* describes the responsiveness of receptors to a drug and the mechanism by which these effects happen (i.e., what the drug does to the body). Individuals respond variably to the same drug, and often these different responses reflect the pharmacokinetics and/or pharmacodynamics among patients (Table 2.1).

Pharmacokinetics (which determines the onset of action and duration of the drug effect) is affected by the route of administration, absorption, and volume of distribution. The *volume of distribution* is influenced by characteristics of the drug including lipid solubility, binding to plasma proteins, and molecular size. Pharmacodynamics and pharmacologic drug effects are described in terms of dose–response curves, which depict the relationship between the dose of a drug administered and the resulting pharmacologic effect. Dose–response curves predict the effect of the drug on the patient with increasing dose. Titration of a medication should proceed based on expected pharmacodynamics of the medication given. Key considerations during titration of drugs are appropriate choice for the patient's condition (e.g., renal failure, liver failure, previous drug exposure, age, physical condition), appropriate choice of incremental dosing (i.e., time and quantity), desired effect, post-procedure pain control requirements, and periodic monitoring. Preexisting diseases also affect elimination half-life, which is an important consideration when administering sedation. The *elimination half-life* is the time necessary for plasma concentration of a drug to decrease to 50% during the elimination phase. Because the elimination half-life is directly proportional to the volume of distribution and inversely proportional to its clearance, renal and hepatic disease (altered volume of distribution and/or clearance) affect the elimination half-life. In obese patients, lipophilic medications (benzodiazepines, opioids) may demonstrate a longer elimination half-time. It is important to understand that the elimination half-life does not reflect the time to recovery from drug effects. The elimination half-life allows for an estimation of the time it will take to reduce the drug concentration in the plasma by half. After about five elimination half-lives, a drug is nearly fully eliminated from the body. Therefore, drug accumulation is likely if dosing intervals are less than this period of time.

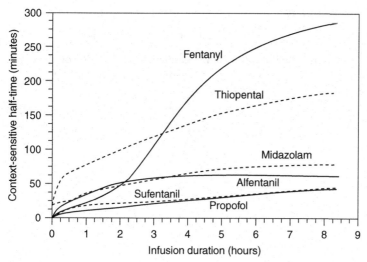

Figure 2.1 Context-sensitive half-lives of drugs used in sedation.

Context-Sensitive Half-Life

The elimination half-life does not always explain the duration of action of all drugs used in sedation, especially if multiple boluses or infusions are used. The *context-sensitive half-life* is defined as the time taken for the blood plasma concentration of a drug to decline by 50% after a drug infusion has been stopped. The "context" refers to the duration of the infusion of the drug. Figure 2.1 shows examples of several types of drugs (benzodiazepines, opioids, barbiturates, propofol) with their context-sensitive half-life (minutes) plotted against the duration of infusion (hours). As shown in this representative graph, several hours of continued infusion or multiple repeated boluses in close succession can result in significant accumulation of the active drug in the patient. This can lead to an increase in side effects (sedation, respiratory depression) and delayed recovery. Therefore, it is prudent to consider the context-sensitive half-life of a drug, especially during longer (> 2-hour) procedures, and also to keep track of the total amount of drug(s) given by adding up all the boluses and/or infusions.

Synergy Effects

Drugs used for sedation can have synergistic (i.e., additive) effects. This presents both advantages and disadvantages for the provider. The advantage is that one can obtain the desired level of sedation by using several agents while minimizing the total amount of each. For example, fentanyl has analgesic properties while midazolam is more useful as a sedative and an anxiolytic drug. However, the synergistic effect of these drugs, when administered together, can lead to exaggerated sedation and respiratory effects. Therefore, titration to effect and close monitoring are required. Table 2.2 displays commonly used drug classes and their relative effects on sedation, anxiety, and pain, and on the cardiovascular and respiratory systems.

Table 2.2 Drug classes commonly used in sedation and their effects

Drug class	Effects				
	Sedation	Anxiolysis	Pain	Cardiovascular system	Respiratory system
Local anesthetic	−	−	++	$+^a$	−
Benzodiazepine	++	++	−	+	$+^a$
Opioid	+	+	++	+	++
Propofol	++	+	−	++	++
Barbiturate	++	+	−	++	++
Ketamine	++	+	++	+	$+^a$
Dexmedetomidine	++	+	+	+	−

Key: −, no effect; +, moderate effect; ++, significant effect.
^{a} Significant effect if overdosed.

Routes of Administration

Routes of medication administration include parenteral (intravenous, intramuscular, inhalational) and enteral (oral, rectal, nasal). Drugs administered by the intravenous (IV) route generally have a more rapid onset than those administered by the intramuscular (IM) route and thus are most useful for moderate and deep sedation. IV sedative/ analgesic drugs should be administered in small, incremental doses titrated to desired end points of sedation and analgesia, with adequate time allowed between doses to achieve those effects.

Preemptive Analgesia

Transmission of pain signals from tissue damage leads to sensitization of both peripheral and central pain pathways. Specifically, injury to nociceptive nerve fibers induces neural and behavioral changes that last long after the injury has healed or the offending stimulus has been removed. This post-injury pain hypersensitivity can result from post-traumatic changes in either the peripheral nervous system or the central nervous system. The noxious stimulus-induced neuroplasticity can be pre-empted by the administration of analgesics or by regional neural blockade. Providing agents prior to surgery to reduce postoperative pain is termed *preemptive analgesia*, and its goal is to prevent sensitization of nociceptors before surgical stimulus. Thus, preemptive analgesia is a treatment that is initiated prior to a surgical procedure to reduce sensitization of pain pathways. Preemptive analgesia, specifically multimodal preoperative analgesia, reduces post-surgical pain and consumption of analgesia in a more effective manner. When appropriately administered just prior to surgery, local anesthetic infiltration, gabapentin, opioids, acetaminophen, *N*-methyl-D-aspartate (NMDA)-receptor antagonists, cyclooxygenase (COX) inhibitors, peripheral nerve blocks, subarachnoid blocks, and epidural blocks have all been shown to provide postoperative pain benefits.

Drug Interactions

Clinicians providing sedation must be cognizant of potential drug–drug interactions, which can lead to morbidity and to mortality. For example, the synergistic effects of two or more sedatives are well described and may result in central nervous system (CNS) and respiratory depression. Anesthesia providers spend years studying and refining their craft, and this is not always the case for a non-anesthesia sedation provider. Therefore, it is recommended that healthcare providers develop an excellent understanding of the side effects as well as potential drug interactions of the agents they are using in the clinical setting. They must also be aware of possible drug interactions with a patient's home medications and even herbals, of which there are over 29,000 available, and many of which can interact in unfavorable ways with conventional sedative medications. For example, St. John's wort can cause a lethal serotonergic crisis with meperidine, and kava-kava can potentiate CNS depression with any sedative. Many of the "G" herbals – including ginger, garlic, ginseng, and ginkgo – can increase the risk of bleeding.

Benzodiazepines

Benzodiazepines are suited for moderate and deep sedation because of their anxiolytic, amnesic, and sedative properties. At recommended doses and with careful titration, this drug class provides hypnosis (sedation) and anterograde amnesia with minimal effect on the cardiovascular and respiratory systems in healthy patients. Benzodiazepines do not provide analgesia. Commonly administered benzodiazepines include midazolam (Versed), diazepam (Valium), and lorazepam (Ativan). Remimazolam is a rapidly metabolized benzodiazepine that has emerged recently as an exciting medication for procedural sedation.

The mechanism of action of benzodiazepines is by enhancing the actions of gamma-aminobutyric acid (GABA) receptors in the brain. GABA is the principal inhibitory transmitter in the CNS. Benzodiazepines are highly lipid-soluble and rapidly enter the CNS, bind to GABA receptors in the brain, and enhance opening of chloride channels (Figure 2.2). Increased chloride conductance produces hyperpolarization of the post-synaptic neuronal cell membrane and reduces excitability.

The clinical effects of the benzodiazepines used during moderate and deep sedation include anxiolysis, hypnosis (sedation), anterograde amnesia, anticonvulsant effects, and spinal-cord-mediated skeletal muscle relaxation. The different clinical effects of each benzodiazepine are due to binding of the GABA receptor at different sites. A large disparity exists between the level of sedation and the degree of amnesia. When given benzodiazepines, patients may seem conscious, but they can be amnesic to events and instructions. To the average patient, benzodiazepines produce minimal changes in hemodynamic parameters (blood pressure, heart rate, cardiac output).

However, dose-related effects of the benzodiazepines range from anxiolysis and amnesia to obtundation of airway reflexes and central respiratory depression. Recommended dose ranges of midazolam, diazepam, and lorazepam and other considerations are shown in Table 2.3.

Midazolam (Versed)

Midazolam is a short-acting, water-soluble benzodiazepine possessing sedative, amnesic, anxiolytic, and anticonvulsant properties. Furthermore, midazolam has replaced

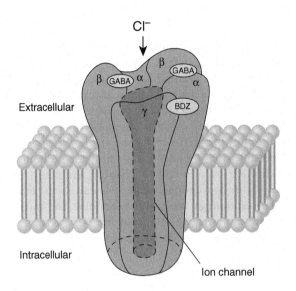

Figure 2.2 Schematic of benzodiazepine–GABA–chloride ion channel complex. BDZ, benzodiazepine.

diazepam for use in moderate and deep sedation. It is two to three times more potent than diazepam and is commonly used in procedural sedation. Midazolam's amnesic effects are more potent than its sedative effects. Midazolam is highly bound to plasma proteins. It is rapidly redistributed from the brain to other tissues and metabolized by the liver. Thus, it has a short duration of action. Midazolam's metabolism in the liver is carried out by hydroxylation, and is excreted by the kidneys after conjugation. The elimination half-life of midazolam is 1–4 hours, and shorter than diazepam. It can be doubled in the elderly as a result of age-related decreases in hepatic blood flow and possibly enzyme activity. Midazolam should be used with caution in the morbidly obese due to their increased volume of distribution and the prolonged half-time of the drug.

Diazepam (Valium)

Diazepam is a water-insoluble benzodiazepine used for procedural sedation as well as in the treatment of anxiety and seizures. Similar to midazolam, it is classified as an anxiolytic, amnesic, anticonvulsant, and sedative. As a result of its high lipid solubility, diazepam is taken up rapidly into the brain. It is then redistributed extensively to other tissues. Because diazepam is highly protein-bound, diseases associated with decreased albumin concentration (e.g., malnutrition, liver disease, renal dysfunction, burns, and sepsis) can increase its effects. Diazepam is metabolized by the liver, which produces two active metabolites: desmethyldiazepam and oxazepam. Desmethyldiazepam is metabolized more slowly and is less potent than diazepam, but contributes to the sustained effects of the drug. In healthy individuals, the elimination half-life is 21–37 hours. This range is greatly increased in those with cirrhosis of the liver and older age, which is consistent with the increased sensitivity of these patients to the drug's sedative effects. Because diazepam is dissolved in propylene glycol and sodium benzoate, another side effect may be pain on injection. Abrupt discontinuation of diazepam after prolonged administration may also result in withdrawal symptoms. These symptoms include anxiety, hyperexcitability, and seizures.

Table 2.3 Commonly used benzodiazepines: dosing and other considerations

Drug (brand name)	Dosing (intravenous)		Onset	Duration	Considerations
	Pediatric	Adult			
All benzodiazepines					Major side effects are respiratory depression and hypotension. Reduce dose by one-third to one-half when used with other CNS-depressing drugs or in the elderly or debilitated.
Midazolam (Versed)	*Incremental bolus*: 0.05–0.1 mg/kg *Titrate*: 0.25mg/kg every 5 min *Max*: 0.2 mg/kg	*Initial*: 0.5–2.5 mg slowly over 2 min *Titrate*: 0.5 mg increments *Max*: 5 mg	1–5 min	1–2.5 h	
Diazepam (Valium)	*Incremental bolus*: 0.1–0.3 mg/kg increments over minimum of 3 min *Max*: 0.6 mg/kg	*Initial*: 2.5–10 mg slowly *Titrate*: 2–5 mg every 5–10 min *Max*: 20 mg	30 s – 5 min	2–6 h	Diazepam is painful on injection. Should not be diluted.
Lorazepam (Ativan)	*Incremental bolus*: 0.05 mg/kg over 2 min; may repeat one-half dose every 10–15 min *Max*: 2 mg	*Initial*: 0.02–0.05 mg/kg over 2 min; may repeat one-half dose every 10–15 min 0.05 mg/kg over 2 min; may repeat one-half dose every 10–15 min *Max*: 2 mg	5–10 min	4–6 h	Lorazepam is painful on injection. Prior to IV use, must be diluted with an equal amount of compatible

Lorazepam (Ativan)

Lorazepam, a long-acting benzodiazepine, has similar properties to midazolam and diazepam, but with more potent amnesic properties. Metabolized in the liver, its byproducts are inactive. Lorazepam has an elimination half-life of 10–20 hours, with urinary excretion accounting for more than 80% of the dose given. It has a slower onset of action and much slower metabolic clearance compared to midazolam. Onset with IV administration is within 1–2 minutes and the peak effect occurs at 20–30 minutes. The duration of action of lorazepam is 6–10 hours. Despite its slower onset of action, lorazepam is occasionally utilized for longer procedures requiring amnesia, sedation, and anxiolysis.

Adverse Effects of Benzodiazepines

Adverse effects may occur when benzodiazepines are administered with other drugs such as opioids. In combination with opioids, hemodynamic perturbations become more significant. Respiratory depressant effects on spontaneous ventilation are enhanced significantly when opioids are used in combination with benzodiazepines. These effects are dose-dependent and can also be exaggerated in patients with comorbidities such as chronic obstructive pulmonary disease or obesity. Furthermore, benzodiazepines exhibit a longer elimination half-life and greater sedative effect in elderly patients. Finally, venoirritation may occur with diazepam and lorazepam.

Remimazolam (Byfavo)

Remimazolam is a novel short-acting benzodiazepine that was approved in several countries, including the United States, in 2020 for general anesthesia and procedural sedation typically as an infusion [1]. A bolus is typically utilized as a loading dose. This ester-based benzodiazepine has a very quick onset of action and is rapidly metabolized by tissue esterases throughout the body, independent of any specific organ system. Studies show that its elimination clearance is 3 times the rate of midazolam and its context-sensitive half-time after 3 hours of continuous infusion is 5 times shorter (7 minutes). Overall, the context-sensitive half-life of remimazolam mostly stays consistent regardless of the infusion time. Therefore, it provides rapidly titratable sedation, anxiolysis, and maintenance of anesthesia regardless of how long it is infused. Thus far, it has proven to be highly effective for procedural sedation in cases such as colonoscopies and upper-gastrointestinal endoscopies. When compared to an agent with similar utility such as propofol, it is touted to cause less hypotension, has less respiratory depression, and has the capability of being reversed with flumazenil. As the use of remimazolam becomes more common, it will likely be integrated into a wider variety of anesthetics and clinical settings in the future.

Opioids

Opioids, also known as narcotics, are potent analgesics commonly used to provide pain relief. Opioids in combination with benzodiazepines provide adequate moderate and/or deep sedation and analgesia for many procedures. Some of the commonly used opioid agonists are morphine, fentanyl (Sublimaze), hydromorphone (Dilaudid), meperidine (Demerol), and remifentanil (Ultiva) (Table 2.4).

Opioids include all exogenous substances, natural or synthetic, that function to bind to opioid receptors and produce some agonist effects. Opioids act as agonists of opioid receptors at presynaptic and postsynaptic sites inside and outside the CNS. Binding of opioid receptors results in increased potassium conductance, calcium channel inactivation, or both, which produces an immediate decrease in neurotransmitter release. Opioid receptor activation results in mostly presynaptic inhibition of neurotransmitters (i.e., acetylcholine, dopamine, norepinephrine, and substance P). Opioid effects are

Table 2.4 Commonly used opioid agonists: dosing and other considerations

Drug (brand name)	Dosing (intravenous)		Onset	Duration	Considerations
	Pediatric	Adult			
All opioids					Reduce dose by one-third to one-half when given with other CNS-depressing drugs, or in the elderly or debilitated. May cause CNS and/or respiratory depression, nausea, vomiting, hypotension, dizziness.
Morphine	*Incremental bolus:* 0.05–0.15 mg/kg slowly *Titrate:* to desired effect Max: 3.0 mg single dose	*Initial:* 1–2 mg slowly *Titrate:* 1–2 mg slowly every 5–10 min Max: 15 mg	5–10 min	3–4 h	
Hydromorphone (Dilaudid)	Not recommended outside critical care areas in pediatrics	*Initial:* 0.1–0.2 mg *Titrate:* 0.1–0.2 mg Max: 2.5 mg	3–5 min	2–3 h	
Fentanyl (Sublimaze)	Not recommended outside critical care areas in pediatrics	*Initial:* 0.05–2 µg/kg slowly over 3–5 min *Titrate:* 1 µg/ kg at 30 min intervals Max: 4 µg/kg	30–60 s	30–60 min	Fentanyl and meperidine are contraindicated in patients who have received monoamine oxidase (MAO) inhibitors within last 14 days.
Meperidine (Demerol)		*Initial:* 10 mg *Titrate:* 10 mg increment Max: 150 mg	1–5 min	1–3 h	
Remifentanil (Ultiva)	*Bolus:* 0.5–1 µg/kg infusion: 0.05–1.0 µg/kg per minute	*Bolus:* 0.5–1 µg/kg infusion: 0.05–2.0 µg/kg per minute	0.5–2 min	10–20 min, typically utilized as infusion	Major side effects are bradycardia, respiratory depression, nausea, and muscular rigidity

dose-dependent and occur as a result of opioid binding at receptor sites. These receptor sites, located primarily in the CNS, include the mu, kappa, delta, and sigma receptors. The affinity of most opioid agonists for receptors corresponds well with their analgesic potency. Desired clinical effects of opioids are analgesic, sedative, antitussive, and antishivering effects. Agonist action through the mu receptor is responsible for analgesia, euphoria, and sedation. Kappa-receptor activation leads to sedation and weak analgesia. Agonist action at the delta receptor also produces weak analgesia. The analgesic effect from systemic administration of opioids likely occurs from receptor activity at several sites. These include sensory neurons in the peripheral nervous system, the dorsal horn of the spinal cord, the brainstem medulla, and the cortex of the brain. Each of these sites plays a crucial role in opioid-induced analgesia. The dorsal horn of the spinal cord provides analgesia by inhibiting transmission of nociceptive information. The medulla potentiates descending inhibitory pathways that modulate ascending nociceptive signals. The cerebral cortex decreases the perception and emotional response to pain.

However, because of the widespread distribution of opioid receptors, many varied and unwanted effects may occur. Respiratory depression, physical dependence, pruritus, and bradycardia result from agonist activity at the aforesaid receptor sites. Furthermore, agonism of the sigma receptor results in hypertension, tachycardia, delirium, and dysphoria. Other undesirable side effects of opioid agonists include orthostatic hypotension, skeletal muscle rigidity, nausea and vomiting, constipation and delayed gastric emptying, urinary retention, pupillary constriction, and sphincter of Oddi spasm.

Morphine

Morphine is the prototype opioid agonist with which other opioids are compared. Morphine causes analgesia, euphoria, and sedation. The cause of pain may persist, but even low doses of morphine increase the pain threshold and modify the perception of pain. In general, continuous, dull pain is relieved by morphine more effectively than sharp, intermittent pain. Analgesia is most effective when morphine is administered before the painful stimulus occurs. In the absence of pain, morphine can produce dysphoria rather than euphoria. When morphine is given IV, onset of the clinical effects occurs within a few minutes, and they peak within 15–30 minutes. The elimination half-life is 2–4 hours. Morphine is also well absorbed when administered IM with an onset of effect in 15–30 minutes; peak effect occurs in 45–90 minutes, and the duration of action is 4 hours. However, repeat doses of IM morphine are not recommended because absorption becomes unpredictable. Morphine is metabolized by conjugation with glucuronic acid at both hepatic and extrahepatic sites, especially the kidney. Its active metabolite, morphine-6-glucuronide, produces analgesia and ventilatory depression by way of agonism of the mu receptors. Elimination of morphine in patients with renal failure can be impaired, causing an accumulation of metabolites and unexpected depression of ventilation even with small doses of opioids. Morphine also causes significant venodilation and histamine release.

Hydromorphone (Dilaudid)

Hydromorphone is a semisynthetic opioid derivative of morphine with five to six times the potency of morphine. Hydromorphone can be used to relieve moderate to severe pain, and can be administered via oral, IM, or IV routes. It has a slightly faster onset of action and slightly shorter duration of action than morphine. Unlike morphine, it is metabolized to inactive compounds and results in less histamine release. Adverse side effects of hydromorphone are similar to those of other potent opioid analgesics such as morphine and meperidine, but it may be a useful alternative in patients with contraindications or allergies to other opioids.

Fentanyl (Sublimaze)

Fentanyl is a phenylpiperidine-derivative synthetic opioid agonist structurally similar to meperidine. Analgesic effects of fentanyl are 75–125 times more potent than those of morphine (Table 2.5). Fentanyl is frequently used as the analgesic component in moderate and deep sedation because of its rapid onset and minimal histamine release. A dose of fentanyl IV has a more rapid and shorter duration of action than morphine. The greater lipid solubility of fentanyl compared to morphine contributes to its more rapid onset and greater potency. The short duration of a single dose of fentanyl associated with a rapid fall in plasma concentration reflects its rapid redistribution into inactive tissue sites such as muscle and fat. However, when multiple IV doses of fentanyl are administered, or with continuous infusion, progressive saturation of inactive tissues can occur. As a result, the duration of analgesia and depression of ventilation may be prolonged. Metabolism of fentanyl takes place in the liver. IV fentanyl administration results in clinical effects within 30 seconds to 1 minute. Peak effects occur within 10 minutes and duration of action is 30–120 minutes following a single dose. Analgesic concentrations of fentanyl strongly potentiate the effects of midazolam and decrease the dose requirements of propofol. Synergism of opioids and benzodiazepines plays a critical role in achieving hypnotic states for potentially painful procedures. However, the combination can easily result in ventilatory depression. Chest wall rigidity has also been reported in adults receiving analgesic doses of fentanyl and is best avoided by slow injection of low doses.

Table 2.5 Equianalgesic opioid dosage table for a 70-kg adult

Drug	Duration (hours)	Oral dosage	Parenteral dosage	Half-time
Codeine	4–6 h	200 mg	120 mg IM	3 h
Morphine	3–6 h	30–60 mg	10 mg IM/IV	1.5–2 h
Hydromorphone	4–5 h	7.5 mg	1.5 mg IM/IV	2–3 h
Meperidine	2–4 h	300 mg	75 mg IM/IV	3–5 h
Fentanyl	1–2 h	N/A	0.1 mg IM/IV	1.5–6 h
Oxycodone	4–6 h	20 mg	N/A	N/A
Methadone	4–6 h	10–20 mg	10 mg IM/IV	15–40 h
Oxymorphone	3–6 h	N/A	1 mg IM/IV	
Levorphanol	6–8 h	4 mg	2 mg IM/IV	
Hydrocodone	3–4 h	30 mg	N/A	

Source: Adapted from Urman and Vadivelu [2].

Meperidine (Demerol)

Meperidine is a synthetic opioid agonist and phenylpiperidine derivative similar in structure to fentanyl. Overall, meperidine is about one-tenth as potent as morphine. It is shorter-acting than morphine with a duration of action of about 2–4 hours. Meperidine causes sedation and euphoria similar to that of morphine in equal analgesic doses. Metabolism is primarily through the liver. The primary metabolite, normeperidine, produces CNS stimulation in high concentrations. Urinary excretion is the principal route of elimination. The elimination half-time of meperidine is 3–5 hours. Impaired renal function can predispose to an accumulation of the active metabolite of meperidine, normeperidine. Structurally, meperidine has similarities to atropine and possesses atropine-like effects, which may result in a dry mouth, tachycardia, and pupillary dilatation. Myocardial depression can occur with meperidine at clinically relevant doses. In patients taking antidepressant drugs (MAO inhibitors, fluoxetine), meperidine may precipitate serotonin syndrome (autonomic instability with hypertension, tachycardia, diaphoresis, hyperthermia, agitation, and hyperreflexia) or potentiate side effects of serotonin reuptake inhibitors. In addition, meperidine may cause seizures in patients with renal insufficiency or a history of seizures, or when used in repeated or high doses. Normeperidine-induced seizures are more likely in patients who have received high chronic meperidine therapy, large doses of meperidine over a short period, and/or have an impaired ability to eliminate the metabolite. Elderly patients manifest decreased protein binding of meperidine, resulting in increased free drug in the plasma and an apparent increased sensitivity to the opioid. Because of its unique and extensive side-effect profile, meperidine is recommended as a second-line analgesic.

Remifentanil (Ultiva)

Remifentanil is an esterase-metabolized piperidine mu-receptor opioid agonist that is useful as an infusion and bolus for its rapid onset and offset actions. The drug displays potent mu-receptor agonist activity, leading to analgesia and sedation. Its adverse effects are ventilatory depression, nausea, vomiting, muscular rigidity, bradycardia, and pruritus. However, it does not release histamine upon injection, and therefore has fewer hemodynamic adverse effects than an opioid such as morphine. It has a wide range of clinical applications to provide analgesia and sedation, including intraoperatively, in the intensive care unit (ICU), and on labor and delivery. It is also possible to utilize remifentanil to maintain spontaneous breathing at low infusion rates, but does necessitate adequate monitoring. Remifentanil is 100–200 times more potent than morphine and, similar to other opioids, has widely variable effects in patients. In terms of pharmacokinetics, the package insert reports that with IV doses administered over 60 seconds, the pharmacokinetics of remifentanil fit a three-compartment model with a rapid distribution half-time of 1 minute, a slower distribution half-time of 6 minutes, and a terminal elimination half-time of 10–20 minutes. When administered as an infusion, it's short context-sensitive half-lives of 3–6 minutes allows for rapid offset despite long infusion times. This is a result of its esterase metabolism. The pharmacokinetic profile of remifentanil is not significantly changed with renal or hepatic impairment. While remifentanil has high utility because of its rapidly titratable analgesic and sedative effects, one must take into account the rapid decline of opioid concentration following its use. This leads to higher postoperative pain scores likely because of the rapid cessation of an analgesic state and opioid-induced hyperalgesia. Thus, another analgesic agent should be utilized at the end of a remifentanil-based anesthetic, especially if significant postoperative pain is expected.

Adverse Effects of Opioids

Opioids have a direct effect on the respiratory center in the brain. This results in a dose-dependent depression of the ventilatory response to carbon dioxide. Opioids also blunt the increase in ventilation that typically occurs in response to hypoxia They can produce generalized skeletal muscle rigidity. At clinically relevant doses, morphine and fentanyl do not cause significant myocardial depression. However, morphine and fentanyl can reduce cardiac output by causing a dose-dependent bradycardia. Other undesirable effects include nausea and vomiting, constipation, biliary spasm, and urinary retention.

Other Drugs for Deep Sedation

Other drugs used for deep sedation include propofol (Diprivan), ketamine (Ketalar), dexmedetomidine (Precedex), and etomidate (Amidate) (Table 2.6).

Propofol (Diprivan)

Propofol is a substituted isopropylphenol with rapid, short-acting sedative hypnotic properties. The mechanism of action involves potentiation of the GABA receptor complex. Propofol is highly lipid-soluble, which explains the drug's fast onset with bolus administration and makes it a readily titratable drug for IV sedation. The concentration of propofol decreases quickly after an IV bolus due to redistribution. Propofol is suited for deep sedation because it allows for fast recovery without residual sedation and a low incidence of nausea and vomiting. Dosing for sedation and amnesia effects is typically 25–100 μg/kg per minute. Analgesic effects of propofol are uncertain and remain up for debate. Metabolism of propofol is hepatic and non-hepatic (pulmonary uptake and first-pass elimination, renal excretion). Hepatic metabolism is rapid, resulting in metabolites that are excreted in the urine. The elimination half-life is 0.5–1.5 hours. Despite its hepatic metabolism, there is no evidence of impaired elimination in patients with cirrhosis. Even at low doses, propofol may cause decreased oxygen levels, increased carbon dioxide levels, and inhibit airway reflexes. Because of its respiratory depressant effects and narrow therapeutic range, propofol should only be administered by individuals trained in airway management.

Propofol is popular for sedation of mechanically ventilated patients in the ICU. However, propofol has been implicated in propofol infusion syndrome (PRIS), which typically occurs in critically ill patients requiring long-term (> 24 hours) sedation who develop an otherwise unexplained high anion-gap metabolic acidosis, rhabdomyolysis, hyperkalemia, acute kidney injury, elevated liver enzymes, and cardiac dysfunction. Risk factors for PRIS include inappropriately high propofol doses and durations of administration, carbohydrate depletion, severe illness, and concomitant administration of catecholamines and glucocorticosteroids. Propofol may also cause pain and irritation upon IV injection. Mixing of propofol with any other drug is not recommended. For example, mixing of propofol with lidocaine to prevent pain with IV injection may result in coalescence of oil droplets, which may pose a risk of pulmonary embolism. The

Table 2.6 Other drugs: dosing and considerations

Drug (brand name)	Dosing (intravenous) Pediatric	Dosing (intravenous) Adult	Onset	Duration	Considerations
Propofol (Diprivan)	–	Bolus: 10–50 mg Titrate: 25–100 µg/kg per minute	Within 30 s	2–4 min	Contraindicated in patients with egg or soybean oil allergy. Does not have any analgesic properties. Pain on injection may be reduced by lidocaine. May cause respiratory depression, hypotension, hiccoughs, wheezing, coughing.
Ketamine (Ketalar)	Initial: 1–2 mg/kg IV (IM dose: 2 mg/kg)	Initial: 10 mg, or 0.2–0.75 mg/kg	1 min	5–15 min	Consider concurrent midazolam. Contraindicated in patients with increased intracranial pressure. May cause hypertension, confusion, delirium, hallucinations, nystagmus, nausea, hypersecretions, respiratory depression, agitation.
Dexmedetomidine (Precedex)	–	Loading dose: 1 µg/kg per hour over 10–20 min Titrate: 0.2–0.7–1 µg/kg per hour	10–15 min	2–4 h	Reduce loading dose by one-half for patients 65 years or older, and for those with impaired renal or hepatic function. May cause bradycardia, hypotension, and dry mouth. Concomitant use of other CNS depressants will result in increased levels of sedation.
Etomidate (Amidate)	0.2–0.3 mg/kg (ketamine preferred)	0.2 mg/kg over 30–60 s	< 1 min	3–5 min (up to 10 min)	Effects may be prolonged in liver failure. May cause nausea and vomiting, muscle twitching, respiratory depression.

formulation of propofol contains soybean oil, glycerin, yolk lecithin, and sodium edentate. Therefore, it should be avoided in patients with allergies to the aforesaid ingredients. Risk of infection and hypertriglyceridemia is also a concern. As supplied, it should be handled with an aseptic technique and disposed of once open for 6 hours.

Water-soluble preparations of propofol exist, including *fospropofol*, which is a pro-drug that is metabolized to propofol, formaldehyde, and phosphate. Lusedra (fospropofol disodium injection) has been discontinued; however, generic brands may be available. Fospropofol has a slower onset and longer duration of action when compared to propofol. Advantages of a water-soluble preparation are reduced pain at the site of IV administration and reduced chance for bacteremia and hyperlipidemia. Initial dosing of fospropofol is 6.5 mg/kg followed by 1.6 mg/kg supplemental doses. Fospropofol's peak levels are lower than for equipotent doses of propofol, and the drug has a longer-lasting effect. Dosing regimens are adjusted for sedation in elderly patients and those with severe systemic disease.

Ketamine (Ketalar)

Ketamine, a phencyclidine derivative, differs from other hypnotic drugs in that it produces a cataleptic state in which a patient's eyes remain open with a slow nystagmic gaze. Ketamine is a CNS depressant that produces a dissociative state and analgesia. Hypertonus and purposeful skeletal muscle movements may also occur with ketamine administration. The main effect of ketamine is thought to be produced through inhibition of the NMDA-receptor complex. Ketamine also interacts with opioid, nicotinic, and muscarinic receptors. Ketamine's onset of action is rapid and reaches peak plasma concentrations within 1 minute after IV administration and 5 minutes after IM administration. Intense analgesia can be produced with subanesthetic doses of ketamine at 0.2–0.5 mg/kg IV. Ketamine's clinical effects occur rapidly, with a return to consciousness typically within 15 minutes after a single dose.

Ketamine is not significantly bound to plasma proteins and exits the blood rapidly, to be distributed into the tissues. Ketamine is extremely lipid-soluble, which explains the rapid effects on the brain following administration. It undergoes hepatic metabolism and has a large volume of distribution, resulting in an elimination half-life of 2–3 hours. Ketamine's active metabolite, norketamine, is one-third as potent as ketamine. Chronic administration of ketamine produces enzyme induction and tolerance to subsequent doses. In addition to its CNS effects, ketamine produces bronchodilation. It also produces sympathetic nervous system stimulation with increases in blood pressure, heart rate, and cardiac output. Therefore, it should be utilized with caution in patients with hypertension and coronary artery dis- ease. Critically ill patients can experience the opposite effects, including hypotension and decreased cardiac output as a result of depletion of catecholamine stores and exhausted sympathetic nervous system compensatory mechanisms.

Ketamine does not cause significant ventilatory depression or affect airway tone. However, secretions are increased with ketamine administration. Patients also remain at risk for nausea and vomiting. Pre-treatment with glycopyrrolate may help combat hypersalivation. Unpleasant emergence reactions typically limit the use of ketamine outside of the operating room. Combinations of ketamine and benzodiazepines limit these unwanted reactions and also increase amnesia.

Ketamine and Propofol ("Ketofol")

The combination of ketamine and propofol, or "ketofol," is being studied for use in procedural sedation. Synergistic benefits of these two drugs may allow for lower doses and reduce the risk of potential side effects including propofol-induced hypotension and ketamine-induced vomiting and emergence reactions. Benefits of adding ketamine to propofol may include less respiratory depression requiring intervention, fewer episodes of apnea and oxygen desaturation, smaller cumulative doses of propofol, more consistent sedation, good recovery, and potent post-procedural analgesia. Multiple propofol–ketamine mixture ratios have been investigated. The safety and efficacy of ketofol as a sedative–analgesic are dependent on the dose and ratio of the mixture.

Dexmedetomidine (Precedex)

Dexmedetomidine is a highly selective alpha-2-adrenergic agonist, which is utilized for its sedative properties in numerous settings. Hypnosis arises from stimulation of the alpha-2 receptors in the locus ceruleus, and the analgesic effect originates at the level of the spinal cord. Overall, dexmedetomidine produces sedation, pain relief, anxiety reduction, stable respiratory rates, and predictable cardiovascular responses.

Dexmedetomidine facilitates patient comfort, compliance, and comprehension by offering sedation with the ability to rouse patients. This makes it a great medication for sedation in the ICU. Dexmedetomidine also produces sedative and analgesic effects without respiratory depression, making it an attractive agent for short-term procedural sedation. It has been safely utilized for sedation in a variety of procedures (i.e., transesophageal echocardiography, colonoscopy, shockwave lithotripsy, percutaneous tracheotomy). Rapid administration of dexmedetomidine (loading dose of 1µg/kg per hour if given in less than 10 minutes) can cause transient hypertension, but hypotension and bradycardia may also occur with ongoing therapy. Dexmedetomidine (0.2–1.0 µg/kg per hour) is useful for postoperative critical care patients requiring mechanical ventilation. It does not cause clinically significant ventilatory depression, and sedation mimics natural sleep. The elimination half-life of dexmedetomidine is 2–4 hours. Dexmedetomidine is highly protein-bound and undergoes rapid and extensive metabolism in the liver. Dose adjustments are necessary in patients with hepatic failure because of the lower rate of metabolism. Dexmedetomidine's metabolites are excreted in the urine. Moderate decreases in heart rate can occur with dexmedetomidine infusion. Other adverse effects are probably due to unopposed vagal stimulation and include heart block, severe bradycardia, hypotension, and sinus arrest. Should it become necessary to reverse the sedative and cardiovascular effects of IV dexmedetomidine, atipamezole (Antisedan) is a specific and selective alpha-2-receptor antagonist that rapidly reverses these effects.

Etomidate (Amidate)

Etomidate is an IV medication with hypnotic but not analgesic properties. It causes minimal hemodynamic effects and maintains cardiovascular stability at clinically relevant doses. Etomidate is a carboxylated imidazole derivative of which one isomer has hypnotic qualities. Etomidate appears to have GABA-like effects, producing hypnosis through potentiation of GABA-mediated chloride currents. Etomidate is metabolized by hydrolysis via hepatic enzymes and plasma esterases. It is primarily cleared via the urine and has a short elimination half-life of 2–5 hours. Involuntary myoclonic movements are common with etomidate use and may reduce the rate of procedural success. The myoclonic-like activity can be attenuated by prior administration of an opioid. Awakening after a single injection of etomidate is rapid, and typically occurs without residual depressant effects. Etomidate has a high incidence of pain on injection. Strategies to reduce pain with injection of etomidate are similar to those used with propofol. Nausea and vomiting after administration is also common. Respiratory depression occurs at comparable rates to that of propofol. Another side effect of etomidate use is that it causes dose-dependent adrenal suppression via inhibition of 11-beta-hydroxylase, which may be harmful in critically ill patients.

Adjunct Medications

Diphenhydramine (Benadryl)

Benadryl is a sedating antihistamine with anticholinergic properties and is available in oral, IV, and IM formulations. As a *first-generation* histamine 1 (H_1) antihistamine, it crosses the blood–brain barrier because of its lipophilic molecular structure, leading to sedation. Providers should be aware that adverse reactions may be due to its inhibition on muscarinic, serotoninergic, and adrenergic receptors. Toxicity with overdose has been reported. Clinically relevant uses can extend beyond the treatment of allergic symptoms to the treatment of vestibular disorders, as sedatives, as sleeping aids, and as antiemetics. In this regard, diphenhydramine, typically in a dose of 25–50 mg IV, provides safe and effective sedation in most patients. Potential side effects include a dry mouth, drowsiness, dizziness, nausea and vomiting, constipation, headaches, photosensitivity, and urinary retention.

Scopolamine

Scopolamaine is a muscarinic antagonist well known for possesses sing antiemetic effects, often in the context of motion sickness. However, it also possesses sedative properties. Historically, from the 1940s to the 1960s it was commonly used to induce twilight sleep in laboring mothers to eliminate the memory of pain. Today, it is more rarely utilized to provide amnesia and sedation, and more commonly used prophylactically for postoperative nausea and vomiting. Rare side effects are confusion, rambling speech, agitation, hallucinations, paranoid behaviors, and delusions. Preparations include oral, subcutaneous, IV, transdermal patch, and ophthalmic.

Non-Steroidal Anti-Inflammatory Drugs

Prostaglandins were first discovered from semen, prostate, and seminal vesicles by Goldblatt and von Euler in the 1930s [3]. The identification of the COX reaction, the identification of the COX enzyme, and the demonstration by Sir John Vane that aspirin, indomethacin, and NSAIDs were all inhibitors of COX, all occurred in the early 1970s. Works by Habenicht in 1985 and Needleman in 1990 ultimately demonstrated that an endogenous COX-1 and an inducible enzyme COX-2 existed [4].

Non-steroidal anti-inflammatory drugs (NSAIDs) have served as analgesics, anti-inflammatory, and antipyretic medicines since 1898 and are effective in mild to moderate surgical pain. One benefit of this class of drugs is that they lack many of the adverse effects of opioids, including respiratory depression. Common NSAIDs available include ibuprofen, naproxen, aspirin, indomethacin, and meloxicam. NSAIDs are not without risk. They can be nephrotoxic, cause adverse gastrointestinal events, and lead to surgical bleeding via platelet dysfunction.

Pharmaceutical companies in the 1990s invested billions of dollars to develop more selective NSAIDs, namely COX-2 inhibitors (e.g., celecoxib). These selective agents worked differently than older NSAIDs. Extensive research nearly 20 years ago identified the COX-2 site as an inducible enzyme that is the location for the mediation of pain, inflammation, and fever pathways. Although these agents work well for pain relief and combating inflammation while avoiding gastrointestinal side effects, their long-term use is limited by adverse cardiac effects.

Overall, these agents are widely used for mild to moderate pain relief. Ketorolac (Toradol) and ibuprofen (Caldolor) are used as IV preparations. Parecoxib is a COX-2 selective inhibitor used in Europe. It is not approved for use in the United States. Multimodal analgesia is two or more analgesic agents acting by different mechanisms to provide analgesia. Combinations of NSAIDs, COX-2-specific inhibitors, opiates, and acetaminophen are routinely used for prevention and treatment of pain.

Intravenous Acetaminophen

Acetaminophen is widely utilized to reduce pain and fever. IV acetaminophen is available in the United States as acetaminophen injection (Ofirmev). IV acetaminophen is indicated to treat mild to moderate pain and moderate to severe pain with adjunctive opioid analgesics. When used for acute post-surgical pain management, IV acetaminophen, produces pain relief and opioid dose-sparing effects. In conjunction with other non-opioid analgesics, IV acetaminophen plays a crucial role in preemptive analgesia. It inhibits prostaglandin synthesis in the CNS and works peripherally to block pain signal generation. It also acts on the hypothalamus to produce antipyresis.

IV acetaminophen is metabolized by the liver and is contraindicated in patients with severe hepatic impairment. Dosing for adults larger than 50 kg is 1,000 mg every 6 hours and should not exceed 4 g/day. IV infusion of acetaminophen should be administered over at least 15 minutes. Renal-impaired adjusted doses and timing are dependent on creatinine clearance. Care should be taken when prescribing other acetaminophen-containing products to avoid exceeding maximum daily limits.

IV acetaminophen infusion for procedural sedation has been reported to reduce pain and the risk of intraoperative respiratory events such as upper airway obstruction in high-risk cardiac patients when compared to fentanyl during implantation of cardiac devices. However, further studies are needed to support this conclusion.

Clonidine

Clonidine is a central alpha-2-receptor agonist, and is typically utilized as an antihypertensive medication. As a depletory of free and total catecholamine levels, it inhibits the release of norepinephrine. It can be used for many treatments beyond elevated blood pressure, including opioid withdrawal, other hyperarousal states, insomnia, and neuropathic pain. This is related to its sedative, anxiolytic, and analgesic properties. It is used in numerous preparations, including oral, transdermal, and epi- dural, to prolong the effects of analgesia when used together with local anesthetics (LAs). Since clonidine is a mild sedative, it can also be used as a premedication before surgery or procedures. Significant side effects include lightheadedness, dry mouth, dizziness, and constipation.

Local Anesthetics

Local anesthetics prevent the generation and the conduction of nerve impulses. Their primary site of action is the cell membrane. The major mechanism of action of these drugs involves their interaction with one or more specific binding sites within the sodium channel. The degree of blockade produced by a given concentration of LA depends on how the nerve has been stimulated and on its resting membrane potential. Therefore, a resting nerve is much less sensitive to an LA than one that is repetitively stimulated; a higher frequency of stimulation and more positive membrane potential cause a greater degree of anesthetic block. These frequency- and voltage-dependent effects of LAs occur because the LA molecule in its charged form gains access to its binding site within the pore when the sodium channel is in an open state, and because the LA binds more tightly to and stabilizes the inactivated form of the sodium channel. As a general rule, small nerve fibers are more susceptible to the effects of local anesthetics than are large fibers.

Under typical conditions of administration, the pH of the LA solution rapidly equilibrates to that of the extracellular fluids. Although the unprotonated species of the LA is necessary for diffusion across cellular membranes, the cationic species interacts preferentially with sodium channels. Changes in pH of the injected LA solution can produce a shortening of onset time, with marked decreases paralleling significant pH changes. The limiting factor for the pH adjustment is the solubility of the base form of the drug. For each LA, there is a pH at which the amount of base in solution is maximal (a saturated solution).

Another method to shortening onset time for producing surgical anesthesia has been through the use of carbonated LA solutions. The LA salt is the carbonate, and the solution contains large quantities of carbon dioxide to maintain a high concentration of the carbonate anion. Combinations of LA with an opioid are increasingly used in scenarios where one desires sensory blockade without significant motor block, as in obstetrical anesthesia and pain management. The addition of epidural and intrathecal opioids allows use of lower concentrations of LA.

Plasma concentrations of LAs are dependent on:

- the dose of the drug administered
- the absorption of the drug from the specific site injected, which depends on the vasoactivity of the drug, site vascularity, and whether a vasoconstrictor such as epinephrine has been added to the anesthetic solution
- biotransformation and elimination of the drug from the circulation

Undesired Effects of Local Anesthetics

Table 2.7 shows the toxic dose of several LAs.

Central Nervous System

Following absorption, LAs can cause stimulation of the CNS, producing restlessness and tremor that may proceed to clonic convulsions. In general, the more potent the

Table 2.7 Local anesthetics: duration of action and toxic dose

Local anesthetic (brand name)	Concentrations	Maximum total recommended dose	Volume of maximum total recommended dose	Average onset and duration of action
Procaine (Novocaine)	0.25–0.5%	350–600 mg	140–240 mL of 0.25% 70–120 mL of 0.5%	Onset: 2–5 min Duration: 15–60 min
Chloroprocaine (Nesacaine)	1–2%	≤ 800 mg	80 mL of 1% 40 mL of 2%	Onset: 6–12 min Duration: 30 min
Lidocaine, plain (Xylocaine)	1–2%	3–5 mg/kg; ≤ 300 mg	30 mL of 1% 15 mL of 2%	Onset: 1–2 min Duration: 30–60 min
Lidocaine, with epinephrine	1–2% lidocaine: epinephrine: 1: 100,000 or 1:200,000	5–7 mg/kg; ≤ 500 mg	50 mL of 1% 25 mL of 2%	Onset: 1–2 min Duration: 60–240 min
Bupivacaine, plain (Marcaine, Sensorcaine)	0.25–0.5%	2.5 mg/kg; ≤ 175 mg	70 mL of 0.25% 35 mL of 0.5%	Onset: 5 min Duration: 120–240 min
Bupivacaine, with epinephrine	0.25–0.5% Bupivacaine: epinephrine: 1:200,000	≤ 225 mg	90 mL of 0.25% 45 mL of 0.5%	Onset: 5 min Duration: 180–360 min
Mepivacaine (Polocaine)	1%	≤ 400 mg	40 mL of 1%	Onset: 3–5 min Duration: 45–90 min

Source: Adapted from Windle [5].

anesthetic the more readily convulsions may be elicited. Alterations of CNS activity are thus predictable from the LA agent in question and the blood concentration achieved. Central stimulation is followed by depression; death is usually caused by the resulting respiratory failure.

Cardiovascular System

Following systemic absorption, LAs may act on the cardiovascular system. The primary site of action is the myocardium, where LAs can decrease electrical excitability, conduction rate, and force of contraction. In addition, LAs can cause arteriolar dilatation. The cardiovascular effects are usually only seen when high systemic concentrations are attained and effects on the CNS are produced. However, on rare occasions lower doses can cause cardiovascular collapse and death, due to either an action on the conduction of the heart or the sudden onset of ventricular fibrillation. However, it should be noted that ventricular tachycardia and fibrillation are very uncommon consequences of LAs other than bupivacaine. Finally, it should be stressed that unwanted cardiovascular effects of LA agents are often a result of inadvertent intravascular administration, especially if epinephrine is also present.

Lidocaine

Lidocaine (Xylocaine), introduced in 1948, is currently the most commonly used LA.

Pharmacologic Actions

The pharmacologic actions that lidocaine shares with other LA drugs have been described extensively. Lidocaine is an amide LA that produces faster, more intense, longer-lasting, and more extensive anesthesia than does an equal concentration of procaine. It is a good choice for individuals sensitive to ester-type LAs.

Absorption, Fate, and Excretion

Lidocaine is absorbed rapidly after parenteral administration and from the gastrointestinal and respiratory tracts. Although it is effective when utilized without any vasoconstrictor, in the presence of epinephrine, the rate of absorption and the toxicity are decreased, and the duration of action usually is prolonged. Lidocaine is dealkylated in the liver by mixed-function oxidases to monoethylglycine xylidide and glycine xylidide, which can be metabolized further to monoethylglycine and xylidide. Both monoethylglycine xylidide and glycine xylidide retain LA activity. In human beings, about 75% of xylidide is excreted in the urine [6].

Toxicity

The side effects of lidocaine seen with increasing doses are drowsiness, tinnitus, dysgeusia, dizziness, and twitching. As the dose increases, seizures, coma, and respiratory depression and arrest can occur. Clinically significant cardiovascular depression typically occurs at serum lidocaine levels that produce significant CNS effects. The metabolites monoethylglycine xylidide and glycine xylidide may contribute to some of these adverse effects.

Clinical Uses of Lidocaine

Lidocaine has a wide range of clinical uses as an LA. It has utility in almost any application where an LA of intermediate duration is needed. Lidocaine can also be used as an IV infusion as an antiarrhythmic and analgesic agent.

Bupivacaine

Bupivacaine (Marcaine, Sensorcaine), introduced in 1963, is a commonly utilized amide LA. Its structure is comparable to that of lidocaine, except that the amine-containing group is a butyl piperidine. It is known for its potency and ability to produce prolonged anesthesia. Its long duration of action and tendency to provide more sensory than motor blockade has made it a popular drug for providing prolonged analgesia during labor or the postoperative period. By utilizing indwelling catheters and continuous infusions, bupivacaine can be used to provide several days of effective analgesia.

Bupivacaine has made contributions to regional anesthesia second in importance only to that of lidocaine. It is one of the first of the clinically used LA drugs that is able to provide good separation of motor and sensory blockade after its administration. The onset of analgesia and the duration of action are long and can be further prolonged by the addition of epinephrine in areas with a low fat content. Only minimal increases in duration are seen when bupivacaine is injected into areas with a high fat content. For instance, a 50% increase in duration of brachial plexus blockade (an area of low fat content) follows the addition of epinephrine to bupivacaine solutions; in contrast, only a 10–15% increase in duration of epidural anesthesia is seen from the addition of epinephrine to bupivacaine solutions, since the epidural space has a high fat content.

Toxicity

Bupivacaine is more cardiotoxic than equi-effective doses of lidocaine. Clinically, this presents as severe ventricular arrhythmias and myocardial depression usually after inadvertent intravascular administration of large doses of bupivacaine. The enhanced cardiotoxicity of bupivacaine is due to multiple factors. Lidocaine and bupivacaine block cardiac sodium channels rapidly during systole. However, bupivacaine dissociates significantly more slowly than does lidocaine during diastole, so a large fraction of sodium channels remains blocked at the end of diastole (at physiologic heart rates) with bupivacaine [7]. Therefore, the block by bupivacaine is cumulative and substantially more than would be predicted by its LA potency. At least a part of the cardiac toxicity of bupivacaine may be mediated centrally, as direct injection of small quantities of bupivacaine into the medulla can produce malignant ventricular arrhythmias [8]. Bupivacaine-induced cardiac toxicity can be extremely difficult to treat, and its severity is enhanced in the presence of acidosis, hypercarbia, and hypoxemia.

Clinical Uses of Bupivacaine

In the United States, bupivacaine has been used mostly for obstetric anesthesia and postoperative pain control when analgesia without significant motor blockade is desirable, as this is achievable with low bupivacaine concentrations. In contrast to lidocaine, bupivacaine has a poorer therapeutic index in producing electrophysiologic toxicity of the heart [9]. Although bupivacaine metabolism is slower in the fetus and newborn than in the adult, active biotransformation is accomplished by the fetus and newborn.

A second major use of bupivacaine is in subarachnoid anesthesia. It produces very reliable onset of anesthesia in 5 minutes, and the duration of anesthesia is approximately 3 hours. In many ways, it is similar to tetracaine; however, the dose of bupivacaine required is larger – specifically, 10 mg of tetracaine is approximately equal to 12–15 mg of bupivacaine. The initiation of sympathetic blockade following spinal anesthesia appears to be more gradual with bupivacaine than with tetracaine. Also, the sensory blockade created by bupivacaine lasts longer than the motor blockade, which is in contrast to what occurs with etidocaine and tetracaine.

Bupivacaine Liposome Injectable

Bupivacaine incased in a liposomal membrane (Exparel) is indicated for single-dose infiltration into the surgical site to produce post-surgical analgesia in non-pregnant adults. This technology allows for sustained drug delivery over longer periods of time. Dosing is based on the size of the surgical site, the volume required to cover the area, and individual patient factors impacting the safety of amide LAs. The maximum dose is

266 mg or 20 mL. Local infiltrations of bupivacaine liposome injection result in significant systemic plasma levels of bupivacaine and can persist for up to 96 hours. Other formulations of bupivacaine should not be administered within 96 hours after administration of liposomal bupivacaine injection. The rate of systemic absorption of bupivacaine is dependent on the total dose of the drug, the route administered, and the vascularity at the site of administration. After bupivacaine has been released from the liposome and is absorbed systemically, distribution, metabolism, and excretion of bupivacaine is the same as any bupivacaine hydrochloric acid (HCl) solution formulation.

Compatibility considerations of bupivacaine liposome injectable include administration with bupivacaine HCl, altered pharmacokinetics/physiochemical properties, additive toxic effects, and direct contact with certain drugs (i.e., lidocaine, non-bupivacaine-based LAs). Specific recommendations from the manufacturer should be reviewed prior to use of liposomal bupivacaine with other drugs. Warnings and precautions regarding monitoring for cardiovascular and neurologic status and vital signs during and after administration of bupivacaine liposome injection are the same as that of other LAs. As an amide LA, it is metabolized by the liver and excreted by the kidney and should be used with caution in patients with hepatic and renal disease. Bupivacaine liposome injection is not recommended for epidural use, intrathecal use, regional nerve blocks, or intravascular or intra-articular use at the moment.

Ropivacaine

The cardiac toxicity of bupivacaine created interest in developing a less toxic long-lasting LA. The result of that investigation was the development of a new amino ethylamine, ropivacaine, the S-enantiomer of 1-propyl-2′,6′-pipecolocylidide. The S-enantiomer, like most LAs with a chiral center, was selected because it has a lower toxicity than the R isomer. This is thought to be due to slower uptake, resulting in lower blood levels for a given dose. Ropivacaine is not as potent as bupivacaine in producing anesthesia. However, compared to bupivacaine, clinically adequate doses of ropivacaine have a lower propensity for motor block and reduced potential for CNS toxicity and cardiotoxicity. Ropivacaine appears to be suitable for both epidural and regional anesthesia, with a duration of action similar to bupivacaine. Overall, ropivacaine is an important option for regional anesthesia and management of post-surgical and labor pain.

Clinical Uses of Local Anesthetics

Local anesthesia is the loss of sensation in a body part without loss of consciousness or impairment of central control of vital functions. It offers two major advantages. The first is that the physiologic stresses associated with general anesthesia are avoided. The second is that neurophysiologic responses to pain and stress can be modified, as described earlier in the chapter under the section on preemptive analgesia. As discussed earlier, LAs also have the potential to produce deleterious side effects. The choice of an LA and care in its use are the determinants of such toxicity. There is a variable relationship between the amount of LA injected and peak plasma levels in adults. The serum level depends greatly on the area of injection. It is highest with IV injection and interpleural or intercostal block and lowest with subcutaneous infiltration. Thus, recommended doses serve only as general safety guidelines.

Treatment of Local Anesthetic Systemic Toxicity

Symptoms of local anesthetic systemic toxicity (LAST) include tinnitus, metallic taste in the mouth, lip numbness or tingling, lightheadedness, seizures, arrhythmias, and finally cardiovascular collapse. If suspicion for LAST is high, prompt airway management is crucial in preventing hypoxia and acidosis, which are known to potentiate LAST. The following advice for treatment of LAST is adapted from Weinberg [10].

If a seizure occurs, it should be rapidly treated with benzodiazepines. Small doses of propofol or thiopental may also be utilized. Although propofol can stop seizures, large doses can further depress cardiac function. Thus, propofol should be avoided when there are signs of cardiovascular compromise.

If cardiac arrest occurs, initiate advanced cardiac life support . Avoid calcium channel blockers and beta-receptor blockers. If ventricular arrhythmias develop, amiodarone is the preferred treatment. (Lidocaine or procainamide are not recommended.)

Lipid emulsion therapy should be initiated at the first signs of LAST, but after airway management. Dosing consists of a 1.5 mL/kg 20% lipid emulsion bolus, followed by an infusion of 0.25 mL/kg per minute, continued for at least 10 minutes after circulatory stability is attained. If circulatory stability is not obtained, consider giving another bolus and increasing infusion to 0.5 mL/kg per minute. Approximately 10 mL/kg lipid emulsion over 30 minutes is recommended as the upper limit for the initial dose. Propofol is not a substitute for lipid emulsion. Failure to respond to lipid emulsion and vasopressor therapy should prompt initiating cardiopulmonary bypass. Because there can be considerable delay in beginning cardiopulmonary bypass, it is reasonable to notify the closest facility capable of providing it when cardiovascular compromise is first identified during LAST.

Reversal Agents for Benzodiazepines and Opioids

The benzodiazepine and opioid antagonists are important drug classes to consider when administering moderate and/or deep sedation. Reversal agents provide a method to quickly restore sensorium following short procedures. In addition, these drugs can be used to restore airway reflexes and/or reverse respiratory depression due to benzodiazepine and/or opioid administration. Reversal agents exist (Table 2.8) and should be readily available to treat apnea and hypoxemia, in appropriate scenarios. If required, the use of reversal agents warrants an extended recovery observation period.

Flumazenil (Romazicon)

Flumazenil is a specific benzodiazepine-receptor antagonist that reverses most of the CNS effects of benzodiazepines. It is a competitive antagonist that prevents or reverses all agonist effects of benzodiazepines in a dose-dependent manner. It reverses the sedative–hypnotic effects of benzodiazepines as well as the ventilatory depression that can occur when benzodiazepines are used in combination with opioids. Titration of flumazenil dosing to the desired level of consciousness is recommended (Table 2.8). Lower total doses of flumazenil, 0.3–0.6 mg IV, are typically adequate to decrease the degree of sedation, whereas doses of 0.5–1.0 mg IV abolish the therapeutic effects of benzodiazepines. Because the duration of action of the benzodiazepines is longer (up to 6 hours) than flumazenil's duration of action (30–60 minutes), supplemental doses may be required to

Table 2.8 Reversal agents

| Drug (brand name) | Dosing (intravenous) | | Onset | Duration | Considerations |
	Pediatric	Adult			
Flumazenil (Romazicon)	0.005–0.1 mg/kg, with 0.01 mg/kg most used dose	0.2 mg over 15 s, repeat at 0.2 mg every 60 s to 1 mg *Max*; may repeat at 20-min intervals. *Max*: 3 mg in 30 min	30–60 s	30–60 min	Can precipitate seizures in those with history of seizures and tricyclic overdose. If seizures occur, they may be refractory until flumazenil is metabolized. May cause visual disturbances, diaphoresis, arrhythmias.
Naloxone (Narcan)	Less than 5 years or 20 kg: 0.001–0.1 mg/kg, may repeat every 2–3 min *Max*: 2 mg; Greater than 5 years or 20 kg: 2 mg dose, may repeat as needed	0.4 mg every 2–3 min *Max*: 10 mg	2 min	45 min	Can precipitate ventricular tachycardia and fibrillation in those with cardiovascular disease or receiving cardiotoxic drugs. May cause nausea and vomiting, sweating, tachycardia, hypertension, pulmonary edema.

maintain antagonist activity. A continuous low-dose infusion of flumazenil of 0.1–0.4 mg/hour may be used rather than administering repeated doses to maintain wakefulness. There are risks to reversal of benzodiazepines. In patients with a history of seizures, flumazenil can precipitate withdrawal seizure activity. Therefore, flumazenil is not recommended for use in patients taking antiepileptic drugs for seizure control. Flumazenil antagonism does not generally cause acute anxiety, hypertension, or tachycardia when reversing the sedative effects of benzodiazepines. The drug is also not associated with alterations in coronary hemodynamics in patients with coronary artery disease. Presumably, flumazenil's weak intrinsic agonist activity attenuates effects of abrupt reversal of the benzodiazepines.

Naloxone (Narcan)

Naloxone is a non-selective antagonist at all three opioid receptors. It is a competitive opioid antagonist, which reverses opioid-induced analgesia and depression of ventilation. The short duration of action of naloxone (45 minutes) is thought to be the result of its rapid removal from the brain. The return of opioid effects (re-narcotization) such as delayed respiratory depression can occur unless supplemental doses of naloxone are administered. Alternatively, a continuous IV infusion of naloxone (3–5 μg/kg per hour) may be initiated rather than additional IV boluses of the drug. Providers must also be aware that rapid reversal of analgesia occurs with administration naloxone. However, slow titration of naloxone may reverse the unwanted respiratory effects while allowing for partial agonism of opioid receptors and some analgesia. Naloxone is primarily metabolized in the liver. Other adverse reactions may occur with reversal of opioid activity, including tachycardia, hypertension, dysrhythmias, nausea, vomiting, and diaphoresis. Nausea and vomiting appear to be related to the dose and speed of injection and may be attenuated by administration of the drug over 2–3 minutes. Cardiovascular stimulation after IV administration of naloxone is thought to result from the sudden perception of pain and sympathetic nervous system stimulation. Furthermore, withdrawal symptoms may occur with reversal of both benzodiazepines and/or opioids in patients dependent on them.

Clinical Pearls

- *Sedating to a desired effect.* To provide sedation safely requires an understanding of drug pharmacokinetics such as half-time, context-sensitive half-life, and common side effects. However, sedating to a desired effect is often more of an art than a science. It also requires experience and understanding of both the procedure and of patient characteristics. If the patient has had sedation before, it is important to review prior records for documentation of drugs given, total dosages used, and reported patient comfort.

- *Desired characteristics of the drugs* used in moderate and deep sedation include: rapid onset; easily controlled depth of sedation and possibility for reversal, if necessary; rapid recovery; minimal respiratory effects; amnesic and analgesic effects, cardiovascular stability; non-allergic and with no active metabolic by-products.

- Unfortunately, none of the drugs used in moderate or deep sedation has *all* of the desired characteristics outlined afore. Therefore, a combination of drugs is often employed to achieve many of the desired effects while minimizing the unwanted side effects.

- *Common objectives of sedation include*:

  1. Managing patient anxiety: This is best accomplished with benzodiazepines.
  2. Increasing pain threshold: Pain can be preempted and treated with acetaminophen and/or NSAIDs such as ibuprofen (oral, IV) and ketorolac (IV). Short- and long-acting opioid medications can provide effective pain control, but can be associated with several side effects.
  3. Imposing some level of amnesia: Benzodiazepines are the most effective agents for this purpose.
  4. Maintaining minimal variation of vital signs: such as blood pressure, heart rate, and oxygen saturation. Some of the medications used can lead to hypotension (propofol, opioids), bradycardia (dexmedetomidine, high-dose opioids), and decreased respiratory rate (propofol, opioids). Using a combination of drugs from multiple classes can help achieve desired sedation end points while resulting in fewer unwanted side effects.

- *Slowly titrate medication(s) to desired effect.* It is important to remember that patients may respond differently to a given amount of medication, and that one may observe delayed side effects, such as respiratory depression. Carefully titrating to desired effects and setting limits on total dose that can be given can help prevent unintended over-sedation (see the American Society of Anesthesiologists' continuum of depth of sedation, Table 1.2 [11]).

- *Drug dosing adjustments* may be required to account for the patient's body habitus (obesity can lead to increased drug volume of distribution), cardiac status (decreased cardiac output), nutritional status (drug protein binding), liver and/or kidney dysfunction (reduced drug metabolism and excretion), extremes of age, concurrent use of other drugs (a patient's regularly taken drugs can interact with the administered drugs and result in increased side effects), and allergies.

- *Have I given enough sedation and analgesia?* As mentioned previously, slowly titrating to the desired effect is prudent. Administer drugs appropriate for the given level of stimulation during the procedure. Also, it is important to be familiar with the procedure and anticipate a more/less stimulating period before it occurs. Another useful end point is observing changes in vital signs such as blood pressure and heart rate in response to the medications you have just administered to counteract the discomfort/pain caused by the procedure. Another useful end point is the change in respiratory rate in response to the drugs given and the procedure stimulation.

Summary

The safe and effective administration of moderate and deep sedation by non-anesthesia providers occurs frequently in a variety of locations within and outside of the hospital setting. Providing sedation and analgesia for the many different types of patients and procedures requires knowledge of commonly used medications. An understanding of the pharmacology of the benzodiazepines and opioids as well as their reversal agents is crucial to assure patient safety. Other drugs used in sedation, such as propofol, ketamine, etomidate, and dexmedetomidine, require similar attention prior to their use to maintain safety. Furthermore, techniques to obtain the desired end point with drug administration while avoiding undesirable side effects should be kept in mind. Slow titration of a medication while monitoring the patient's response (level of consciousness, respiratory rate, blood pressure, etc.) should dictate dosing. Drug choice should be based on the procedure. Painful procedures require analgesia and possibly sedative–hypnotics, whereas non-painful procedures may only require sedation. Dose requirements vary based on patient characteristics (e.g., height, weight, age) and body habitus. Comorbidities such as hepatic and/or renal failure also affect dose requirements, as does a history of alcohol and/or drug use. Generally, decreased doses are required when combining benzodiazepines and/or opioids with other CNS-depressive drugs. Decreased doses should also be utilized in the elderly and the debilitated.

References

1. Kim KM. Remimazolam: pharmacological characteristics and clinical applications in anesthesiology. *Anesth Pain Med.* 2022;17(1):1–11. doi: 10.17085/apm.21115

2. Urman R, Vadivelu N. Acute and postoperative pain management. In *Pocket Pain Medicine.* Philadelphia, PA: Lippincott, Williams & Wilkins, 2011.

3. Flower RJ. Prostaglandins, bioassay and inflammation. *Br J Pharmacol.* 2006;147(Suppl 1):S182–92. doi: 10.1038/sj.bjp.0706506

4. Habenicht A, Salbach P, Goerig M. et al. The LDL receptor pathway delivers

arachidonic acid for eicosanoid formation in cells stimulated by platelet-derived growth factor. *Nature.* 1990;345;634–6. doi: 10.1038/345634a0

5. Windle ML. Infiltrative administration of local anesthetic agents. *Medscape emedicine,* 2011. emedicine.medscape.com/article/149178-overview (updated 2022)

6. Arthur GR. Pharmacokinetics. In Strichartz GR, ed., *Handbook of Experimental Pharmacology,* vol. 81. Berlin: Springer-Verlag, 1987, 165–86.

7. Clarkson CW, Hondeghem LM. Mechanism for bupivacaine depression of cardiac conduction: fast block of sodium channels during the action potential with slow recovery from block during diastole. *Anesthesiology.* 1985;62:396–405.

8. Thomas RD, Behbehani MM, Coyle DE, Denson DD. Cardiovascular toxicity of local anesthetics: an alternative hypothesis. *Anesth Analg.* 1986;65: 444–50.

9. Nath S, Häggmark S, Johansson G, Reiz S. Differential depressant and electrophysiologic cardiotoxicity of local anesthetics: an experimental study with special reference to lidocaine and bupivacaine. *Anesth Analg.* 1986;65: 1263–70.

10. Weinberg GL. Treatment of local anesthetic systemic toxicity (LAST). *Reg Anesth Pain Med.* 2010;35:188–193.

11. American Society of Anesthesiologists Task Force on Sedation and Analgesia by Non-Anesthesiologists. Practice guidelines for sedation and analgesia by non-anesthesiologists. *Anesthesiology.* 2002;96:1004–17.

Additional Reading

Barash PG, Cullen BF, Stoelting RK, Cahalan MK, Stock MC, eds. *Clinical Anesthesia,* 6th ed. Philadelphia, PA: Lippincott Williams & Wilkins, 2009.

Faust RJ, Cucchiara RF, Rose SH, et al. *Anesthesiology Review,* 3rd ed. Philadelphia, PA: Churchill Livingstone, 2002.

Hospira. Dosing guidelines for Precedex®: nonintubated procedural sedation and ICU sedation. https://aamsn.org/wp-content/uploads/2010/02/Precedex_Dosing_Guide.pdf

Mirrakhimov AE, Voore P, Halytskyy O, et al. Propofol infusion syndrome in adults: a clinical update. *Crit Care Res Pract.* 2015;15:1–10.

Morgan GE, Mikhail MS, Murray MJ. *Clinical Anesthesiology,* 4th ed. New York, NY: McGraw-Hill, 2006.

Orlewicz MS. Procedural sedation. *Medscape emedicine,* September 14, 2015. https://emedicine.medscape.com/article/109695-overview?form=fpf (updated 2022).

Riker RR, Shehabi Y, Bokesch PM, et al. Dexmedetomidine vs midazolam for sedation of critically ill patients: a randomized trial. *JAMA* 2009; 301:489–99.

Stoelting RK, Hillier SC. *Pharmacology and Physiology in Anesthetic Practice,* 4th ed. Philadelphia, PA: Lippincott Williams & Wilkins, 2006.

Stoelting RK, Miller RD. *Basics of Anesthesia,* 5th ed. Philadelphia, PA: Churchill Livingstone, 2007.

Watson DS, Odom-Forren J. *Practical Guide to Moderate Sedation/Analgesia,* 2nd ed. New York, NY: Mosby, 2005.

Chapter 3

Pain Assessment and Management Considerations

K. Elliott Higgins, Renata M. Miketic,
Eugenie S. Heitmiller, and Emmett E. Whitaker

Introduction

A comprehensive pain management strategy is needed through the entire peri-procedure period for effective and safe patient care. Assessments and interventions pre-procedure, peri-procedure, and post-procedure are codependent. For example, failure to recognize an opioid-dependent patient during the initial pre-procedure screening may result in ineffective analgesia strategies. This chapter deals with important considerations with regard to pre-procedure, peri-procedure, and post-procedure patient assessment and pain management strategies. For a detailed discussion of patient evaluation and procedure selection, see Chapter 4.

Considerations and Patient Assessment Prior to Procedural Sedation

The primary goal of a comprehensive pain plan for sedation should be maximizing both patient safety and patient comfort. There are a multitude of adverse outcomes, including the life-threatening, that can accompany sedation. It is paramount that, before the start of any procedure, practitioners evaluate patient characteristics, patient preferences, appropriateness of sedation given the invasiveness of the procedure, and special considerations during the procedure (e.g., risk to the patient with movement during the procedure).

All practitioners who administer sedatives should be able to manage, or immediately identify someone who can manage, complications in patients whose level of sedation is deeper than originally intended. Thus, practitioner training and experience in administering sedation and the resources surrounding a procedure involving sedation are important considerations because it is often difficult to predict how an individual patient will respond to a given dose of sedative medications. The American Society of Anesthesiologists' (ASA) consensus guidelines entitled "Practice guidelines for moderate procedural sedation and analgesia 2018" indicate that a practitioner should be able to recognize sedation that is deeper than anticipated and be authorized to seek additional help in order to rescue a patient from deeper-than-moderate sedation. Additionally, especially when using drugs intended for general anesthesia, providers should be able to reliably rescue patients as necessary from the consequences of unintentionally deep sedation [1].

Comprehensive perioperative risk stratification is beyond the scope of this chapter. However, regarding patient characteristics, pre-procedural evaluation is a necessary step prior to sedation [1]. This evaluation should include, but not be limited to, a review of the patient's medical records, focused physical examination, review of available laboratory data, and assessment for any changes in the patient's health in the time since the pre-sedation evaluation [1]. Additionally, regarding patients with underlying medical conditions felt to be significant, expert advice from the appropriate consultant specialist should be sought prior to administering sedation. The sedation provider should always consider the following important patient factors when formulating a sedation plan: past experiences/complications with sedation and/or anesthesia, expectations, pain tolerance, anxiety levels, ability to cooperate with the procedure, drug allergies, time and nature of last oral intake, current drugs that may amplify sedation, and overall health (Box 3.1).

Regarding evaluating the patient's overall health, it would be prudent to seek consultation with an expert skilled in perioperative management for patients who have significant organ-system abnormalities and/or those who would be assigned an ASA physical status of III or higher (Table 3.1). Sedative drugs and medications can cause critical cardiovascular and hemodynamic perturbations in deeper states of sedation.

For patients with preexisting pain, it is useful to perform an initial pain assessment prior to the procedure to establish a baseline for post-procedure comparison. When evaluating pain characteristics, questions should address a pain rating, location, quality,

---

Box 3.1 Important patient history aspects for pre-sedation patient evaluation

Details of past experiences with sedation and/or anesthesia:

- Previous effective and ineffective sedation and pain control regimens
- Drug allergies
- Adverse reactions to any medications

Patient expectations:

- Anxiety levels/ability to cooperate

Risk and consequences of movement during the procedure
Time and nature of last oral intake:

- Overall health

Organ-system abnormalities:

- Airway or respiratory problems or predictors of complications
- History of drug or alcohol abuse
- History of chronic pain and/or chronic opioid use

onset, duration, pattern, alleviating/aggravating factors, and any related symptoms (Box 3.2). A focused physical examination of the pain site should also be performed. Any unusual factors including erythema, swelling, temperature changes, skin changes, pain with non-noxious stimuli, muscle atrophy, and hair growth patterns at the pain site should be noted and discussed with all involved proceduralists prior to proceeding with sedation.

Box 3.2   Criteria for assessing pain

Pain rating (using an appropriate assessment scale)
Location
Quality (sharp, dull, burning, shooting)
Onset (sudden, gradual)
Duration
Pattern (continuous, intermittent)
Alleviating/aggravating factors
Related symptoms

Table 3.1 American Society of Anesthesiologists physical status classification system

ASA physical status	Definition
I	A normal healthy patient
II	A patient with mild systemic disease that is medically well controlled
III	A patient with severe systemic disease or poorly controlled systemic disease
IV	A patient with severe systemic disease that is a constant threat to life
V	A moribund patient who is not expected to survive without the operation
VI	A declared brain-dead patient whose organs are being removed for donor purposes

Table 3.2 Pain scale comparison for various patient populations

Patient population	General population scales used*
Normal adult/mature child	NRS preferred by most adults; FPS
Elderly adult	FPS most preferred; VAS least preferred
Mild–moderate cognitive impairment	FPS most preferred; VAS least preferred
Psychomotor impairment	VNS commonly used
Visual impairment	VNS commonly used
Low educational level	FPS most preferred, reading ability not required

*NRS, Numeric Rating Scale; VNS, Verbal Numeric Scale; VAS, Visual Analog Scale; FPS, Faces Pain Scale.

For most patients, pain assessments and establishment of pain treatment goals can be performed by a non-anesthesiologist. However, consultation should be sought for special populations, including the elderly, patients with a history of substance abuse, chronic pain patients, pediatric patients, patients with indwelling pain pumps/catheters, and those patients at increased risk from respiratory depression (e.g., sleep apnea, history of airway problems, or difficult airway). It is well known that opioid-tolerant patients can be challenging to sedate [2]. While definitions are evolving on which opioid-tolerant patients are at greatest risk of peri-sedation complications, patients who regularly use 50 or greater oral morphine equivalents daily are at increased risk of harm from their opioid tolerance and prescribed opioids [3]. Furthermore, opioid-tolerant patients are sometimes also prescribed various additional medications with implications for sedation. These include anxiolytics, antidepressants, anticonvulsants, and muscle relaxants, all of which can unpredictably impact targeted levels of sedation compared to the typical patient. Unless an adverse drug interaction is foreseen, baseline pain medications should not be withheld ahead of any procedure. Consider having these patients, along with patients on methadone or buprenorphine, reviewed for excessive risk by an anesthesiologist prior to any planned sedation. Of particular note, to decrease the risk of relapse and death, buprenorphine should not be routinely discontinued in any peri-procedural setting [4]. Managing patients on buprenorphine, as well as patients who may benefit from buprenorphine initiation in the setting of acute pain, is best done by an acute pain specialist.

Previously discussed peri-procedural pain assessment relies heavily on verbal communication. However, adequate pain assessments may not be possible during moderate or deep sedation. In these situations, behavioral pain assessments are useful (see Tables 3.3 and 3.4). Behaviors that indicate pain include facial grimacing, writhing or shifting, moaning, agitation, and/or withdrawal from a painful stimulus. In addition, changes in physiologic parameters can also be sensitive indicators of pain or nociception. Specifically, increases in respiratory rate, heart rate, and/or blood pressure can indicate inadequate analgesia or depth of sedation. Often, all three physiologic parameters are increased.

Table 3.3 The FLACC scale

	0	1	2
Face	No particular expression or smile	Occasional grimace or frown, withdrawn, disinterested	Frequent or constant frown, clenched jaw, quivering chin
Legs	Normal position or relaxed	Uneasy, restless, tense	Kicking or legs drawn up
Activity	Lying quietly, moves easily	Squirming, shifting back and forth, tense	Arched, rigid, or jerking
Cry	No cry	Moans or whimpers, occasional complaint	Crying steadily, screams, or sobs
Consolability	Content, relaxed	Reassured by occasional touching or talking to, distractible	Difficult to console or comfort

Table 3.4 The Behavioral Pain Scale (BPS)

Item	Description	Score
Facial expression	Relaxed	1
	Partially tightened	2
	Fully tightened	3
	Grimacing	4
Upper limbs	No movement	1
	Partially bent	2
	Fully bent with finger flexion	3
	Permanently retracted	4
Compliance with ventilation	Tolerating movement	1
	Coughing but tolerating ventilation for most of the time	2
	Fighting ventilator	3
	Unable to control ventilation	4

In addition to complex oral pain regimens, chronic pain patients may also have advanced pain adjuncts such as intrathecal pain pumps and/or spinal cord stimulators. These devices should be continued through the peri-procedural period. If this cannot be done for procedural reasons, an advanced pain specialist, ideally the provider who manages the advanced pain adjunct(s), should be contacted to develop a peri-procedural pain plan. It is imperative that the proceduralist and the sedation provider know the placement of these devices to avoid damaging a catheter or dislodging a lead. Interrogation may also be prudent to determine baseline settings and battery power. In all instances, it is imperative for the chronic pain patient to form an acceptable perioperative sedation and pain management strategy with the healthcare delivery team during the evaluation phase. In most instances a chronic pain expert should be consulted.

Regional anesthesia techniques (epidural, spinal, and peripheral nerve blocks with or without catheters) can also be employed in conjunction with a regional anesthesia specialist and an acute pain service to spare opioids and minimize or eliminate procedural pain. While these techniques can be deliberately employed for any patient for certain procedures, opioid-tolerant patients perhaps stand to benefit most from such interventions. These systems deliver analgesia (usually local anesthetics and/or opioids) directly to target nerves (peripheral nerve catheters) and/or dermatomal regions (neuraxial catheters or injections). In hospitalized patients with established, well-working neuraxial or peripheral nerve catheters, the catheters should be continued through the procedure phase, with recommendations from a regional anesthesia and acute pain specialist.

Existing patient-controlled analgesia (PCA) intravenous systems may also need adjustments or titrations in the procedure phase. In many centers, PCA adjustments are made only with input from an acute pain specialist. If a patient on PCA presents concerns for difficult procedural sedation, strongly consider seeking guidance from an acute pain specialist prior to providing sedation.

Overview of Pain Assessment Scales

In 2020, the International Association for the Study of Pain (IASP) updated its definition of *pain* to "an unpleasant sensory and emotional experience associated with, or resembling that associated with, actual or potential tissue damage" [5]. Appropriate assessment of pain increases caregiver awareness of pain status, allows for the delivery of appropriate interventions, decreases patient and caregiver frustration, and improves patient satisfaction.

Effective, targeted, and deliberate pain management can prevent harm and facilitate recovery. Broadly, it is well understood that effective analgesia mitigates many adverse physiologic effects of pain including decreased respiratory function (e.g., atelectasis, hypercapnia, and pneumonia), deleterious cardiovascular effects (e.g., hypertension, tachycardia, and myocardial ischemia), poor wound healing, coagulopathy, and delayed return of bowel function. Clinical practice guidelines issued by the Agency for Healthcare Research and Quality recommend reassessing pain intensities 30 minutes after parenteral drug administration, 60 minutes after oral drug administration, and with each report of new or changed pain [6].

No single all-encompassing method of pain assessment can ensure adequate awareness of a patient's experience of pain in every clinical situation as the cognitive functionality, intellectual development, level of alertness, and ability to participate in a pain assessment can vary dramatically among individual patients. To address this, a wide range of pain assessment tools have been developed and validated over the past 30 years. The following sections expound upon the most common pain assessment tools in current use in (1) general and (2) special populations. When using any of these tools, it is important to keep in mind that a trend in pain scores is more useful than a single pain score by itself.

General Population Scales

In the general population, which includes mature children, adults, and the cognitively intact elderly, the use of self-report scales has been validated as the most reliable indicator of pain. The most common self-report scales include the Numeric Rating Scale (NRS), the Verbal Numeric Scale (VNS), the Visual Analog Scale (VAS), and the Faces Pain Scale (FPS). Although these scales are most commonly used, they only measure the intensity of pain and do not evaluate the multifactorial aspects of pain described previously.

Numeric Rating Scale

The NRS is the most commonly used pain scale. With this scale, patients quantify their pain by pointing to a number on a 0–5 or 0–10 scale, where 0 represents the absence of pain and 5 or 10 represents the worst pain imaginable. This assessment is easy to administer and score, resulting in its popularity. Validated in multiple studies, the NRS is preferred by most adults [7, 8]. However, certain populations may have difficulty with the NRS (e.g., the elderly or those with physical functional limitations) [6].

Verbal Numeric Scale (VNS)

The VNS is a variation of the NRS that requires the patient to verbally rate pain on a scale of 0–10. This scale is the one most commonly utilized in clinical practice; like the

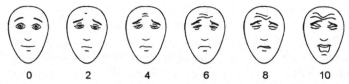

0   2   4   6   8   10

Figure 3.1 Faces Pain Scale (FPS) [15]. This Faces Pain Scale-Revised has been reproduced with the permission of the International Association for the Study of Pain.

NRS, the VNS is easy to use and is especially useful with patients who have psychomotor or visual impairment [6]. The VNS is also useful for virtual or remote pain evaluations.

Visual Analog Scale (VAS)

Similar to the NRS, the VAS is a horizontal or vertical 10-cm line with "no pain" written at one end and "the worst imaginable pain" at the other end [6]. Patients mark a point on the line correlating with pain intensity. The practitioner then measures the distance from "no pain" to the patient's mark to determine a score based on length. The VAS is highly sensitive to change in pain intensity [9, 10]. Like the NRS, this scale is not preferred for use with elderly patients, particularly those with mild to moderate cognitive impairment.

Faces Pain Scale

The FPS is a categorical scale that uses visual descriptors. The FPS has been validated for use in adults and children [11, 12, 13]. Patients are shown a scale with six faces that display different expressions ranging from neutral to grimacing (Figure 3.1). Patients then point to the face that corresponds to their level of pain. Each face correlates with a score between 0 (no pain) and 10 (terrible pain). As the FPS does not require reading ability, this scale is well suited for many populations including children. The FPS has been validated across multiple cultures and has a strong positive correlation with other pain scales [11, 14]. Disadvantages include the need for comprehension of the faces, which can be lacking in very young children, and that the faces could convey, instead of pain, misery, discomfort, depression, or anxiety.

When deciding which pain scale to choose, Table 3.2 offers a comparison between various patient demographics.

Special Population Scales

Pain Assessment in the Young Child

The Premature Infant Pain Profile (PIPP) and the Neonatal/Infant Pain Scale (NIPS) are commonly used in infants. These scales compute a pain score using variables such as heart rate, oxygen saturation, facial expressions, crying, and breathing patterns. For children who cannot communicate (because of either sedation or cognitive impairment), the Faces, Legs, Activity, Cry, Consolability (FLACC) scale and the Children's Hospital of Eastern Ontario Pain Scale (CHEOPS) are often used. Logistics permitting, parents should also be asked to help assess pain levels [16].

The FLACC scale is one of the most commonly used assessments during sedation (Table 3.3). It is an observer report-based scale that has been validated with low interrater variability [17]. A score of 0–2 is given in each of five categories (face, legs, activity, cry, and consolability). These point values are added together to provide a pain score between 0 and 10. The CHEOPS is another behavioral scale that has an observer evaluate and score parameters such as crying, facial expressions, verbal, torso position, touch, and leg position to arrive at a cumulative pain score. Pediatric sedation is discussed in Chapters 23 and 24.

Pain Assessment in the Non-Verbal but Cognitive Patient

A practitioner may have to manage the pain of a patient unable to verbalize. Examples include the intubated patient, the patient with neurologic deficits (acute stroke), or any patient with a pathologic condition that influences phonation. Because these patients are alert and aware of their surroundings and condition, most critical care practices recommend the use of self-report scales to assess pain [18, 19]. For this subset of patients, a few of the validated self-report scales described earlier are particularly helpful. These include the NRS, the VAS, and the Verbal Descriptor Scale (VDS).

For the VDS, also known as the Pain Thermometer, patients choose the expression that best describes their pain from a written list, which contains "no pain," "mild pain," "moderate pain," "severe pain," "extreme pain," and "pain as bad as it could be." The usefulness of the VDS is limited in the case of patients of lower education levels and those with poor eyesight. Of the NRS, VAS, and VDS, the one found to best correlate with correct assessment of pain is the NRS [20].

Pain Assessment in the Delirious or Sedated Patient

With delirious and/or sedated patients, direct verbal communication is not possible. Assessment tools should thus aim to address the sensory and behavioral dimensions of pain. These scales rely on behavioral indicators such as restlessness, muscle tension, frowning, grimacing, and vocalizations. Several different pain scales have been validated, including the Behavioral Pain Scale (BPS) [21, 22, 23]. To use the BPS, a patient is observed for 1 minute. Evaluation of pain status is based on the sum of three subscales: facial expression, upper limb movement, and compliance with mechanical ventilation (Table 3.4). Each subscale is scored from 1 to 4 based on the response. Thus, the cumulative BPS score is between 3 (no pain) and 12 (maximal pain).

Pain Assessment in the Intellectually and Developmentally Delayed

Assessing pain in individuals with intellectual and/or developmental delay can be particularly challenging. Two commonly used scales in this population include the Non-Communicating Children's Pain Checklist (NCCPC) in the pediatric population and the Non-Communicating Adult Pain Checklist (NCAPC) in the adult population.

In brief, the NCCPC is based on a 27-item scale representing six subcategories of pain behavior, which include vocal reaction, emotional reaction, facial expression, body language, protective reaction, and physiologic reaction. The total score ranges from 0 to 81. The NCAPC is a modified version of the NCCPC, which is based on an 18-item scale with a total score that ranges from 0 to 54. In general, the use and interpretation of these assessment tools requires special training, and they are beyond the scope of this chapter.

Recovery and Discharge

Common post-sedation factors that result in discharge delay include pain, postoperative nausea and vomiting, drowsiness, and lack of a patient escort. Concern over inadequate pain control is a major source of anxiety for patients undergoing procedures. Moreover, uncontrolled pain itself is associated with increased complaints of nausea, vomiting, delirium, admission to the hospital, and delayed resumption of normal activities upon discharge [24]. Broadly speaking, until a patient is felt to be ready for discharge, they should be evaluated at regular intervals (5–15 minutes) [1].

The American Society of PeriAnesthesia Nurses (ASPAN) has published clinical guidelines for dealing with post-sedation pain [25]. Care is broken down into three phases: *assessment, intervention,* and *expected outcomes.* The assessment portion should include a history of any pre-procedure pain and any previous interventions with clinical outcome. With any patient intervention, vigilance with proper monitoring for adverse effects is critical.

Familiarity with the procedure requiring sedation can also help guide therapy and outcomes. For example, a patient complaining of arm pain after an abdominal procedure might have had a positioning injury or existing arthritis prior to the procedure.

When treating post-sedation patients, ASPAN suggests the use of non-opioid medications for patients experiencing mild to moderate pain. For moderate to severe pain, multimodal therapy is often necessary. Different classes of effective analgesics used may include opioids, non-steroidal anti-inflammatory drugs, tricyclic antidepressants, and anticonvulsants. A full explanation of multimodal analgesia as it pertains to postprocedural pain is beyond the scope of this chapter. However, by leveraging distinct analgesics of different medication classes, classes which target different receptors involved in nociception, side effects of any single drug can be limited while taking advantage of the analgesic benefits of each medication class. When using non-traditional therapies, classes of medications that are unfamiliar, or dealing with refractory pain, a pain expert should be consulted. Buss and Melderis [26] offer a practical pain treatment algorithm for pain in the post-anesthesia care unit (PACU) (Figure 3.2). If no contraindications exist, pre-procedure baseline pain regimens should always be continued in the recovery period. Taking care of psychosocial needs (allowing visitation from family members) may also be beneficial for recovery.

In general, the use of opioid medications (both during sedation and in the recovery phase) must be thoughtful and incorporate caution regarding their side effects (in particular, respiratory depression). Overuse of opioids may in fact significantly prolong recovery times because of their side effects.

Comprehensive post-procedure discharge criteria are beyond the scope of this chapter; patient recovery and discharge considerations are discussed in Chapter 13. However, specific considerations for discharge readiness from a pain management perspective include: allowance of sufficient time to elapse (2 hours) after the last administration of sedation reversal agents (naloxone, flumazenil) to ensure patients do not become re-sedated; providing ambulatory patients and their designated escorts with instructions regarding diet, medications, activities post sedation, and a telephone contact number in case of emergency; and counseling parents/guardians on the possibility of airway obstruction in children if the head falls forward when the child is secured in a car seat.

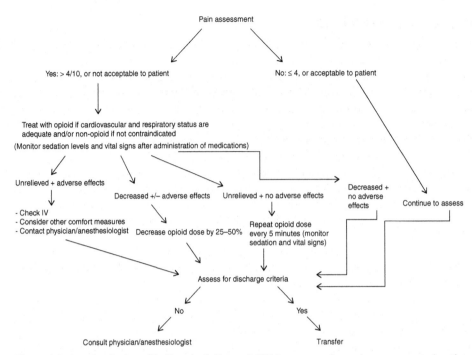

Figure 3.2 American Society of PeriAnesthesia Nurses (ASPAN) post-procedure pain management algorithm. Modified from Buss and Melderis [26].

Summary

Successful pain management in the peri-procedure period is a collaborative team effort between the patient and all involved healthcare team members. The peri-procedure pain experience is a dynamic process that requires constant assessment and adjustment. With appropriate vigilance, planning, and continuous communication between team members, peri-procedural pain management can routinely be both safe and effective..

References

1. Practice guidelines for moderate procedural sedation and analgesia 2018: a report by the American Society of Anesthesiologists Task Force on Moderate Procedural Sedation and Analgesia, the American Association of Oral and Maxillofacial Surgeons, American College of Radiology, American Dental Association, American Society of Dentist Anesthesiologists, and Society of Interventional Radiology. *Anesthesiology.* 2018;128(3):437–79.

2. Shingina A, Ou G, Takach O, et al. Identification of factors associated with sedation tolerance in 5000 patients undergoing outpatient colonoscopy: Canadian tertiary center experience. *World J Gastrointest Endosc.* 2016;8(20):770–6.

3. Centers for Disease Control and Prevention. (n.d.). Calculating total daily dose of opioids for safer dosage. www.cdc.gov/opioids/providers/prescribing/pdf/calculating-total-daily-dose.pdf

4. Kohan L, Potru S, Barreveld AM, et al. Buprenorphine management in the

perioperative period: educational review and recommendations from a multisociety expert panel. *Reg Anesth Pain Med.* 2021;46(10):840–59.

5. Raja SN, Carr DB, Cohen M, et al. The revised International Association for the Study of Pain definition of pain: concepts, challenges, and compromises. *Pain.* 2020;161(9):1976–82.

6. Berry PH, Covington E, Dahl J, Katz J, Miaskowski C. *Pain: Current Understanding of Assessment, Management and Treatments.* Reston, VA: National Pharmaceutical Council and the Joint Commission on Accreditation of Healthcare Organizations, 2006.

7. Gagliese L, Weizblit N, Ellis W, Chan VW. The measurement of postoperative pain: a comparison of intensity scales in younger and older surgical patients. *Pain.* 2005;117:412–20.

8. Herr KA, Spratt K, Mobily PR, Richardson G. Pain intensity assessment in older adults: use of experimental pain to compare psychometric properties and usability of selected pain scales with younger adults. *Clin J Pain.* 2004;20:207–19.

9. Dworkin RH, Turk DC, Farrar JT, et al. Core outcome measures for chronic pain clinical trials: IMMPACT recommendations. *Pain.* 2005;113 (1–2):9–19.

10. Peters ML, Patijn J, Lamé I. Pain assessment in younger and older pain patients: psychometric properties and patient preference of five commonly used measures of pain intensity. *Pain Med.* 2007;8(7):601–10.

11. Bieri D, Reeve RA, Champion GD, Addicoat L, Ziegler JB. The Faces Pain Scale for the self-assessment of the severity of pain experienced by children: development, initial validation, and preliminary investigation for ratio scale properties. *Pain.* 1990;41: 139–50.

12. Taylor LJ, Harris J, Epps CD, Herr K. Psychometric evaluation of selected pain intensity scales for use with cognitively

impaired and cognitively intact older adults. *Rehabil Nurs.* 2005;30:55–61.

13. Stuppy DJ. The Faces Pain Scale: reliability and validity with mature adults. *Appl Nurs Res.* 1998;11:84–9.

14. Matsumoto D. Ethnic differences in affect intensity, emotion judgments, display rule attitudes, and self-reported emotional expression in an American sample. *Motiv Emotion.* 1993;17:107–23.

15. Hicks CL, von Baeyer CL, Spafford PA, van Korlaar I, Goodenough B. The Faces Pain Scale – Revised: toward a common metric in pediatric pain measurement. *Pain.* 2001;93:173–183.

16. Stallard P, Williams L, Lenton S, Velleman R. Pain in cognitively impaired, non-communicating children. *Arch Dis Child.* 2001;85:460–2.

17. Merkel SI, Voepel-Lewis T, Shayevitz JR, Malviya S. The FLACC: a behavioral scale for scoring postoperative pain in young children. *Pediatr Nurs.* 1997;23:293–7.

18. Jacobi J, Fraser GL, Coursin DB, et al. Clinical practice guidelines for the sustained use of sedatives and analgesics in the critically ill adult. *Crit Care Med.* 2002;30:119–41.

19. Sauder P, Andreoletti M, Cambonie G, et al. Sedation and analgesia in intensive care (with the exception of new-born babies). French Society of Anesthesia and Resuscitation. French-speaking Resuscitation Society. *Ann Fr Anesth Reanim.* 2008;27:541–51.

20. Chanques G, Viel E, Constantin JM, et al. The measurement of pain in intensive care unit: comparison of 5 self-report intensity scales. *Pain* 2010;151:711–21.

21. Payen JF, Bru O, Bosson JL, et al. Assessing pain in critically ill sedated patients by using a behavioral pain scale. *Crit Care Med* 2001;29:2258–63.

22. Aissaoui Y, Zeggwagh AA, Zekraoui A, Abidi K, Abouqal R. Validation of a behavioral pain scale in critically ill, sedated, and mechanically ventilated patients. *Anesth Analg* 2005;101: 1470–6.

23. Ahlers SJ, van Gulik L, van der Veen AM, et al. Comparison of different pain scoring systems in critically ill patients in a general ICU. *Crit Care.* 2008;12:R15.

24. Joshi GP. Pain management after ambulatory surgery. *Ambulat. Surg.* 1999;7:3–12.

25. Krenzischek DA, Wilson L, Newhouse R, Mamaril M, Kane LH. *Clinical evaluation of the ASPAN pain and comfort clinical guideline. J Perianesth Nurs.* 2004;19(3), 150–9. https://paininjuryrelief.com/wp-content/uploads/2021/07/aspan-pain-and-comfort-clinical-guideline.pdf

26. Buss HE, Melderis K. PACU pain management algorithm. *J Perianesth Nurs.* 2002;17:11–20.

Additional Reading

Prabhakar A, Mancuso KF, Owen CP, et al. Perioperative analgesia outcomes and strategies. *Best Pract Res Clin Anaesthesiol.* 2014;28(2):105–15.

Vadivelu N, Mitra S, Kaye AD, Urman RD. Perioperative analgesia and challenges in the drug-addicted and drug-dependent patient. *Best Pract Res Clin Anaesthesiol.* 2014;28(1):91–101.

Chapter

4

Patient Evaluation and Procedure Selection

Emily Goldenberg and Debra E. Morrison

Patient Evaluation

Pre-screening

Patient evaluation for a sedation procedure may begin with the first telephone contact. When the patient first calls to schedule an appointment, an administrative assistant or scheduler may ask screening questions about age, height and weight, the presence of common comorbid diseases such as diabetes, heart and lung disease, snoring/obstructive sleep apnea, and routine use of narcotics or sedatives. Although clerical staff may not have the clinical education to question in detail or follow up on positive findings, initial screening may help determine which patients are good candidates for sedation and those who are not. Categories of sedation include (1) local with minimal to no sedation, (2) moderate sedation, (3) deep sedation, and (4) sedation administered by an anesthesia provider.

A standardized one-page screening tool will allow the person who makes the first telephone contact to ask specific questions, and record yes/no answers or any explanations offered, without going into clinical details. Such a tool may help with the initial triage of patients, or at least identify those who appear to be "too sick" or in "too much pain" to be good candidates for a procedure under sedation. Sedation becomes more dangerous to provide and more likely to fail when patients have significant medical comorbidities and/or baseline pain. These patients, as well as those who must undergo a more complex procedure that would distract the proceduralist and the nurse from caring for the patient, are the categories of patients most associated with sedation complications and failures.

A sedation screening tool is especially helpful when patients are not routinely seen and evaluated until the day of the procedure when it may be too late to provide an alternative to sedation. Physicians who refer to radiology may have an inaccurate impression that diagnostic or interventional radiology modalities and procedures are fairly simple and can be easily performed without discomfort or danger to the patient. The pre-sedation evaluation may need to be completed at extremely short notice in the emergency department or the cardiac catheterization laboratory when a procedure is urgent or emergent.

Patients may be referred by their primary care physician or may be self-referred for elective procedures. The physician who receives the referral may not be able to determine whether the referral is a query alone ("Does this patient need a procedure? There are other unresolved medical issues, so please send the patient back before scheduling anything.") or a query accompanied by a clinical green light to proceed ("If this patient needs a procedure, the patient is optimized to proceed with whatever you think is necessary and the evidence is attached."). It is helpful to request clarification of this issue from referring physicians, but the problem remains when the patient is self-referred.

If time allows, particularly if the procedure is elective, a formal screening questionnaire may be employed. A screening questionnaire filled out by the patient prior to the first encounter (either mailed from home or completed electronically) will facilitate the evaluation. This screening questionnaire can be followed up by a nurse practitioner or an experienced sedation nurse, depending on the urgency of the case and how the unit is typically staffed.

The pre-screening interview should address medical history, surgical history, medication use, allergies, pain, exercise tolerance, social habits, and expectations regarding the procedure and sedation. The interviewer can discover the patient's previous experiences with anesthesia, sedation, and other procedures. It is important to uncover intolerances to medications, positioning issues (ability to lie flat, neck range of motion), snoring/obstructive sleep apnea, difficult venous access, difficult intubation, or any history of adverse events during prior procedures. The patient will not always know what historical information is important. If an experienced provider asks the right questions in a kind, non-threatening and non-judgmental way, clinical experience may guide further investigation if necessary. The physician can be notified of patients who present more of a clinical challenge and must be evaluated further or scheduled differently.

History and Physical

Patients may be referred to their primary care physician for a pre-procedure history and physical (H&P) or medical clearance between the date of initial encounter and the day of the procedure. If appropriate, the physician who is to perform the procedure may complete the H&P, which should be documented within 30 days of the planned procedure and sedation. If completed prior to the day of the procedure, a brief update to the H&P should be documented within 4 hours of the procedure.

Patient Instructions

It is important that the patient be at their baseline "steady state" for the procedure. Patients should take their required medications with a sip of water on the day of their procedure to ensure that blood pressure, heart rate, and other medical conditions are controlled prior to the procedure. The phrase "NPO [nothing by mouth] after midnight" should always be accompanied by the statement "except for the following necessary medications (to be clarified in advance of procedure, see below) to be taken with a sip of water or other clear liquid."

It is acceptable for patients to continue to drink clear liquids until 2 hours before they arrive at the facility. This allows for bowel preps to be completed, adequate hydration, improved patient satisfaction, and maintenance of adequate blood glucose for diabetic patients. Clear liquids may include black tea or coffee without milk or cream, clear juices and sodas without particulate matter, fat-free broth, water, or bowel prep.

Any procedure can be an anxiety-producing event. If the patient takes medication for baseline anxiety or pain, these medications should be continued on the day of the procedure. Diabetic patients should hold oral diabetic medications and/or the usual dose of short or intermediate-acting insulin in order to avoid hypoglycemia. The dose of long-acting non-peaking insulin (glargine or detemir) should be adjusted to cover only basal requirements. Patients may require the assistance of their primary care physician to adjust insulin doses appropriately. They may bring short- or intermediate-acting insulin to the facility to be administered as needed during the peri-procedure period.

Clerical staff members may do simple initial screenings or give straightforward instructions, such as location and time of procedure and routine arrival information. However, clinically experienced staff should be responsible for giving any other medical instructions. Lack of critical information or incorrect instruction may result in a procedure being canceled or rescheduled, or worse, an adverse event may occur during or after the procedure. Patients should be medically optimized and adequately informed in advance, so that all aspects of the procedure can go ahead as planned.

Initial Evaluation on the Day of Procedure

The procedural nurse will likely perform the initial evaluation on the day of the procedure. Much of the information may have already been gathered based on the screening questionnaire, follow-up discussion, and/or H&P. Essential elements to be collected include: medical history, surgical history, social history, medications, and drug allergies and/or intolerances. If not already discussed and documented, previous experiences with anesthesia and sedation, positioning limitations, or any history of unexpected events during procedures should also be covered. The pre-procedural assessment will also address whether the patient has a ride home (if applicable), who to call in an emergency, code status, and discharge planning.

Baseline data recorded should include height, weight, blood pressure, heart rate, respiratory rate, temperature, oxygen saturation and amount of supplemental oxygen if indicated, and pain score (0–10). Pertinent laboratory tests, including immediate pre-procedure glucose for diabetics or potassium for renal failure patients, should also be documented.

The initial assessment should include a baseline level of consciousness or sedation score, which will be monitored and documented during sedation (Table 4.1). This baseline score may be used for comparison when the patient is in the recovery area and being evaluated for discharge from post-sedation monitoring (Table 4.2).

Physician Exam, Informed Consent, and Attestation

The US Centers for Medicare and Medicaid Services requires that the procedural physician participates in the pre-procedure evaluation. A licensed physician or allied health professional (fellow, resident, physician assistant, or nurse practitioner) may complete the initial assessment. If an H&P has already been completed, a simple update

Table 4.1 Richmond Agitation–Sedation Scale

Score	Description
+4	Combative, violent, danger to staff
+3	Pulls or removes tube(s) or catheter(s); aggressive
+2	Frequent non-purposeful movement, fights ventilator
+1	Anxious, apprehensive, but not aggressive
0	Alert and calm
−1	Awakens to voice (eye opening/contact) > 10 seconds
−2	Light sedation, briefly awakens to voice (eye opening/contact) < 10 seconds
−3	Moderate sedation, movement or eye opening; no eye contact
−4	Deep sedation, no response to voice, but movement or eye opening to physical stimulation
−5	Unarousable, no response to voice or physical stimulation

Table 4.2 Adult Aldrete Score (modified)[a]

Variable		Pre	Post
Activity: can move voluntarily or on command	Four extremities	2	2
	Two extremities	1	1
	No extremities	0	0
Respiration	Can deep breathe/cough freely	2	2
	Dyspnea/shallow or limited breathing	1	1
	Apneic/mechanical ventilator	0	0
Circulation (preoperative blood pressure [BP], mmHg)	BP ± 20% of pre-sedation level	2	2
	BP ± 20–49% of pre-sedation level	1	1
	BP ± 50% of pre-sedation level	0	0
Consciousness	Fully awake	2	2
	Arousable on calling	1	1
	Not responding	0	0
Oxygen saturation %	> 92% on room air	2	2
	Needs oxygen to remain > 90%	1	1
	< 90% with oxygen	0	0
	Total score		

Based on Aldrete JA, Kroulik D. A postanesthetic recovery score. *Anesth Analg.* 1970;49:924–934.
[a] A minimum score of 10 (or baseline), with no score less than 1 in any category, is required for discharge from sedation monitoring.

Table 4.3 A guide to airway examination

Non-intubated patient	Intubated patient
	☐ **Endotracheal tube** ☐ **Tracheostomy**
☐ Cooperative patient ☐ Uncooperative patient	☐ Cooperative patient ☐ Uncooperative patient
Mouth opening/temporomandibular joint excursion ☐ < 3 cm ☐ 3–4 cm ☐ > 4 cm	*Anatomy externally* ☐ Normal ☐ Abnormal
Mallampati class ☐ 1 ☐ 2 ☐ 3 ☐ 4	*History of airway problems* ☐ No ☐ Yes
Thyromental distance/chin ☐ < 6.5 cm ☐ 6.5–7 cm ☐ > 7 cm ☐ beard	
Teeth ☐ Intact/Normal for age ☐ Poor repair ☐ Loose ☐ Missing	
Denture ☐ in ☐ Out	
Neck extension/range of movement ☐ Full ☐ Limited ☐ Thick obese short neck	
Remarks:	

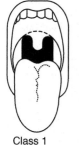 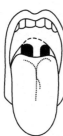 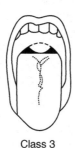 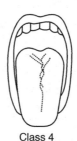

Figure 4.1 Mallampati classification of mouth opening.

Class 1   Class 2   Class 3   Class 4

is required the day of the procedure. If the H&P was completed more than 30 days prior to the procedure, a new one is needed. This should include a physical examination: heart, lungs, neurologic, and any other pertinent physical abnormalities. An airway examination (Table 4.3), including a Mallampati score (Figure 4.1), should be documented. The physician's assessment should also include a plan for sedation.

A high Mallampati score, a short distance between chin and thyroid cartilage (small chin/recessed mandible), poor mouth opening, short thick neck, and other abnormalities predict difficult intubation and/or difficult mask ventilation and should alert the procedural physician that the patient may be a poor candidate for moderate or deep sedation because it may be difficult to manage and secure the airway in an emergency. Other indicators include but are not limited to the presence of a beard (which may cover a small chin or make mask ventilation difficult), protruding upper teeth (maxilla relatively large, making mandible relatively small, is predictive of a difficult airway), narrow jaw, history of head and neck radiation, and loose teeth. If the patient is uncooperative, the airway examination must be based on external appearance alone. If the patient has an established airway (tracheostomy or endotracheal tube), airway patency is more or less assured under most circumstances.

An American Society of Anesthesiologists (ASA) score should be assigned, and the implications of the assigned score should be considered before proceeding with sedation. Even if the procedure is simple or short, a moribund patient with a difficult airway who has a massive deep venous thrombosis may not be a candidate for an inferior vena cava (IVC) filter under minimal or moderate sedation in the radiology suite. The ASA score predicts the possibility of adverse events:

- *Class 1* patients are healthy with no systemic disease, and the pathologic process for which the operation is to be performed is localized, without systemic effect. *Example*: a healthy athlete scheduled for knee surgery.
- *Class 2* patients have mild to moderate systemic dysfunction caused by a coexisting systemic disease or by the pathologic process for which the operation is to be performed. *Examples*: controlled hypertension, controlled diabetes, upper respiratory infection, smoking, thyroid tumor that does not threaten the airway. Pregnancy and extremes of age are sometimes included in this category.
- *Class 3* patients have multi-system diseases or a controlled severe disease that affects activity. *Examples*: chronic obstructive pulmonary disease, chronic stable angina, obesity, end-stage renal disease on regular dialysis, lung tumor that decreases pulmonary function, pheochromocytoma after medical optimization.
- *Class 4* patients have severe systems disorders that are life-threatening and may not be correctable by medical management or operation. *Examples*: congestive heart failure, unstable angina, severe pulmonary or hepatic dysfunction, major trauma, prematurity with respiratory distress and necrotizing enterocolitis, pheochromocytoma prior to medical optimization.
- *Class 5* patients are moribund, with little chance of survival with surgery, and no chance of survival without surgery. *Examples*: ruptured aortic aneurysm, major trauma, massive intracerebral injury.
- *Class 6* is used to denote a brain-dead organ donor.
- *E* is used as a modifier to denote an emergency operation, with no time to optimize medical condition. A healthy patient with an acute appendicitis would be classified as 1E. "E" implies increased risk.

Class 4 and 5 patients are at increased risk for morbidity and mortality. Emergency does not mean that an unstable patient should be rushed to a procedure under sedation. If a patient's condition cannot be optimized, dedicated anesthesia care with a managed airway and the ability stabilize the patient may be the most appropriate plan of care.

The attending physician is required to review the assessment and examination, talk to the patient and/or the patient's surrogate about the procedure and the sedation plan (including a contingency plan in the event of failed sedation, which may include consent for anesthesia), and declare that the patient is an appropriate candidate for the procedure and sedation planned.

Final Review

The procedural physician and the sedation nurse should confer briefly as a final review, stating specific plans and any concerns before commencing with sedation and the procedure.

Patient and Procedure Selection

Patient Selection

Before moving on to the procedure selection, it must be restated that patient selection and procedure selection go hand in hand. After patients are screened, and even after evaluation on the day of the procedure, only those patients who are appropriate candidates for sedation should go ahead with procedures under sedation. It is never too late to change plans when new information or findings become evident.

Avoid complications and sedation failure by selecting patients who are amenable to sedation. A good candidate for sedation is a person with good overall health status. Adverse events that occur during sedation most often involve respiratory or cardiovascular complications. Consider scheduling patients with key characteristics under anesthesia rather than moderate sedation, unless the procedure is amenable to local anesthesia with minimal sedation.

The following characteristics may trigger concerns, even if discovered at the last moment:

- obesity
- difficult airway/significant craniofacial abnormalities
- sleep apnea
- history of malignant hyperthermia
- coagulopathy
- heart or lung disease that is a threat to life
- significant neurological disease
- history of anesthesia/sedation complications or sedation failure
- intolerance of medications routinely used for sedation
- routine medications or drugs that may react with sedation agents
- chronic pain or anxiety with a baseline need for analgesics or anxiolytics
- pediatric patients, who are not obligated to cooperate

Another option is to schedule patients for moderate sedation with anesthesia backup immediately available after having discussed, planned, and consented for it prior to sedation.

Procedure and Location Selection

Both the procedural physician's scope of practice and the individual facility's capabilities will ultimately determine the range of possible procedures available. The setting may be quite flexible (i.e., an operating room) or very specifically designed and equipped (i.e., interventional radiology or gastroenterology suite, pulmonary laboratory, or cardiac catheterization laboratory).

Procedures should be scheduled in the setting equipped for the specific requirements and complexity of the procedure, specifics of the recovery, and the anticipated length of recovery/time to discharge. Within the hospital itself, there is a range of immediate access to the highest level of care. Outpatient surgery centers on a medical center campus may have access to hospital recovery facilities or 23-hour observation units, as well as inpatient floors and intensive care units (ICUs). Some outpatient surgical centers are equipped for overnight recovery and observation, although most are equipped only for same-day procedures. Office practice locations may be equipped only for recovery in the procedure room itself, allowing procedures to be scheduled no sooner than the end of the recovery period of the previous patient.

A facility should establish designated locations where procedures and/or sedation can take place, with designated recovery areas for each location, even if the setting is the physician's private office. Benefits of designating locations include the ability to monitor quality of care and the ability to direct rescue personnel quickly when needed. Potential locations include the following:

- Hospital operating rooms are perfect for procedures under sedation; however operating room space and/or time may be limited, thus moving sedation procedures elsewhere in the facility.
- Post-anesthesia care units (PACUs) or pre-operative holding areas may have small monitored procedure rooms for a lumbar puncture, echocardiogram, or bone marrow biopsy under moderate sedation.
- Emergency department.
- Hybrid angiography–operating suites adjacent to or part of the main operating room may be sites for diagnostic angiography under local anesthetic with minimal or moderate sedation. An IVC filter might be placed in a very sick patient with local anesthetic alone, with a sedation nurse to monitor, comfort, and reassure the patient.
- ICUs are suitable for procedures such as chest tube placement, wound debridement, bronchoscopy, and endoscopy. A patient who is intubated and sedated in the ICU may safely undergo a wider range of procedures in the ICU as compared to a patient who is not intubated or who lacks an established airway (i.e., tracheostomy). For some ICU patients, the indication for a particular procedure (i.e., upper gastrointestinal bleed requiring endoscopy with cauterization and simultaneous blood transfusion) may make the operating room a better and safer location to undergo that procedure since anesthesia care may be needed.
- Clinic procedure rooms are used for lesion excision, cystoscopy, ultrasound-guided biopsy, Mohs procedure, or vasectomy as appropriate.
- Echocardiography laboratories are used for transesophageal echocardiography, which may be completed under local anesthesia after the patient gargles viscous lidocaine. Cardiac catheterization laboratories are suitable for a range of diagnostic and interventional procedures such as angiography and percutaneous coronary intervention, pacemaker, or automated implantable cardioverter defibrillator placement.
- Interventional radiology is the site of a range of procedures including CT- and fluoroscopy-guided biopsies, cryotherapy, placements of drains and stents, embolization of damaged or abnormal blood vessels, ablation of tumors, and neuro-interventional procedures.
- Diagnostic radiology is the site of many routine procedures (CT, MRI, nuclear medicine/PET scans, ultrasound) and is tolerated by most consenting adults, but

some patients may require minimal sedation in the form of one dose of an oral medication.

- Interventional gastroenterology may perform both simple diagnostic procedures (i.e., upper and lower endoscopies) and complex diagnostic and interventional procedures (i.e., endoscopic ultrasound, endoscopic retrograde cholangiopancreatography, or stent placement). Even a simple diagnostic procedure done with moderate sedation may quickly become hazardous for a fragile patient or someone who is obese or has obstructive sleep apnea. To avoid cases of failed sedation or adverse events, it is prudent to consider both the patient and the planned procedure when selecting moderate sedation or anesthesia care.
- A chronic pain clinic may be the site of procedures, but these patients are often known to the practitioners and therefore pre-screening has been done. Any medications that these patients take chronically should be continued on the day of a procedure. Patients who are unlikely to tolerate a pain procedure should be scheduled with anesthesia in the appropriate location.
- An outpatient laser facility may use local anesthesia with minimal or moderate sedation to perform procedures on eyes or skin. Patients who are unable to cooperate (i.e., pediatric patients or demented patients) will likely require other arrangements for sedation.
- In the pulmonary laboratory, flexible bronchoscopies are performed under moderate sedation by the pulmonologist. Rigid bronchoscopies and flexible bronchoscopies with bronchial ultrasound are usually performed with patients under general anesthesia.
- An outpatient surgery center likely has both anesthesia services as well as moderate sedation capabilities. Some centers may be staffed and equipped for 23-hour overnight observation; however, most patients are expected to recover and be discharged home the same day. At this location, it may be possible to schedule patients for sedation but also discuss and consent for anesthesia in the event that care must be escalated to complete the procedure safely.

Additional Considerations

Consider the length of each procedure: How long can a patient comfortably lie still in a given position? What is the anticipated cumulative dose of local anesthetic, sedative, and/ or opioid that will be required before the procedure is completed?

Schedule procedures in locations equipped for both the procedure and for administering the necessary sedation. Always consider the patient who is having the procedure when choosing the location. If a procedure may involve blood loss or a patient may require a transfusion, the procedure should be scheduled where blood transfusion is feasible.

For procedures where it is critical that the patient does not move, either minimal sedation or anesthesia should be employed. A significantly sedated patient may not be relied upon to cooperate; a patient cannot be guaranteed to stay still unless he or she is cooperative. More sedation is rarely the solution to restlessness, agitation, or lack of cooperation.

If a procedure may be safely performed under moderate sedation in certain but not all patients, it is reasonable to schedule when both sedation and anesthesia options may be available. Communicate in advance with the appropriate personnel, evaluate patients, and obtain their consent for both contingencies. This may allow for a wider range of options without aborting the procedure and being forced to reschedule.

Summary

Preparation for a sedation procedure begins with pre-screening, followed by a thorough history and physical and further evaluation on the day of the procedure. Reevaluation of the patient on the day of the procedure should include an examination by the proceduralist physician, informed consent, and a final affirmation that all is in order prior to initiating sedation. The selection criteria discussed here help ensure that the patient, the procedure, and the location are appropriate for sedation.

Additional Reading

American Society of Anesthesiologists Task Force on Preanesthesia Evaluation. Practice advisory for preanesthesia evaluation. *Anesthesiology.* 2002;96:485–96.

American Society of Anesthesiologists Task Force on Moderate Procedural Sedation and Analgesia. Practice guidelines for moderate procedural sedation and analgesia 2018. *Anesthesiology.* 2018;28:437–79.

Association of periOperative Registered Nurses. Position statement on allied health care providers and support personnel in the perioperative practice setting. www.aorn .org/guidelines-resources/clinical-resources/position-statements

Association of periOperative Registered Nurses. Position statement on one perioperative registered nurse circulator dedicated to every patient undergoing a surgical or other invasive procedure. www .aorn.org/guidelines-resources/clinical-resources/position-statements

Chang B, Urman RD. Non-operating room anesthesia: the principles of patient assessment and preparation. *Anesthesiol Clin.* 2016 Mar;34(1): 223–40. PMID: 26927750.

Frank RL. Procedural sedation in adults. *UpToDate* 2011. www.uptodate.com/ contents/procedural-sedation-in-adults

Morrison DE, Harris AL. Preoperative and anesthetic management of the surgical patient. In Wilson SE, ed. *Educational Review Manual in General Surgery*, 8th ed. New York, NY: Castle Connolly, 2009.

Ogg M, Burlingame B. Clinical issues: recommended practices for moderate sedation/analgesia. *AORN J* 2008;88: 275–7.

Ogg M, Burlingame B. *University Health System Consortium Consensus Group on Deep Sedation: Deep Sedation Best Practice Recommendations*. Oak Brook, IL: UHC, 2006.

Ogg M, Burlingame B. *University Health System Consortium Consensus Group on Moderate Sedation: Moderate Sedation Best Practice Recommendations*. Oak Brook, IL: UHC, 2005.

Patient Monitoring, Equipment, and Intravenous Fluids

Harish Siddaiah, Shilpa Patil, and Deniz Gungor

Patient Monitoring and Equipment

The term "monitoring" is derived from the Latin word monere, which means "to warn." Patient monitoring is important during sedation to ensure patient safety and decrease adverse events [1]. The standards for basic anesthetic monitoring as set forth by the American Society of Anesthesiologists (ASA) are intended to encourage quality patient care in all general anesthetics, regional anesthetics, and monitored anesthesia care. The standards are as follows [2]:

Standard I: Qualified anesthesia personnel shall be present in the room throughout the conduct of all general anesthetics, regional anesthetics, and monitored anesthesia care.

Standard II: During all anesthetics, the patient's oxygenation, ventilation, circulation, and temperature shall be continually evaluated.

Sedation is best viewed as a continuum because individuals vary in their response to the sedative agents. A well-trained and experienced healthcare provider is considered indispensable for safe practice of sedation.

Monitors have become routine and indispensable in supporting the healthcare provider during patient care encounters [3]. Consequently, every healthcare provider involved in patient care during any procedure requiring sedation must be clinically competent in the practice of resuscitation and monitoring. Healthcare providers must be familiar with monitoring equipment and be able to interpret data obtained from instrument readings.

The monitoring process involves vigilant observation of the patient's vital signs and symptoms as well as interpretation of data provided by the monitors. If any parameters are found to be significantly out of range, initiation of corrective action and timely therapeutic intervention are required. The healthcare provider should be aware that monitors may give false alarms, display distorted data, or malfunction. In addition to understanding clinical signs, digital literacy regarding monitor interpretation is imperative [4]. Monitors amplify and quantify clinical information, and despite increasing technological sophistication of monitors, they cannot be a substitute for a trained healthcare provider who can appreciate nuances of clinical signs.

Monitoring devices range from basic to sophisticated, with the choice of device determined by the condition of the patient and the procedure being performed. Whether in the operating room or ambulatory outpatient setting, it is imperative to have appropriate and standardized monitoring of patients. The basic physiologic monitors recommended by the ASA, termed "standard ASA monitors," include pulse oximetry (pulse ox), ECG, blood pressure monitoring, and temperature monitoring. Other ASA monitoring standards include end-tidal carbon dioxide (CO_2), inspired oxygen (O_2) concentration, volume of expired gas, and alarms for low oxygen and disconnected ventilator. Additionally, monitoring may be classified as prolonged without interruption (continuous) or repeated frequently (continual) [2].

This chapter provides a brief review of various monitors that are commonly used during sedation, which are as follows

1. Cardiovascular and hemodynamic monitoring

   • ECG
   • arterial blood pressure (BP) monitoring: non-invasive (NIBP) and invasive (IBP)

2. Respiratory monitoring

   • contact-based:

      ◦ movement, volume, and tissue composition detection: transthoracic impedance, inductance plethysmography, fiber-optic plethysmography, strain-gauge transducers, electromyography, photoplethysmography
      ◦ airflow sensing: temperature sensing, humidity sensing, carbon-dioxide sensing, sound detection
      ◦ blood gas concentration measurement: pulse oximetry, end-tidal O_2 and CO_2 monitors, transcutaneous O_2 and CO_2 monitors

   • non-contact-based:

      ◦ movement of chest wall: radar based, optical based, thermal imaging

3. Temperature monitoring

   • core and near core temperature monitors

4. Brain function monitoring

   • bispectral index (BIS) monitoring

Cardiovascular and Hemodynamic Monitoring

Cardiovascular monitoring is one of the standards recommended by the American Society of Anesthesiologists (ASA) that applies to all anesthesia care. This includes general anesthesia, regional anesthesia, and monitored anesthesia care. The standard perioperative cardiovascular monitors are ECG, heart rate, and NIBP [5, 6].

Electrocardiography

Precise interpretation of the ECG is essential because hemodynamic changes are common in the perioperative period. An indirect method of measuring cardiac electric activity by means of a visual display, an ECG provides information regarding heart rate, myocardial ischemia, arrhythmias, conduction abnormalities, and the presence of pacemaker function, and aids with placement of intracardiac catheters. Proper electrode placement is the most critical aspect for obtaining an accurate ECG. The standard 10-electrode, 12-lead ECG is not employed in the operating room. Rather, 3- or 5-lead ECGs are used [7].

Leads II and V5 are commonly selected for continuous simultaneous monitoring in the operating room. Lead II is used to monitor P waves and detect arrhythmias. Lead V5 is sensitive for the detection of myocardial ischemia, manifested by ST depression. The standard monitoring package (with a 3-lead ECG system) utilizes leads II and V5, which detect 80% of ischemic episodes with a sensitivity of 90–96% [8].

Blood Pressure Monitoring

General anesthesia and moderate to deep sedation can significantly influence cardiovascular function. Early detection and intervention of cardiovascular events reduce the risk of complications. BP monitoring should be tailored to the individual patient. The ASA practice guidelines for sedation recommends monitoring neurological, cardiovascular, spontaneous respiration, and airway for all cases [3].

According to the 2017 guidelines of the American College of Cardiology/American Heart Association (ACC/AHA), normal BP is systolic < 120 mmHg and diastolic < 80 mmHg. Systolic 120–129 mmHg and diastolic > 80 mmHg is considered elevated BP. Hypertension is considered in two stages: stage 1 being systolic 130–139 mmHg or diastolic 80–89 mmHg; stage 2 being systolic > 140 mmHg or diastolic > 90 mmHg. As BP increases, the odds of having a cardiovascular event also increase [9]. Hypertension increases the risk of patients developing cardiac arrhythmias, increased myocardial oxygen consumption, bleeding, and increased systemic vascular resistance [10].

On the other hand, if the patient is hypotensive, they are at increased risk of having shock due to inadequate perfusion [11]. BP may fluctuate in patients perioperatively not only due to inadequately controlled hypertension but also because of the psychological stimuli surrounding the clinic or operative setting [12]. Therefore, the goal is to avoid both hypertension and hypotension during the perioperative period. Episodes of hyper- or hypotension require prompt treatment, which can be achieved with antihypertensive and sedative medications or pressors, respectively. In healthy patients, the goal is to keep mean arterial pressure (MAP – normal 70–100 mmHg) greater than 65 mmHg, while in chronic hypertensive patients, MAP should be 75% above the baseline (autoregulatory curve shifted to right) [13].

For most cases, BP is monitored with an NIBP machine. In more complex cases requiring quicker detection of BP fluctuations, IBP monitoring may be used.

Non-Invasive Arterial Blood Pressure Monitoring

NIBP monitoring is an indirect method of monitoring adequate organ perfusion, used in a variety of procedures and levels of sedation [14]. NIBP includes intermittent varieties like manual auscultatory and automated oscillometric techniques, as well as continuous varieties like the volume clamp method and arterial applanation tonometry.

The auscultation technique requires a sphygmomanometer, BP cuff, and stethoscope. The cuff is placed over the patient's upper arm (removing or rolling sleeve if necessary), with the arm rested on a level surface. The stethoscope is placed over the approximate location of the brachial artery, verified by detection of the pulse. The cuff is inflated to the point where the pulse is no longer audible, and slowly deflated until the pulse reappears, indicating systolic blood pressure (SBP). Deflation of the cuff continues until the pulse is inaudible once again, indicating diastolic blood pressure (DBP). SBP and DBP measurements can be used to calculate MAP [15].

The automated oscillometric BP monitor is the standard device for intraoperative NIBP, with a manual sphygmomanometer available if needed. Oscillometric BP devices detect the magnitude of oscillations in BP caused by blood flow during various stages of inflation and deflation of the cuff. Just like the auscultatory sphygmomanometer, an inflatable cuff is placed over the proximal part of the arm or lower limb, the standard location for BP measurement being the brachial artery. The cuff is inflated to occlude blood flow and is deflated gradually, allowing the arterial pressure to return. As the occlusion is released, a sensor detects changes in amplitude of pressure pulses – oscillations – created by the changing blood flow. The device reports the SBP and DBP as well as MAP. The main difference between auscultatory and oscillometric techniques is that the former uses sound waves while the latter uses oscillation waves to detect changes in pressure [16].

The volume clamp method, or vascular unloading technology, takes continuous BP measurements using an inflatable cuff containing a photodiode placed at the finger. The pressure in the cuff adjusts itself to keep the diameter of the artery in the finger constant, which is sensed by the photodiode. Using the pressure changes of the cuff, a BP curve can be calculated and inferred as brachial artery BP. ClearSight is a device that uses this method [17].

Arterial applanation tonometry is another method for NIBP, which uses a transducer to continuously measure arterial BP. The transducer is held in place, which must be at an artery immediately proximal to a bone, to obtain an arterial pulse wave. MAP, SBP, and DBP can then be calculated. The transducer must be held in place manually, or as part of an automated device such as the T-Line system [17].

BP measurement errors can be due to a variety of factors: movement by the patient, such as shivering or flexing the arm, cardiac arrhythmias, air leakage or kinks in the tubing, inadequate cuff size, deflating the cuff too rapidly (recommended cuff deflation rate is 3–5 mmHg/second), changes in posture, and changing the location of the cuff as it is working [15]. The more distal the artery, the more the systolic pressure increases and the diastolic pressure decreases [14].

Overall, NIBP monitors are automated and have replaced the auscultatory method of BP monitoring. The NIBP monitors can provide periodic BP measurements, which can be scheduled or timed according to the frequency required by the healthcare provider. The ASA Task Force on Sedation and Analgesia by Non-Anesthesiologists recommends that BP should be measured at a minimum of 5-minute intervals during the procedure unless such monitoring interferes with the procedure [6].

Advantages of NIBP include that it is non-invasive, simple to use, does not require critical care, and does not need to be zeroed. Limitations of NIBP are that measurements are intermittent rather than continuous, inaccuracies are more likely, there is potential for neural injury or tissue damage, and discomfort to the patient. NIBP may also have

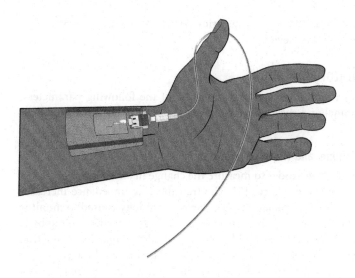

Figure 5.1 Illustration of an arterial catheter inserted in the left radial artery. (https://commons.wikimedia.org/w/index.php?curid=114186838)

inaccuracies stemming from incorrect cuff size, movement of patient or tubing, external compression, hypotension, or arrhythmias [18].

Invasive Arterial Blood Pressure Monitoring

Invasive arterial BP monitoring is a method of direct arterial pressure monitoring by means of a peripheral arterial catheter that connects to an external transducer. Because of its higher accuracy and continuous beat-by-beat monitoring, IBP is considered the gold standard for arterial pressure monitoring. However, NIBP is used more often due to it being less invasive and having more straightforward application. The most often used arteries for IBP are radial, femoral, and brachial (see Figure 5.1) [18].

IBP is performed under sedation. Hemodynamic instability caused by arrhythmias or coronary and valvular heart diseases may compromise the readings from the arterial line. Arterial cannulation for IBP is the clinical standard for high-risk surgery and intensive care. However, this method requires more time and training, and has a risk of major complications such as embolism, neurovascular trauma, or ischemia [18].

Respiratory Monitoring

Respiration, or breathing, is a critical physiological requirement for survival in virtually all living organisms. Continuous respiratory monitoring is crucial for anticipating and/or identifying high-risk situations in patients such as acute respiratory failure, including acute respiratory distress syndrome, which can lead to immediate cardiovascular arrest and death [19].

Respiratory monitoring aims to surveil inhalation, exhalation, and oxygenation. Techniques of respiratory monitoring are continuously advancing thanks to technological improvements and an increasing understanding of the pathophysiology of respiratory failure [20]. Various invasive and non-invasive devices are available for monitoring the patient's respiratory rate (or respiratory frequency), tidal volume, and gas exchange (minute ventilation). Respiratory frequency is an important early indicator of physiological deterioration and can predict potentially serious adverse events such as cardiac arrest, acidosis/alkalosis, and shock.

Devices can be classified into one of two categories: contact-based respiratory devices and non-contact-based respiratory devices.

Contact-Based Respiratory Monitors

Contact-based respiratory monitors usually measure one of the following parameters: respiratory-related abdominal and chest wall movements, respiratory airflow, and blood gas measurement.

Detection of Movement, Volume, and Tissue Composition

Transthoracic impedance uses electrodes to measure the change in air volume within the lungs with variations in thoracic pressures [5]. The transthoracic impedance increases with inhalation and decreases with exhalation [21]. Plethysmography is used to monitor changes in volume in a specific organ or body part [22]. Inductance plethysmography is a non-invasive technique in which two bands or wires made of pliable conducting material measure the respiration rate with a thoracic band placed around the chest wall and abdominal band placed over the abdomen at the level of the umbilicus. The inductive sensor measures the change in inductance of the bands as abdominal wall and chest wall circumference change with respiration [5]. Fiber-optic plethysmography and strain-gauge transducers both measure changes in abdominal and thoracic circumferences. Electromyography measures diaphragmatic muscle activity via skin electrodes. Photoplethysmography measures changes in venous return during respiration. Accelerometers measure acceleration caused by gravity or motion, which may help indicate abnormalities in breathing. Gyroscopes record angular velocity, typically used in conjunction with an accelerometer, which may also aid in the detection of abnormal breathing movements. Magnetometers (magnetic field sensors) detect variation in the magnetic vector in order to estimate breathing-related chest wall movements [23]. These devices are summarized in Table 5.1.

Airflow Sensing

Airflow sensing is helpful in respiratory monitoring because expiratory air is warmer, has higher humidity, and contains more CO_2 than inspiratory air. Variations in these variables can be used for calculating the respiratory rate (Table 5.2). Microphones, though not often used clinically, may be useful to monitor breathing by sound detection. Flowmeters and hot wire anemometers detect temporal trends of air being inhaled and exhaled during breathing. Different fiber-optic sensors have also been proposed to measure flow rates [23].

Blood Gas Concentration

Respiratory monitoring can be achieved indirectly by monitoring of O_2 and CO_2 concentration in arterial blood using pulse oximetry, end-tidal O_2 and CO_2 measurements, and transcutaneous O_2 and CO_2 measurements (Table 5.3). Pulse oximetry is described further in "Monitoring of Oxygenation" section.

Non-Contact-Based Respiratory Monitors

Non-contact-based respiratory monitors include radar-based, optical-based, and thermal-imaging based respiratory monitoring (Table 5.4).

Table 5.1 Contact-based respiratory monitors for the detection of movement, volume, and tissue composition

Method/device	Measuring parameter	Sensor type and placement
Transthoracic impedance sensor	Transthoracic impedance	Skin electrodes or defibrillator pads on chest wall
Inductive sensors (plethysmography)	Abdomen and thoracic circumference	Embedded coils around abdomen and chest wall
Fiber-optic sensors (plethysmography)	Abdomen and thoracic circumference	Fiber-optic strain gauge around abdomen and chest wall
Strain-gauge transducers	Abdomen and thoracic circumference (resistance and capacitance)	Resistive strain gauge around abdomen and chest wall
Electromyography	Muscle activity	Skin electrodes (diaphragm and intercostal muscles)
Modulation cardiac activity - photoplethysmography	Venous return via light intensity	Fiber-optic sensor
Accelerometer, gyroscope, magnetometer	Chest wall movement analysis	Motion/movement detection at chest wall

Table 5.2 Contact-based respiratory monitors for airflow sensing

Method/device	Measuring parameter	Sensor type and placement
Temperature sensing (thermistor, thermocouple, pyroelectric sensory, fiber optic sensor)	Temperature	Temperature sensor (thermometer) in or in front of nasal/oral region
Humidity sensing (capacitive, resistive, nanoparticle, and fiber optic sensors)	Humidity	Hygrometer or fiber-optic sensor in or in front of nasal/oral region
CO_2 sensing (infrared and fiber optic sensors)	CO_2	Infrared absorption, mass spectrometry, or acoustic sensing of gas from nasal/oral sampling
Sound detection (microphone)	Flow of air	Acoustic measuring of nasal/oral airflow
Flowmeters (differential and turbine), hot wire anemometers, fiber optic sensors	Flow of air	Sensor placed near airway to detect air flow

Table 5.3 Contact-based respiratory monitors for blood gas concentration

Method/device	Measuring parameter	Sensor type and placement
Pulse oximetry	O_2 saturation in arterial blood	Fiber-optic sensor on peripheral extremities/skin
End-tidal O_2 measurement	O_2 concentration of expired air	Mass spectrometry, electric analyzer, or paramagnetic O_2 sensor on gas from nasal/oral sampling
End-tidal CO_2 measurement	CO_2 concentration of expired air	Infrared absorption, mass spectrometry, or acoustic measurement of gas from nasal/oral sampling
Transcutaneous O_2 measurement	Transcutaneous O_2 concentration	Heated electrode
Transcutaneous CO_2 measurement	Transcutaneous CO_2 concentration	Heated electrode

Table 5.4 Non-contact-based respiratory monitors of movement of chest wall

Method/device	Measuring parameter	Sensor type
Radar-based	Change in Doppler signals	Sound
Optical-based	Change in infrared signals	Visual
Thermal-imaging based	Change in temperature	Thermal

Radar-based respiratory monitors detect chest wall movements using the "Doppler" phenomenon. Optical-based respiratory monitors detect respiratory movements through infra-ed light. Thermal-based respiratory monitors use sensors that detect temperature changes induced by respiration.

Still in the nascent stage of development, the use of these devices involves concerns regarding patient safety and electromagnetic interference with other medical equipment. Non-contact devices are complex to use, preventing these devices from being employed routinely in the clinical settings. However, with future technological advancements, non-contact devices will one day effectively complement contact-based respiratory monitors [24].

Monitoring of Oxygenation

Developed in the early 1980s, pulse oximetry is the primary source of oxygen saturation monitoring in any clinical setting. It has been shown to be effective to detect desaturation and hypoxemia in a patient sooner than clinical observation alone. Pulse oximeters detect arterial oxygen saturation (SaO_2) by measuring the light absorption of arterial blood at two specific wavelengths: 660 nm, corresponding to oxyhemoglobin; and 940 nm, corresponding to deoxyhemoglobin. The ratio of absorbencies at these two wavelengths is calibrated using an algorithm to generate an estimate of SaO_2 known as SpO_2 when detected by the pulse oximeter [25].

Box 5.1   Limitations of pulse oximetry

1. *Physiologic limitations*

   Shape of oxyhemoglobin dissociation curve

2. *Interference from substances dyes*

   Dyshemoglobins: carboxyhemoglobin, methemoglobin, acrylic nails, skin pigmentation

3. *Limitations in signal processing*

   Low perfusion states: decreased cardiac output, vasoconstriction, hypothermia, motion artifacts

4. *Limitations in knowledge of the technique*

Limitations of Pulse Oximetry

Since the hemoglobin dissociation curve is a sigmoid shape, oximetry is relatively insensitive in detecting hypoxemia in patients with high baseline levels of arterial oxygen pressure (PaO_2). Intravenous (IV) dyes such as indigo carmine, indocyanine green, and methylene blue can cause falsely low SpO_2 readings [26]. Acrylic nails and skin pigmentation can also affect readings, since the measurement is based on light-wave transmission that is modified by skin color [27]. Additionally, low perfusion states such as low cardiac output, vasoconstriction, and hypothermia may decrease peripheral perfusion, affecting readings. Pulse oximeters can detect only two wavelengths (oxyhemoglobin and deoxyhemoglobin); therefore, elevated carboxyhemoglobin and methemoglobin can cause inaccurate readings. Motion artifacts and noise artifacts – from the use of surgical electrocautery or other electrical devices in the operating room – can also interfere with readings [26]. The limitations of pulse oximetry are summarized in Box 5.1.

Clinical Applications of Pulse Oximetry

Pulse oximetry has helped to increase detection of hypoxemia in critically ill patients. However, changes in SpO_2 may not accurately reflect changes in PaO_2. For example, a patient with carbon monoxide poisoning will have a normal SpO_2 reading due to the redness of their skin although they are truly hypoxemic [28]. Pulse oximetry has also been inaccurate in assessing abnormal pulmonary gas exchange, which is defined as an elevated alveolar–arterial O_2 difference [29].

Temperature Monitoring

The normal human core body temperature is about 37 °C. It is the dominant input for autonomic thermoregulatory control and a major determinant of temperature-related complications. Temperature, ideally of the core, can be monitored at several anatomical sites: pulmonary artery, distal esophagus, nasopharynx, tympanic membranes, axilla, bladder, rectum, and skin. It is advised to monitor temperature during general or neuraxial anesthesia exceeding 30 minutes. However, sedation and peripheral nerve blocks do not significantly impair thermoregulatory control or trigger malignant hyperthermia and thus do not require temperature monitoring. Unwarmed surgical patients can become hypothermic, which can lead to complications, so it is important to monitor temperature [30].

Core Temperature Monitoring

The thermal core is made up of highly perfused central tissues, mainly the head and trunk [31]. Especially in patients undergoing general anesthesia it is important to monitor the core temperature to detect malignant hyperthermia and to quantify hyper- or hypothermia. For example, one of the signs of malignant hyperthermia is an out of proportion increase in $PaCO_2$ relative to minute ventilation [31], and detecting an increase in core temperature aids in this diagnosis. The most common perioperative heat-related disturbance is inadvertent hypothermia, which can have numerous post-surgical consequences, thus establishing the need for maintaining normothermia. Core temperature can be evaluated using the pulmonary artery (preferred), distal esophagus, nasopharynx, or tympanic membrane, which are well perfused. Although rarely used, the core temperature may also be obtained continuously over many days via ingested capsules that transmit temperatures to a nearby antenna, usually in a vest worn by the patient [30].

Near-Core Temperature Monitoring

Reasonable estimates of the core temperature can be obtained using oral and axillary temperatures, such as in patients recovering from anesthesia. Less reliable sites include bladder and rectal temperatures due to low perfusion from the core, and thus lag during thermal perturbations. Skin surface temperature is significantly lower than the core, and tends to vary among individuals and over time, making it an inadequate surrogate of the core temperature.

Although not all patients undergoing sedation are exposed to the potent inhalation agents used for general anesthesia, it is still important to monitor temperature. Patients undergoing minor surgical procedures who are exposed to the ambient environment without warming are prone to hypothermia: core heat loss by redistribution effects and peripheral heat loss through physical mechanisms of heat transfer (radiation, conduction, convection, and evaporation). Hypothermia can impact patient recovery and outcomes, including impaired wound healing and coagulation. Shivering can increase oxygen demand, BP, and heart rate [30, 32].

Carbon Dioxide Measurement

Carbon dioxide is produced as a waste product during cellular metabolism, as oxygen is used up. CO_2, dissolved in the blood (measured by partial pressure: $PaCO_2$), is transported to the right heart and then to the pulmonary artery where it exchanges with O_2 and is exhaled from the body via the lungs [33].

The concentration of CO_2 in exhaled breath (end-tidal CO_2 [$EtCO_2$]) indirectly represents circulatory status (cardiac output or CO). Quantitative $EtCO_2$ monitoring is mandatory for all procedures requiring moderate to deep sedation [34]. $EtCO_2$ is helpful in verifying correct placement of the endotracheal tube. For example, in an esophageal intubation, $EtCO_2$ will be absent. Exceptions are when patients consume carbonated drinks, related to belching (eructation), and ineffective mask ventilation, which may force some exhaled gas into stomach. The latter may produce $EtCO_2$ tracing but will fall to zero after at least five breaths as CO_2 is not being continuously generated. The normal gradient between $PaCO_2$ and $EtCO_2$ is approximately 5 mmHg. This gradient is affected by changes in perfusion and ventilation.

There are many methods that can be used to detect CO_2 levels: infrared spectroscopy, Raman spectroscopy, mass spectrometry, photoacoustic spectroscopy, and chemical colorimetric analysis [35]. Capnography (or waveform capnography) is the graphical representation of CO_2 released during the respiratory cycle [36], while capnometry is the measurement and numerical display of CO_2 expressed as $PaCO_2$ in mmHg, but no waveform.

Waveform capnography enables detection of a patient's breathing pattern, whether intubated or breathing spontaneously, and is critical to assess changes in ventilatory pattern. Any change in waveform alerts the practitioner of possible apnea or hypoventilation. By keeping track of changes in the shape or frequency of the CO_2 waveform, capnography can be used to monitor the adequacy of ventilation, help guide sedation, and prevent drug overdosing and hypoventilation [37]. Furthermore, it can be used to verify placement of the endotracheal tube, assess ventilation, and monitor for complications such as airway obstruction, displacement into the esophagus, and pulmonary embolism. Capnography can also help detect problems with the ventilator or endotracheal tube, whether this is caused by obstruction due to secretions or by the presence of leaks in the circuit [38]. Thus, it is a valuable monitoring tool for patients undergoing any type of sedation and can be lifesaving to reduce potential morbidity and mortality, especially in higher-risk populations [39, 40]

The infrared method of CO_2 detection is most common. Capnography and capnometry are based on CO_2's property of absorbing infrared radiation. Infrared rays are given off by all warm objects and are absorbed by non-elementary gases (i.e., those composed of dissimilar atoms), while certain gases absorb specific wavelengths producing absorption bands on the IR electromagnetic spectrum [41]. The intensity of infrared radiation projected through a gas mixture containing CO_2 is diminished by absorption; this allows the CO_2 absorption band to be identified and is proportional to the amount of CO_2 in the mixture. The higher the amount of CO_2, the less light that passes through the sensor. Infrared rays have a wavelength greater than 1 mm, lying beyond the visible spectrum (0.4–0.8 mm). CO_2 shows strong absorption in the far infrared region at 4.3 mm and so this wavelength in the far infrared range is used.

The measurement of exhaled CO_2 can be accomplished by using either a mainstream or a sidestream capnograph method. The mainstream method involves the sensor being placed directly on the patient's air passage to obtain $EtCO_2$ levels. It is considered invasive and non-diverting, since it measures $EtCO_2$ at the airway, and may only be used in non-intubated patients [42]. In the mainstream capnograph, a cuvette containing the source of infrared light and the photodetector is inserted between the breathing circuit and the endotracheal tube. The infrared rays traverse the respiratory gases to an infrared detector within the cuvette, and CO_2 analysis is performed within the airway. To prevent condensation of water vapor, which can cause falsely high CO_2 readings, all mainstream sensors are heated above body temperature [37]. One major disadvantage of using the mainstream capnograph is that the device is heavy and must be supported to prevent endotracheal-tube kinking and/or disconnection. It also contains a heated sensor that comes into direct contact with the patient's skin and can cause burns.

In the sidestream method, air exchange takes place via a circuit placed in the patient's air passage with the sensor collecting values from a connected sampling port. This method is considered non-invasive and diverting, since the $EtCO_2$ is analyzed at a sample cell slightly distant from the airway, as the gas is transported through a plastic tube. The sidestream method may be used in both intubated and non-intubated patients [42]. A sidestream capnography sample of exhaled gas is diverted from patient's breathing circuit to the capnography through a sampling tube to the sensor for analysis and display. The sampling tube is lighter, and allows for greater flexibility, but the sample is subject to variations in water content, humidity, and temperature. One advantage of sidestream capnography is the ability to monitor non-intubated patients, since the sampling of expiratory gases can be obtained from the nasal cavity using nasal adaptors or cannula. The disadvantage is that there is a delay in recording CO_2 measurement, because the exhaled gas needs to travel through the long sampling tubing, and the tubing is subject to disconnection or occlusion [43].

Raman spectroscopy uses the principle of "Raman scattering" for CO_2 measurement [44]. The gas sample is aspirated into the analyzing chamber, where the sample is illuminated by a high-intensity monochromatic argon laser beam. When light collides with gas molecules, the photons lose energy. This produces changes in the wavelength which are converted to an $EtCO_2$ reading. Mass spectrometry can also be used for capnography. Mass spectrometers analyze ions based on mass-to-charge ratio [45]. CO_2 content in the breathing circuit of an anesthesia machine can be reliably determined by using a mass spectrometer with a closed ion source consisting of a tungsten cathode [46].

Photoacoustic spectroscopy uses acoustic detection to measure the effect of absorbed electromagnetic energy, like light, on matter [47]. Gases undergo thermal expansion upon absorbing infrared light [48]. Ambient CO_2 can be determined by the sound made by CO_2 molecules when illuminated with infrared light [49]. Finally, chemical colorimetric analysis involves a pH-sensitive chemically treated foam indicator contained in a plastic housing that functions as an endotracheal tube elbow adapter. The color of the foam adapter changes from purple to yellow when it is exposed to exhaled CO_2.

In summary, capnography can be used to monitor the adequacy of ventilation in both intubated patients and non-intubated patients breathing spontaneously. Methods other than capnography are also available to measure respiration, such as the Linshom thermodynamic sensor [50].

Brain Function Monitoring

Measurement of the electrophysiologic activity of the cerebral cortex has been correlated to the depth of anesthesia. Cerebral cortex activity and sedation depth in patients undergoing anesthesia can be objectively measured using the bispectral index (BIS), which has been proposed as a guide to reduce the risk of intraprocedural oversedation and intraoperative awareness [51]. The BIS is most frequently used in general anesthesia but can be used during both moderate and deep sedation. Values range from 0, denoting no brain activity, to 100, indicating the patient is fully awake. Maintaining the BIS value below 60 decreases the incidence of anesthesia awareness [52], with 40–60 being the recommended range to maintain adequate general anesthesia depth and prevent awareness and 70–90 for moderate sedation [53, 54, 55].

The sedation depth can be monitored using several clinical tools. Widely accepted sedation tools include the Sedation Agitation Scale, the Ramsay Sedation Scale, and the Richmond Agitation Sedation Scale.

The BIS is measured using electrodes placed on the forehead, with the monitor displaying the BIS number, trend graph of BIS values over time, raw EEG waveforms in real time, signal quality index (SQI), electromyography, and alarm indicators. The SQI is positively correlated with the reliability of the BIS number. Electromyography reflects muscle activity [56]. BIS values have an unclear relationship with clinical sedation assessment tools, with some studies finding a correlation [55], while others have deemed the correlation unreliable [57]. In a large prospective observational study examining sedation practice and incidence of adverse events as well as the impact of BIS-guided sedative drug administration, Yang et al. concluded that the use of BIS did not significantly change the mean level of sedation, although the number of adverse events appeared to be lower with BIS utilization [51]. Another potential disadvantage of the BIS is the lack of standardization regarding the interpretation and correlation of all the various measurements provided by the different monitors. Regarding moderate and deep sedation, the role of brain function monitoring has not been established and routine monitoring with the BIS is not recommended. With advancing technology, however, the future landscape of brain monitoring is anticipated to change.

Intravenous Fluids

The three major uses of IV fluids are for maintenance, manipulation, and resuscitation. Obtaining IV access allows for safe and immediate delivery of fluids and medications directly into the patient's bloodstream. This is particularly useful when a patient is unable to consume anything by mouth, or when a medication is not meant for oral administration. IV fluids are an essential part of treatment, especially in trauma situations where high-volume fluid resuscitation and blood product therapy are required. IV fluids can also be used for the administration of life-saving vasopressor and inotropic medications. Additionally, IV access is essential for providing adequate sedation and anesthesia to patients as the anesthesia provider is dependent on IV administration for many of the medications needed to provide an appropriate level of anesthetic care [58].

Several supplies may be required for placing an IV catheter [59, 60]:

- disposable gloves
- topical antiseptic (e.g., povidone-iodine, alcohol)
- tourniquet
- angiocatheter
- tape
- infusion set
- transparent dressing (e.g., Tegaderm)
- labels

A local anesthetic such as lidocaine may be used around the IV site, or topical EMLA cream may be applied to reduce discomfort and improve patient tolerance of the procedure, particularly in the pediatric population [61]. Upon selecting an appropriate vein for access, several factors must be accounted for [60]:

1. Surgical site: an angiocatheter should not be placed in the surgical field, or in a limb that may have drainage affected by a previous lymph node dissection.
2. Patient positioning: during administration of sedation, the provider should have easy access to the IV site for troubleshooting in the event of a malfunction during the procedure.
3. Post-procedure activity level.
4. Anticipated duration of the need for IV access.

After accessing the desired vein, flushing, securing the angiocatheter, and connecting the infusion tubing, the infusion can be started. The site should be closely monitored and periodically checked for fluid infiltration or extravasation both at the beginning and throughout the procedure. If there is no extravasation or infiltration and fluids flow easily, the IV line should be safe to use [59, 60]. The success rate of IV placement in patients with difficult peripheral venous access can be effectively improved with skilled ultrasound use, thereby reducing the need for central line placement and associated complications [62].

Complications of Intravenous Access

There are several potential complications of IV access that should be monitored for throughout the duration of peripheral IV angiocatheter use. These complications may lead to the failure of the catheter or cause severe tissue damage; thus, early identification of these problems is of great importance. Some of the most common complications are infection, thrombophlebitis, infiltration/extravasation, and hematoma:

1. Infection: catheter-related infection is a risk associated with peripheral IV placement. Per the Centers for Disease Control and Prevention guidelines, the risk can be reduced by taking the following careful steps [63, 64]:

   - disinfection of the site prior to catheter placement
   - using an upper-extremity site for catheter placement in adults
   - using an upper- or lower-extremity site in children
   - using the scalp as insertion site in young infants or neonates
   - avoiding steel needles if the administered fluid or agent could cause tissue necrosis in the event of extravasation
   - if peripheral IV access will be needed for more than 6 days, the use of a midline or peripherally inserted central catheter is recommended
   - inspecting and evaluating the catheter site daily, both visually and by palpation
   - removing the catheter immediately if there are signs of phlebitis (local venous inflammation), infection, or if the catheter is not functioning correctly

2. Thrombophlebitis is characterized by local inflammatory signs such as pain, erythema, swelling, and venous thrombosis. Although its cause is not well understood, the risk may be reduced by the following measures [65, 66]

   - careful catheter placement
   - catheter replacement and rotation every 48–72 hours
   - catheter removal within 24 hours if initially placed in the emergency department

- changing the IV tubing within 24 hours if used to deliver blood products or lipid emulsion
- replacing dressings that have become damaged, removed, or loose and ineffective
- proper hand hygiene and disinfection of the intended insertion site
- ensuring proper training of staff to cannulate
- limiting the number of insertion attempts to minimize tissue trauma
- avoiding the administration of drugs and IV fluids with low pH or high flow rates

3. Infiltration and extravasation involve leakage of fluids and medications into the surrounding tissue. Depending on the amount and type of fluid that has infiltrated/extravasated, surrounding tissue may be compressed, leading to pain, swelling, cold and pale skin, reduced mobility of the affected limb, and ischemia. Further complications include necrosis, compartment syndrome, and potential indication for amputation [67]. The site should thus be evaluated for this complication regularly. If extravasation or infiltration is suspected, the IV catheter should be removed immediately, and a dressing applied. Depending on the type of medication being delivered to the tissue, a more advanced intervention, such as surgery, may also be needed [60, 68]

4. A hematoma is a collection of blood that can form within the tissue around where the IV catheter has been placed. If this occurs, it is recommended that the catheter is removed and that a pressure dressing is applied [60, 69].

Intravenous Fluids and Physiology

Compartments

The total body water is estimated at 60% of total body weight, which, in a 70-kg male, is about 42 L. The total body water is further split into intracellular and extracellular fluid compartments. The intracellular fluid comprises approximately two-thirds of total body water while the extracellular fluid makes up the additional one-third. The extracellular fluid is further divided into interstitial fluid, which comprises approximately three-quarters of the compartment, and plasma, which comprises the remaining one-quarter. Classically, intracellular fluid has been described as a portion of the extracellular fluid; however, a more accurate description delineates intracellular fluid into plasma (truly extracellular) and blood volume (includes both intracellular and extracellular components). There is another small compartment referred to as transcellular fluid, normally 1–2 L, which is comprised of fluids in the gastrointestinal tract, collagenous connective tissues, serous and synovial cavities, cerebrospinal space, lower urinary tract, and bile ducts. Transcellular fluid is typically considered extracellular although its composition may differ markedly from interstitial or intracellular fluid [70, 71, 72].

Intracellular Compartment

The intracellular fluid compartment is separated from the extracellular fluid compartment by a membrane that is highly permeable to water but not to most electrolytes. It plays a significant role in maintaining and regulating volume and composition. The primary driver of water movement is osmolal concentration. This concentration is called osmolality when expressed as osmoles per kilogram of water and osmolarity when expressed as osmoles per liter of solution. The higher the osmolality or osmolarity, the more concentrated the solution and thus the higher the osmotic pressure driving water into the concentrated compartment [71]. A membrane-bound adenosine triphosphate (ATP)-dependent pump exchanges three sodium (Na^+) ions out for two potassium (K+) ions in to maintain its electrochemical gradient. The major player in determining intracellular osmotic pressure is K^+. Because the cell membranes are impermeable to most proteins, there is also a high intracellular protein concentration [73]. The Na^+/K^+ ATPase pump is key in preventing intracellular hyperosmolality due to these proteins. Other significant components of the intracellular fluid compartment include magnesium, phosphates, and organic anions.

Extracellular Fluid Compartment

The major player in determining extracellular fluid volume and distribution is Na^+, whereas chloride (Cl^-) and bicarbonate (HCO_3^-) contribute to a lesser degree. The two major components of extracellular fluid – interstitial fluid and plasma – are separated by highly permeable capillary membranes. For this reason, their ionic compositions are extremely similar, except for proteins, which are concentrated in the plasma. The composition of the extracellular fluid is regulated by various systems, arguably the most important being the renal system. When alterations of extracellular components occur, pathologic states can develop, leading to an increase in the volume of the interstitial compartment – seen clinically as tissue edema. Keeping in mind that the extracellular fluid includes most of the intravascular volume – plasma – maintenance of this compartment is crucial to ensuring adequate tissue perfusion and oxygenation [70, 71, 72].

Supplementation of Volume
Tonicity

The terms hypotonic, isotonic, and hypertonic refer to the effect solutions have on cell volume. Hypotonic solutions are less concentrated and therefore increase cell volumes as water moves into the cell to provide balance. Isotonic solutions have relatively equal concentration with cells and have negligible effects on cell volumes. Lastly, hypertonic solutions are more concentrated and cause a movement of water out of cells to maintain balance, therefore decreasing cell volumes [72].

Choice of Intravenous Fluid

IV fluid supplementation exerts its therapeutic effect by expanding fluid compartments. Electrolyte composition and particle size contained in these fluids affect fluid distribution, acid/base status, renal function, and coagulation. The two major categories of available IV solutions are crystalloids and colloids. Crystalloids contain minerals/salts of organic acids while colloids contain oncotic macromolecules that largely remain in the intravascular space, thereby generating an oncotic pressure gradient. There is currently no clear consensus regarding choice of IV fluids on best clinical outcome in the perioperative setting [72].

Crystalloids

The benefits of crystalloid solutions are that they are safe, effective, non-toxic, non-reactive, easy to store, free of religious disagreement concerning their use –Jehovah's Witnesses, for example, will accept crystalloids but not blood products [74] – and

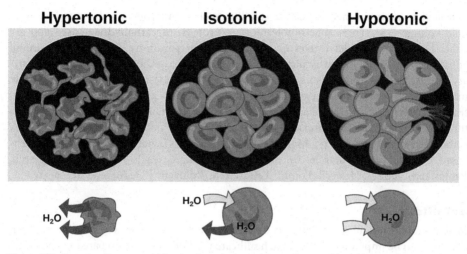

Figure 5.2 Osmotic effects on red blood cells under hypertonic, isotonic and hypotonic states.

inexpensive. There are two major categories of crystalloids, unbalanced and balanced, which refer to their similarity with plasma.

Unbalanced Crystalloids

Normal (0.9%) saline is the most used IV fluid worldwide. It is rapidly distributed between extracellular compartments after administration: in healthy patients approximately 60% of the administered volume is redistributed from the intravascular space to the interstitial space. However, due to its ionic composition, superfluous administration can produce a hyperchloremic normal anion gap metabolic acidosis.

Saline is also available in lower (hypotonic) concentrations (one-half and one-quarter normal) used primarily to replace/prevent free water deficits and hypertonic concentrations used to replace sodium deficits. Dextrose solutions contain glucose dissolved in water with or without sodium chloride, each in varying concentrations. They are hypotonic and used to replace free water losses and maintain blood glucose levels. Sodium bicarbonate ($NaHCO_3$) quickly dissociates to provide Na^+ and HCO_3^- ions and buffers excess hydrogen ions [73].

Balanced Crystalloids

Balanced (isotonic) solutions are more like plasma than 0.9% saline. Some examples of commonly used balanced crystalloid solutions include Ringer's lactate (also called lactated Ringer's solution), Hartmann's solution, Plasma-Lyte, and Sterofundin.

Lactated Ringer's solution can cause a small reduction in plasma osmolality. Hartmann's solution is a slightly modified form of lactated Ringer's. Plasma-Lyte and Sterofundin are composed of electrolyte concentrations very closely mimicking human plasma [73].

Colloids

Colloids are crystalloid solutions that contain oncotic macromolecules that remain in the intravascular space and generate an oncotic pressure gradient [72]. Colloid solutions are indicated to maintain hemodynamic stability, such as intraoperatively to reduce total fluid volume [75]. These macromolecules are protein- or carbohydrate-based and are either human plasma derivatives or semisynthetic preparations. Although they are all effective at expanding intravascular volume, often they have short half-lives and temporary effects. Colloids have also been associated with allergic reactions and are typically much more expensive than crystalloid solutions. Colloids can be gelatin-based (derived from hydrolysis of bovine collagen; e.g., Gelofusine), human-albumin-based (manufactured from cryo-depleted human plasma, e.g., Albumex), dextran-based (large complex carbohydrate polymers, e.g., Macrodex, Rheomacrodex), naturally occurring starch-based (hydroxyethyl starch in maize and potato, e.g., Hextend, Hetastarch, Pentastarch, Elohes, Hesteril, Lomol, Tetrastarch, Voluven) [73, 76].

Summary

Patient monitoring during sedation is of the utmost importance to a healthcare provider. Sedation can be unpredictable, and the healthcare provider must be prepared to encounter fluctuations in patient vital signs, equipment malfunction, and data output distortion. During sedation, the healthcare provider must monitor respiration, oxygenation, temperature, carbon dioxide, brain activity, and the intravenous delivery of fluids and medications. In this chapter we provided an outline of current methods of patient monitoring.

References

1. Hagan KB, Thirumurthi S, Gottumukkala R, Vargo J. Sedation in the endoscopy suite. *Curr Treat Options Gastroenterol.* 2016;14(2):194–209. doi:10.1007/s11938-016-0089-8

2. American Society of Anesthesiologists Committee on Standards and Practice Parameters. Standards for basic anesthetic monitoring. www.asahq.org/standards-and-guidelines/standards-for-basic-anesthetic-monitoring

3. Merchant R, Chartrand D, Dain S, et al. Guidelines to the practice of anesthesia: revised edition 2015. *Can J Anesth Can Anesth.* 2015;62(1):54–79. doi:10.1007/s12630-014-0232-8

4. Poncette AS, Mosch L, Spies C, et al. Improvements in patient monitoring in the intensive care unit: survey study. *J Med Internet Res.* 2020;22(6):e19091. doi:10.2196/19091

5. Casabianca AB, Becker DE. Cardiovascular monitoring: physiological and technical considerations. *Anesth Prog.* 2009;56(2):53–60. doi:10.2344/0003-3006-56.2.53

6. American Society of Anesthesiologists Task Force on Sedation and Analgesia by Non-Anesthesiologists. Practice guidelines for sedation and analgesia by non-anesthesiologists. *Anesthesiology.* 2002;96(4):1004–17. doi:10.1097/00000542-200204000-00031

7. Sampson M. Continuous ECG monitoring in hospital: part 2, practical issues. *Br J Card Nurs.* 2018;13(3):128–34. doi:10.12968/bjca.2018.13.3.128

8. Nedios S, Romero I, Gerds-Li JH, Fleck E, Kriatselis C. Precordial electrode placement for optimal ECG monitoring: implications for ambulatory monitor devices and event recorders. *J Electrocardiol.* 2014;47(5):669–76. doi:10.1016/j.jelectrocard.2014.04.003

9. Whelton PK, Carey RM, Aronow WS, et al. 2017 ACC/AHA/AAPA/ABC/ACPM/AGS/APhA/ASH/ASPC/NMA/PCNA Guideline for the prevention, detection, evaluation, and management of high blood pressure in adults: a report of the American College of Cardiology/American Heart Association Task Force on Clinical Practice Guidelines. *Hypertens*

Dallas Tex 1979. 2018;71(6):e13–115. doi:10.1161/HYP.0000000000000065

10. Gupta R, Guptha S. Strategies for initial management of hypertension. *Indian J Med Res.* 2010;132(5):531–42.

11. Vincent JL, De Backer D. Circulatory shock. *N Engl J Med.* 2013;369:1726–34. doi:10.1056/NEJMra1208943

12. Koutsaki M, Thomopoulos C, Achimastos A, et al. Perioperative SBP changes during orthopedic surgery in the elderly: clinical implications. *J Hypertens.* 2019;37(8):1705–1713. doi:10.1097/HJH.0000000000002085

13. Geddes LA. The direct measurement of blood pressure. In Geddes LA, ed., *Handbook of Blood Pressure Measurement.* Humana Press, 1991, 1–47. doi:10.1007/978-1-4684-7170-0_1

14. Ogedegbe G, Pickering T. Principles and techniques of blood pressure measurement. *Cardiol Clin.* 2010;28(4):571–586. doi:10.1016/j.ccl.2010.07.006

15. Pickering D, Stevens S. How to measure and record blood pressure. *Community Eye Health.* 2013;26(84):76.

16. Berger A. Oscillatory blood pressure monitoring devices. *BMJ.* 2001; 323:919.

17. Meidert AS, Saugel B. Techniques for non-invasive monitoring of arterial blood pressure. *Front Med.* 2018;4:231. doi:10.3389/fmed.2017.00231

18. Goodman CT, Kitchen GB. Measuring arterial blood pressure. *Anaesth Intensive Care Med.* 2021;22(1):49–53. doi:10.1016/j.mpaic.2020.11.007

19. Folke M, Cernerud L, Ekström M, Hök B. Critical review of non-invasive respiratory monitoring in medical care. *Med Biol Eng Comput.* 2003;41(4):377–383. doi:10.1007/BF02348078

20. Tobin MJ. Respiratory monitoring during mechanical ventilation. *Crit Care Clin.* 1990;6(3):679–709.

21. Redmond C. Transthoracic impedance measurements in patient monitoring.

Analog Devices Inc., 2013. www.analog.com/en/resources/technical-articles/transthoracic-impedance-measurements-in-patient-monitoring.html

22. Criée CP, Sorichter S, Smith HJ, et al. Body plethysmography: its principles and clinical use. *Respir Med.* 2011;105(7):959–71. doi:10.1016/j.rmed.2011.02.006

23. Massaroni C, Nicolò A, Lo Presti D, et al. Contact-based methods for measuring respiratory rate. *Sensors.* 2019;19(4):908. doi:10.3390/s19040908

24. Al-Khalidi FQ, Saatchi R, Burke D, Elphick H, Tan S. Respiration rate monitoring methods: a review. *Pediatr Pulmonol.* 2011;46(6):523–9. doi:10.1002/ppul.21416

25. Brochard L, Martin GS, Blanch L, et al. Clinical review: respiratory monitoring in the ICU: a consensus of 16. *Crit Care.* 2012;16(2):219. doi:10.1186/cc11146

26. Jubran A. Pulse oximetry. *Crit Care.* 1999;3(2):R11–R17. doi:10.1186/cc341

27. Crooks CJ, West J, Morling JR, et al. Pulse oximeter measurements vary across ethnic groups: an observational study in patients with COVID-19. *Eur Respir J.* 2022;59(4):2103246. doi:10.1183/13993003.03246-2021

28. Haymond S, Cariappa R, Eby CS, Scott MG. Laboratory assessment of oxygenation in methemoglobinemia. *Clin Chem.* 2005;51(2):434–44. doi:10.1373/clinchem.2004.035154

29. Tin W, Lal M. Principles of pulse oximetry and its clinical application in neonatal medicine. *Semin Fetal Neonatal Med.* 2015;20(3):192–7. doi:10.1016/j.siny.2015.01.006

30. Sessler DI. Perioperative temperature monitoring. *Anesthesiology.* 2021;134(1):111–18. doi:10.1097/ALN.0000000000003481

31. Larach MG, Gronert GA, Allen GC, Brandom BW, Lehman EB. Clinical presentation, treatment, and complications of malignant hyperthermia in North America from 1987 to 2006. *Anesth Analg.*

2010;110(2):498–507. doi:10.1213/ANE.0b013e3181c6b9b2

32. Kurz A. Thermal care in the perioperative period. *Best Pract Res Clin Anaesthesiol.* 2008;22(1):39–62. doi:10.1016/j.bpa.2007.10.004

33. Crystal GJ. Carbon dioxide and the heart: physiology and clinical implications. *Anesth Analg.* 2015;121(3):610–23. doi:10.1213/ANE.0000000000000820

34. Weaver J. The latest ASA mandate: CO_2 monitoring for moderate and deep sedation. *Anesth Prog.* 2011;58(3):111–12. doi:10.2344/0003-3006-58.3.111

35. Huttmann SE, Windisch W, Storre JH. Techniques for the measurement and monitoring of carbon dioxide in the blood. *Ann Am Thorac Soc.* 2014;11(4):645–52. doi:10.1513/AnnalsATS.201311-387FR

36. Shah R, Streat DA, Auerbach M, Shabanova V, Langhan ML. Improving capnography use for critically ill emergency patients: an implementation study. *J Patient Saf.* 2022;18(1):e26. doi:10.1097/PTS.0000000000000683

37. Casey G. Capnography: monitoring CO_2. *Nurs N Z.* 2015;21(9):20–4.

38. Kerslake I, Kelly F. Uses of capnography in the critical care unit. *BJA Educ.* 2017;17(5):178–83. doi:10.1093/bjaed/mkw062

39. Fukuda K, Ichinohe T, Kaneko Y. Is measurement of end-tidal CO_2 through a nasal cannula reliable? *Anesth Prog.* 1997;44(1):23–6.

40. Scoccimarro A, West JR, Kanter M, Caputo ND. Waveform capnography: an alternative to physician Gestalt in determining optimal intubating conditions after administration of paralytic agents. *Emerg Med J EMJ.* 2018;35(1):62–4. doi:10.1136/emermed-2017-206922

41. Schumacher TE, Smucker AJ. Measurement of CO_2 dissolved in aqueous solutions using a modified infrared gas analyzer system. *Plant Physiol.* 1983;72(1):212–14. doi:10.1104/pp.72.1.212

42. Pekdemir M, Cinar O, Yılmaz S, Yaka E, Yuksel M. Disparity between mainstream and sidestream end-tidal carbon dioxide values and arterial carbon dioxide levels. *Respir Care.* 2013;58(7):1152–56. doi:10.4187/respcare.02227

43. Donald MJ, Paterson B. End tidal carbon dioxide monitoring in prehospital and retrieval medicine: a review. *Emerg Med J EMJ.* 2006;23(9):728–30. doi:10.1136/emj.2006.037184

44. White SN. Qualitative and quantitative analysis of CO_2 and CH_4 dissolved in water and seawater using laser Raman spectroscopy. *Appl Spectrosc.* 2010;64(7):819–27. doi:10.1366/000370210791666354

45. Price P. Standard definitions of terms relating to mass spectrometry: a report from the Committee on Measurements and Standards of the American Society for Mass Spectrometry. *J Am Soc Mass Spectrom.* 1991;2(4):336–48. doi:10.1016/1044-0305(91)80025-3

46. Elokhin VA, Ershov TD, Levshankov AI, Nikolaev VI, Elizarov AYu. Application of a mass spectrometer as a capnograph. *Tech Phys.* 2010;55(12):1814–16. doi:10.1134/S1063784210120194

47. Jones RW, McClelland J. Fourier transform infrared photoacoustic spectroscopy of ageing composites. In Martin R, ed., *Ageing of Composites.* Woodhead Publishing, 2008, 160–85. doi:10.1533/9781845694937.1.160

48. Blohm A, Sieburg A, Popp J, Frosch T. Detection of gas molecules by means of spectrometric and spectroscopic methods. In Baia L, Pap Z, Hernadi K, Baia M, eds., *Advanced Nanostructures for Environmental Health. Micro and Nano Technologies.* Elsevier, 2020, 251–94. doi:10.1016/B978-0-12-815882-1.00006-9

49. Palzer S. Photoacoustic-based gas sensing: a review. *Sensors.* 2020;20(9):2745. doi:10.3390/s20092745

50. Preiss D, Drew BA, Gosnell J, et al. Linshom thermodynamic sensor is a reliable alternative to capnography for monitoring respiratory rate. *J Clin Monit*

Comput. 2018;32(1):133–40. doi:10.1007/
s10877-017-0004-4

51. Yang KS, Habib AS, Lu M, et al.
A prospective evaluation of the incidence
of adverse events in nurse-administered
moderate sedation guided by sedation
scores or bispectral index. Anesth Analg.
2014;119(1):43–8. doi:10.1213/
ANE.0b013e3182a125c3

52. Avidan MS, Zhang L, Burnside BA, et al.
Anesthesia awareness and the bispectral
index. N Engl J Med.
2008;358(11):1097–108. doi:10.1056/
NEJMoa0707361

53. Leslie K, Sessler DI, Smith WD, et al.
Prediction of movement during propofol/
nitrous oxide anesthesia. Performance of
concentration, electroencephalographic,
pupillary, and hemodynamic indicators.
Anesthesiology. 1996;84(1):52–63.
doi:10.1097/00000542-199601000-00006

54. Gelfand ME, Gabriel RA, Gimlich R,
Beutler SS, Urman RD. Practice patterns
in the intraoperative use of bispectral
index monitoring. J Clin Monit Comput.
2017;31(2):281–9. doi:10.1007/s10877-
016-9845-5

55. Bower AL, Ripepi A, Dilger J, Boparai N,
Brody FJ, Ponsky JL. Bispectral index
monitoring of sedation during
endoscopy. Gastrointest Endosc.
2000;52(2):192–6. doi:10.1067/
mge.2000.107284

56. Olson DM, Chioffi SM, Macy GE, Meek
LG, Cook HA. Potential benefits of
bispectral index monitoring in critical
care. A case study. Crit Care Nurse.
2003;23(4):45–52.

57. Gill M, Green SM, Krauss B. A study of
the bispectral index monitor during
procedural sedation and analgesia in the
emergency department. Ann Emerg Med.
2003;41(2):234–41. doi:10.1067/
mem.2003.53

58. Cheung E, Baerlocher MO, Asch M,
Myers A. Venous access. Can Fam
Physician. 2009;55(5):494–6.

59. Milliam DA. How to teach good
venipuncture technique. Am J Nurs.
1993;93(7):38–41.

60. Kost M. Intravenous insertion techniques.
In Manual of Conscious Sedation.
W. B. Saunders, 1998, 162–175.

61. Rogers TL, Ostrow CL. The use of
EMLA cream to decrease venipuncture
pain in children. J Pediatr Nurs.
2004;19(1):33–9. doi:10.1016/
j.pedn.2003.09.005

62. Shokoohi H, Boniface K, McCarthy M,
et al. Ultrasound-guided peripheral
intravenous access program is associated
with a marked reduction in central
venous catheter use in noncritically ill
emergency department patients. Ann
Emerg Med. 2013;61(2):198–203.
doi:10.1016/j.annemergmed.2012.09.016

63. O'Grady NP, Alexander M, Burns LA,
et al. Guidelines for the prevention of
intravascular catheter-related infections.
Clin Infect Dis. 2011;52(9):e162–93.
doi:10.1093/cid/cir257

64. Centers for Disease Control and
Prevention. Background information:
strategies for prevention of catheter-
related infections in adult and pediatric
patients. November 5, 2015. www.cdc
.gov/infectioncontrol/guidelines/bsi/
background/prevention-strategies.html

65. Tagalakis V, Kahn SR, Libman M,
Blostein M. The epidemiology of
peripheral vein infusion
thrombophlebitis: a critical review. Am
J Med. 2002;113(2):146–51. doi:10.1016/
s0002-9343(02)01163-4

66. Singh N, Kalyan G, Kaur S, Jayashree M,
Ghai S. Quality improvement initiative to
reduce intravenous line-related
infiltration and phlebitis incidence in
pediatric emergency room. Indian J Crit
Care Med. 2021;25(5):557–65.
doi:10.5005/jp-journals-10071-23818

67. DosSantos LM, de Jesus Nunes K, Silva
CSGE, et al. Elaboration and validation of
an algorithm for treating peripheral
intravenous infiltration and extravasation
in children. Rev Lat Am Enfermagem.
2021;29:e3435. doi:10.1590/1518-
8345.4314.3435

68. Doellman D, Hadaway L, Bowe-Geddes
LA, et al. Infiltration and extravasation:

update on prevention and management. *J Infus Nurs Off Publ Infus Nurses Soc.* 2009;32(4):203–11. doi:10.1097/NAN.0b013e3181aac042

69. Kagel EM, Rayan GM. Intravenous catheter complications in the hand and forearm. *J Trauma.* 2004;56(1):123–27. doi:10.1097/01.TA.0000058126.72962.74

70. Holte K, Jensen P, Kehlet H. Physiologic effects of intravenous fluid administration in healthy volunteers. *Anesth Analg.* 2003;96(5):1504–9. doi:10.1213/01.ANE.0000055820.56129.EE

71. Roumelioti ME, Glew RH, Khitan ZJ, et al. Fluid balance concepts in medicine: principles and practice. *World J Nephrol.* 2018;7(1):1–28. doi:10.5527/wjn.v7.i1.1

72. Edwards MR., Grocott MPW. Perioperative fluid and electrolyte therapy. In *Miller's Anesthesia*, 9th ed. Elsevier, 2019, 1480–523.

73. Varrier M, Ostermann M. Fluid composition and clinical effects. *Crit Care Clin.* 2015;31(4):823–37. doi:10.1016/j.ccc.2015.06.014

74. Remmers PA, Speer AJ. Clinical strategies in the medical care of Jehovah's Witnesses. *Am J Med.* 2006;119(12):1013–18. doi:10.1016/j.amjmed.2006.04.016

75. Reiterer C, Kabon B, Halvorson S, et al. Hemodynamic responses to crystalloid and colloid fluid boluses during noncardiac surgery. *Anesthesiology.* 2022;136:127–37. doi:https://doi.org/10.1097/ALN.0000000000004040

76. Yunos NM, Bellomo R, Story D, Kellum J. Bench-to-bedside review: chloride in critical illness. *Crit Care.* 2010;14(4):226. doi:10.1186/cc9052

Credentialing, Competency, and Education

Laurie Demeule and Lisa Govoni

Introduction

The safe transition of patients through procedures performed under moderate or deep sedation is a complex and challenging clinical situation. In recognition of the safety risks involved in caring for patients requiring any level of sedation, in the USA the Joint Commission has set specific standards around credentialing, competency assessment, and education [1].

Credentialing

The Joint Commission standard MS.06.01.01 require accredited organizations to collect, verify, and evaluate "data relevant to a practitioner's professional performance" as part of the credentialing and privileging process. Recent revisions to this standard further define three new concepts relevant to credentialing and privileging [1]:

1. Integration of six areas of general competencies (see Box 6.1) developed by the Accreditation Council for Graduate Medical Education (ACGME) and the American Board of Medical Specialties.
2. Focused professional practice evaluation where medical staff focus on a practitioner's performance in situations where the documentation suggests competence but additional information on performance is necessary to confirm competence, or when

---

Box 6.1 ACGME Outcome Project (1999): six general competencies for medical practice [3]

Patient care
Medical/clinical knowledge
Practice-based learning and improvement
Interpersonal and communication skills
Professionalism
Systems-based practice

---

questions arise regarding a practitioner's professional practice during the course of the ongoing professional practice evaluation.

3. Ongoing professional practice evaluation that calls for continuous monitoring and evaluation of professional performance by an organization or staff that provides opportunities to identify and resolve potential problems efficiently as they arise while providing an added evidence base to the traditional privilege renewal process.

The Joint Commission elaborates on this process by noting that the performance-related evidence collected is then presented to the governing body with "the ultimate authority for granting, restricting and revoking privileges."

Defining specific elements for credentialing is left to the institution's credentialing body, based on their assessment of what is required for safe practice at the local level. Most organizations require successful completion of institutionally developed programs specific to the management of moderate and deep procedural sedation. Physicians may obtain certification by an established educational provider such as the American Heart Association or the American College of Surgeons Committee on Trauma as standard for providers of deep sedation. Board certification in anesthesiology, critical care, or emergency medicine may be the minimum requirement for providers of deep sedation in some organizations. Registered nursing certification specific to moderate sedation can be obtained through the American Association of Moderate Sedation Nurses.

Credentials must be renewed at least every 2 years. In many institutions this practice often coincides with license and certification expiration and renewal. The institutions are responsible for determining and reviewing required elements for credentialing. Individuals are responsible for maintaining professional, legal, and organizational credentials on a current basis.

General Competencies

Competence to perform is assessed as an element of the initial credentialing process. Epstein and Hundert, while emphasizing the multidimensional aspects of competency, highlight the importance of basic clinical skills, scientific knowledge, and moral development as the foundations of competency in practice [2]. The six general competencies identified by the ACGME [3] are cited by the Joint Commission as a framework for credentialing and ongoing competency assessment (Box 6.1).

Developing programs that identify and assess knowledge, skill, behavior, and commitment in the context of complex medical treatments and unpredictable patient response is challenging. An initial review of institutional procedures and practice settings should be conducted to define both general and specific competencies. Orientation programs address the minimal requirements and standards for safe practice. Subsequently, the organization must be vigilant and responsive to the need for ongoing competency development as new procedures, medications, and equipment are introduced into practice settings. Annual or biannual competency programs provide an opportunity not only for practitioner competency validation but also for program evaluation. Current quality reports and safety data provide evidence that existing programs incorporate competencies relevant to practice within the organization. Simulation has become a best practice to assess and validate clinical competency. This is often presented utilizing low-, medium-, or high-fidelity scenarios. The application of a multidisciplinary team approach benefits team dynamic and individual skill set confidence for procedural sedation [4].

Sedation-Specific Competencies

Procedural sedation, also described as moderate sedation, is a technique to administer "sedatives or dissociative agents without analgesics to induce a state that allows the patient to tolerate unpleasant procedures while maintaining cardiorespiratory function. Procedural sedation and analgesia are intended to result in a depressed level of consciousness that allows the patient to maintain their oxygenation and airway control independently" [5]. Patient response to pharmaceutical agents is unpredictable and requires that providers "be qualified to manage the patient at whatever level of sedation is achieved either intentionally or unintentionally" [1]. The opinion of the American Society of Anesthesiologists (ASA) Task Force is that the primary causes of morbidity associated with sedation/analgesia are drug-induced respiratory depression and airway obstruction [6]. Therefore, competency programs for providers of moderate and deep sedation must focus on specific knowledge, skills, and behaviors that prevent these complications.

Managing Levels of Sedation

The ability to identify varying levels along the sedation continuum enables providers to successfully intervene when intended levels of sedation are not successfully achieved or inadvertently exceeded. Skillful application of a validated and reliable sedation assessment tool provides an objective measure of when providers should intervene [7].

Medication Management Competencies

Comprehensive knowledge of the pharmacologic agents of procedural sedation, and accuracy in the choice of the right combination of agents for specific patient populations, is an essential competency. The ability to safely administer the medication, monitor for intended and unintended effects, and appropriately use reversal agents provides behavioral evidence of competence in the management of procedural sedation medications.

Hemodynamic and Cardiac Monitoring

An understanding of the effects of pharmacologic agents on hemodynamic and cardiac function is required to safely manage procedural sedation. Skillful initiation and management of hemodynamic and cardiac monitoring equipment and interpretation of the changes in the patient's baseline status are required to anticipate and prevent complications. Knowledge of normal cardiac rhythm, skill in ECG interpretation, and identification of and response to potentially serious dysrhythmias are minimal requirements of providers and monitors of procedural sedation.

Airway Management

Basic and advanced competence in the assessment and management of the patient's airway is required before, during, and following the procedure. Knowledge of normal anatomy and physiology, and skilled assessment of the oral cavity to evaluate the need for anesthesia consultation, should be part of the pre-procedure evaluation.

Skills required to maintain a patient's airway can range from basic repositioning and manipulation of the airway with chin-lift and jaw-thrust maneuvers to the more sophisticated implementation of respiratory adjuncts such as oropharyngeal airways and bag-valve mask devices.

Oxygenation and Ventilation

An understanding of the mechanics of breathing and the physiology of oxygenation and ventilation is required to anticipate, intervene in, and prevent the more serious respiratory and cardiac complications associated with procedural sedation. The use of continuous oxygen saturation monitoring as a reliable tool to supplement the clinical observation and auscultation of breathing and to detect changes in oxygenation has long been supported in clinical practice and strongly recommended by the consultants to the ASA [6].

The standards for basic anesthetic monitoring amended by the ASA House of Delegates in October 2010 state that "during moderate or deep sedation the adequacy of ventilation shall be evaluated by continual observation of qualitative clinical signs and monitoring for the presence of exhaled carbon dioxide unless precluded or invalidated by the nature of the patient, procedure or equipment" [8].

The addition of capnography to standard monitoring has proven beneficial in the early identification of hypoxic events and supports this recommendation [9]. Thus, providers must demonstrate skill in the application and management of both the oximetry and capnography devices to assure the adequacy of the pleth or waveform. The provider must also be competent in the interpretation of the various waveforms and digital readouts and correlate this data to clinical changes in the patient's condition.

Education

The intended audience of educational programs around procedural sedation is the professional healthcare provider. As adult learners, these individuals must be recognized as highly motivated learners who accept responsibility for learning and approach new knowledge and skill acquisition as an extension of previous knowledge and practice experience [10].

The intent of procedural sedation education is to develop and validate knowledge, skills, and behavioral competency in the management of patients requiring pharmacologic intervention during procedures. Traditional classroom instruction and testing is limited to addressing only the cognitive aspects of learning and does not validate competency. The addition of flexible and experiential learning strategies should be considered to address other modalities of learning and skill acquisition.

Significant advances in technology over the past few decades have created the opportunity for organizations to meet the challenges of competency development and validation for healthcare practitioners. Through computer-based tutorials and internet-based learning environments healthcare practitioners can acquire the core cognitive knowledge required for certification in basic and advanced cardiac life support, basic ECG analysis, and airway management. Knowledge acquisition occurs at the individual learner's own pace, at times and in places convenient for the learner. Simulation laboratories have offered safe opportunities for practitioners to integrate their knowledge while honing their skills as they practice using case-based scenarios.

Knowles et al. emphasize the importance of experiential learning for adult learners [10]. Teaching the skills required to translate knowledge into clinical practice is best accomplished in environments that recreate real-life clinical situations. The high-risk, high-stakes practice environment of modern healthcare organizations has forced a shift from knowledge-based to outcomes-based education [11]. The competent application of knowledge and skills in the context of unpredictable patient response must be accomplished using sound clinical reasoning and expert communication skills.

Management of procedural sedation is a complex clinical situation. More than merely knowing (cognitive) or knowing how (psychomotor), the clinician must demonstrate high-level clinical reasoning and decision-making behaviors (affective) around knowing why and when certain actions must be initiated in response to specific patient needs. Such decision making is accomplished within the context of the integrated team. All team members must have the interpersonal and communication skills to clearly articulate the goals of sedation and analgesia, and the confidence and ability to clearly communicate their clinical concerns. Simulation-based education has emerged as a learning and assessment modality that educates, provides practice experience, and validates the competencies required to manage procedural sedation (see Chapter 13). In simulated clinical environments, all learning domains (cognitive, psychomotor, and behavioral) can be assessed in controlled settings where immediate feedback is provided to change or reinforce behaviors. Table 6.1 lists common educational strategies and outcomes that address domains of learning.

The Association of Perioperative Registered Nurses (AORN) has published recommended practices for managing the patient receiving moderate sedation/analgesia [12]. These practice guidelines were developed by the AORN Recommended Practices Committee and have been approved by the AORN Board of Directors, effective January 1, 2002, and reaffirmed April 2016. As the practice guidelines state, "these recommended practices are intended as achievable recommendations representing what is believed to be an optimal level of practice. Policies and procedures will reflect variations in practice settings and/or clinical situations that determine the degree to which the recommended practices can be implemented."

In 2019, the ASA amended the statement on safe use of propofol [13], which emphasizes that sedation is a continuum, and that moderate sedation can inadvertently evolve into deep sedation or general anesthesia. When propofol is used, the patient should "receive care consistent with that required for deep sedation."

In 2010, the American Association of Nurse Anesthetists published "Considerations for Policy Development Number 4.2: Registered Nurses Engaged in the Administration of Sedation and Analgesia" [14]. These considerations are intended to provide registered nurses with the definitions of sedation and analgesia, to establish suggested qualifications, and to provide suggestions for patient management and monitoring practices.

The ASA has published two guideline statements, one addressing educational and competency standards for the practitioner (an MD or DO physician, dentist, or podiatrist) supervising or directly administering moderate sedation, and the other for practitioners participating in deep sedation [15, 16]. Each healthcare facility should establish its own educational standards and guidelines but may choose to incorporate some or all the elements of moderate and/or deep sedation privileging process as out- lined by the ASA and use the guideline information as the basis for the healthcare facility's sedation policy.

The first statement, originally introduced in 2005 and amended October 13, 2021, is the statement on granting privileges for administration of *moderate sedation* to practitioners who are not anesthesia professionals [15]. This statement is intended to offer "a framework for granting privileges that will help ensure competence of individuals who administer or supervise the administration of moderate sedation." This statement is intended as a guide for any type of facility "in which an internal or external credentialing process is required for administration of sedative and analgesic drugs to establish a level of moderate sedation."

Table 6.1 Procedural sedation competencies: learning and assessment modalities

Learning domain	Educational strategies	Outcome and measurement
Cognitive (knowledge)		
1. Levels of sedation 2. Pharmacology of sedation/analgesia 3. Airway assessment 4. Basic hemodynamics and ECG analysis 5. Oxygenation/ventilation	Traditional classroom Computer-based tutorial Interactive web-based module Case study Standardized patient	1. (a) Accurately identifies levels of sedation (b) Applies valid sedation assessment tool 2. (a) Identifies intended/unintended medication effects (b) Initiates use of reversal agents 3. (a) Pre-procedure assessment using Mallampati (b) Appropriate request for anesthesia consult 4. (a) Appropriately identifies changes in patient status (b) Intervenes in response to changes 5. (a) Identifies changes from patient baseline (b) Initiates airway management techniques
Psychomotor (skills)		
1. Levels of sedation 2. Intravenous and medication skills 3. ECG/hemodynamic skills	Traditional classroom Computer-based tutorial Simulation training	1. Responds therapeutically to intended/unintended levels of sedation 2. (a) Establishes and maintains IV access (b) Responds to intended/unintended side effects (c) Appropriately administers reversal agents 3. (a) Effectively troubleshoots monitoring equipment (b) Initiates appropriate intervention in response to changes in patient status

Table 6.1 (cont.)

Learning domain	Educational strategies	Outcome and measurement
4. Airway management 5. Oxygenation management 6. Ventilation management	Low-fidelity simulation Task trainer Virtual-reality trainers High-fidelity simulation	4. (a) Stimulates/repositions patient to maintain airway (b) Effectively uses respiratory adjuncts as needed 5. (a) Identifies normal O_2 saturation pleth (b) Troubleshoots oximetry device (c) Applies supplemental oxygen as needed 6. (a) Identifies normal/abnormal CO_2 waveform (b) Troubleshoots capnography device (c) Initiates use of bag-valve mask device to support ventilation when indicated
Affective (behavioral)		
1. Clinical decision making 2. Interpersonal relationships 3. Communication skills	Case study/role play Group discussion Standardized patient Human patient simulation Simulation technology Moderate-fidelity simulation High-fidelity simulation	1. Appropriate response to variations in patient response 2. (a) Identifies role/responsibilities of team members (b) Understands and functions within scope of practice 3. (a) Effectively communicates as member of the team (b) Timely/clearly articulates changes in patient status (c) Uses closed-loop communication within team

The second guideline statement, introduced in 2010, and amended October 25, 2017, is the statement on granting privileges for *deep sedation* to non-anesthesiologist sedation practitioners [16]. It helps provide a "framework to identify those physicians, dentists, oral surgeons, or podiatrists who may potentially qualify to administer or supervise the administration of deep sedation." The entire guideline statement addresses education, training, licensure, performance evaluation, and improvement.

Summary

Care of patients undergoing procedural sedation is predicated on compliance with state and federal laws governing practice and educational programs that ensure positive outcomes for patients undergoing procedural sedation. It is an organizational and individual commitment to ensure that credentialing, competency, and education requirements are consistently met.

Acknowledgments

The authors wish to acknowledge Ellen K. Bergeron and Jennifer Kales, the authors of the previous version of this chapter in the second edition of this textbook.

References

1. Joint Commission. Joint Commission standards: HR 01.06.01, PC 03.01.01–07 and MS 06.01.01. www.jointcommission.org/standards

2. Epstein RM, Hundert EM. Defining and assessing professional competence. *JAMA* 2002;287:226–35.

3. Accreditation Council for Graduate Medical Education. Outcome Project.

4. Clark, R, Collins-Yoder A. Simulating rescue strategies from procedural sedation: one aspect of competency validation. *J Radiol Nurs.* 2020;39(2): 82–5.

5. American College of Emergency Physicians. Procedural sedation. https://emedicine.medscape.com/article/109695-overview?form=fpf.

6. American Society of Anesthesiologists Task Force on Sedation and Analgesia by Non-Anesthesiologists. Practice guidelines for sedation and analgesia by non-anesthesiologists. *Anesthesiology.* 2002;96:1004–17.

7. Rassin M, Sruyah R, Kahakon A, et al. "Between the fixed and the changing": examining and comparing reliability and validity of 3 sedation–agitation measuring scales. *Dimens Crit Care Nurs.* 2007;26(2):76–82.

8. American Society of Anesthesiologists. Standards for basic anesthetic monitoring (reaffirmed December 13, 2020). www.asahq.org/standards-and-practice-parameters/standards-for-basic-anesthetic-monitoring

9. Deitch K, Miner J, Chudnofsky C, Dominici P, Latta D. Does end tidal CO_2 monitoring during emergency department procedural sedation and analgesia with propofol decrease the incidence of hypoxic events?

A randomized controlled trial. *Ann Emerg Med.* 2010;55:258–64.

10. Knowles M, Holton E, Swanson R. *The Adult Learner,* 5th ed. Woburn: Butterworth-Heinemann, 1998.

11. Michelson J, Manning L. Competency assessment in simulation-based procedural education. *Am J Surg.* 2008;196:609–15.

12. Association of Perioperative Registered Nurses (AORN). Recommended practices for managing the patient receiving moderate sedation/analgesia. *AORN J.* 2002;75:642–6, 649–52.

13. American Society of Anesthesiologists (ASA). Statement on safe use of propofol (amended October 23, 2019). www.asahq.org/standards-and-practice-parameters/statement-on-safe-use-of-propofol

14. American Association of Nurse Anesthetists (AANA). *Considerations for Policy Development Number 4.2: Registered Nurses Engaged in the Administration of Sedation and Analgesia.* Park Ridge, IL: AANA, 2010.

15. American Society of Anesthesiologists (ASA) Statement on granting privileges for administration of moderate sedation to practitioners who are not anesthesia professionals. www.asahq.org/standards-and-practice-parameters/statement-on-granting-privileges-for-administration-of-moderate-sedation-to-practitioners-who-are-not-anesthesia-professionals

16. American Society of Anesthesiologists (ASA). Statement on granting privileges for deep sedation to non-anesthesiologist sedation practitioners. www.asahq.org/standards-and-practice-parameters/statement-on-granting-privileges-for-deep-sedation-to-non-anesthesiologist-physicians

Additional Reading

American Association of Critical-Care Nurses. Considerations for policy guidelines for registered nurses engaged in the administration of sedation and analgesia https://sedationcertification.com/resources/position-statements/aana

American Society of Anesthesiologists (ASA). *Statement on Granting Privileges to Non-anesthesiologist Practitioners for Personally Administering Deep Sedation or Supervising Deep Sedation by Individuals Who Are Not Anesthesia Professionals.* Park Ridge, IL: ASA, 2011.

Eichorn V, Henzler D, Murphy M. Standardizing care and monitoring for anesthesia or procedural sedation delivered outside the operating room. *Curr Opin Anaesthesiol* 2010;23:494–9.

Godwin SA, Caro DA, Wolf SJ, et al. American College of Emergency Physicians. Clinical policy: procedural sedation and analgesia in the emergency department. *Ann Emerg Med* 2005;45:177–96.

Levine A, Swartz M. Standardized patients: the "other" simulation. *J Crit Care.* 2008;23:179–84.

Pisansky AJ, Beutler SS, Urman RD. Education and training for nonanesthesia providers performing deep sedation. *Curr Opin Anaesthesiol.* 2016;29(4):499–505.

Practice guidelines for moderate procedural sedation and analgesia 2018: a report by the American Society of Anesthesiologists Task Force on Moderate Procedural Sedation and Analgesia, the American Association of Oral and Maxillofacial Surgeons, American College of Radiology, American Dental Association, American Society of Dentist Anesthesiologists, and Society of Interventional Radiology. *Anesthesiology.* 2018;128:437–79. https://doi.org/10.1097/ALN.0000000000002043

Tetzlaff J. Assessment of competence in anesthesiology. *Curr Opin Anaesthesiol* 2009;22:809–13.

Chapter 7

Quality, Legal, and Risk Management Considerations: Ensuring Program Excellence

Mary T. Antonelli and David E. Seaver

Procedural Sedation Committee

The goal of a procedural sedation program is to provide guidance to establish the best standard of care, yielding the best outcome for the patient. This ambition starts with the establishment of an institutional procedural sedation committee. Institutional leadership that provides central oversight for sedation practice is required by The Joint Commission (TJC) and the Centers for Medicare and Medicaid Services (CMS). Due to this requirement many hospitals and organizations have a committee that provides oversight for each area and department providing sedation. The committee structure should include all those providing sedation services to facilitate interprofessional team conversations to ensure optimal sedation practices supported by the anesthesia and nursing professional organizations' regulatory agency guidelines.

The committee's membership should include, but not be limited to, anesthesia, nursing, surgery, nurse practitioners, physician assistants, emergency department, quality, risk management, pharmacy, hospital information systems, and other representatives from areas performing moderate or deep sedation by non-anesthesiologists. Chair selection for the team is to be based on the demonstration of strong leadership skills and the ability to move a team toward successful outcomes. It is essential the chair holds a position within the organization that is recognized as expert within the field of sedation practice, as they will need to provide feedback to practitioners to reinforce the standards set by the policy. To foster interprofessional practice, it is recommended to have a member from the department of anesthesia and the department of nursing to jointly chair the committee, since both disciplines are primarily involved in sedation practice. It is imperative that anesthesia is included in the committee's leadership due to the regulatory bodies holding anesthesia accountable over this domain.

Policy Development

Once the committee is established and the members appointed, the development of a comprehensive, practical policy is the first order of business. The policy is critical to set the institutional philosophy for the sedation care standards, followed by the clinical and technical requirements that provide the infrastructure to successfully meet the institutional and regulatory body's goals. It is the policy that establishes the structure of the program and sets the excellence in practice (Figure 7.1).

Though the clinical and technical requirements have similarities between organizations, it is unwise to adapt a policy directly from one organization to another. Policies generally are organizationally specific since the document is an expression of a philosophy of care, which addresses specific patient populations, scope of services offered, professional mix, and educational requirements needed. Since all of these vary from institution to institution, practice will vary. And since policy sets the framework for practice, each hospital needs to develop its own policy.

The first step in policy development is to conduct a literature review and evaluate current nationally endorsed position statements, practice guidelines, research, regulatory requirements, and analysis of "community" standards for the type of facility the practice will occur. This activity establishes the evidence-based foundation for the care practices that are outlined within the policy (Box 7.1). An analysis of all the information is to be completed to determine the mandatory elements required to establish best practice. The mandatory elements and mission concepts are then built into the body of the policy.

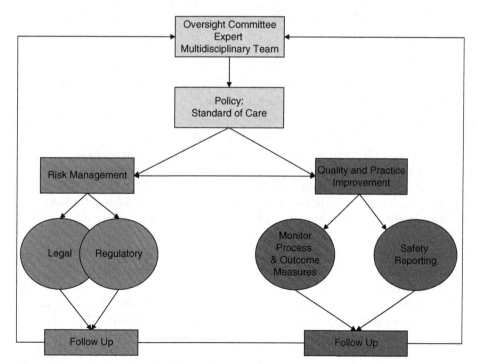

Figure 7.1 Procedural sedation quality and risk program structure.

Box 7.1 Professional and regulatory organizations and their representative practice guidelines and standards for the administration of sedation

American Society of Anesthesiologists	Practice guidelines for sedation and analgesia by non-anesthesiologists
American Association of Nurse Anesthetists	Position statements
American Nurses Association	Position statement on the role of the registered nurse in the management of patients receiving conscious sedation
American Academy of Pediatrics Committee on Drugs	Guidelines for monitoring and management of pediatric patients during and after sedation for diagnostic and therapeutic procedures
American College of Emergency Physicians	Clinical policy: procedural sedation and analgesia in the emergency department
Centers for Medicare and Medicaid	Condition of Participation 482.52
The Joint Commission	Sedation and anesthesia care standards Review of glossary for definitions of key words
State Boards of Medicine	Sedation policy/position statements
State Nursing Practice Acts	Scope of practice
University HealthSystem Consortium	Moderate and deep sedation best practice recommendations

The format of the policies varies and is determined by the specific institution. The following, however, is an example of such a format:

- *Purpose* – intent of the policy and scope of practice.
- *Philosophy/mission statement* – a framework for the development of practice processes. It is suggested the framework includes a patient-centered focus.
- *Definitions* – a list of key definitions that provides a basis for interpretation and application of the policy. Examples: procedural sedation, levels of sedation, what is meant by a rescue. It is suggested to use the American Society of Anesthesiologists (ASA) definitions, since the definitions are endorsed by most regulatory agencies.
- *Governance* – structure for overall accountability.
- *Personnel/education/competency* – expectations for education and competency for the healthcare professionals involved in the moderate/deep sedation procedure and recovery.
- *Care elements* – required supplies and equipment, medication guidelines, assessment and monitoring requirements from pre-procedure through recovery, discharge criteria, and documentation expectations.
- *Quality and system assessment* – outlines the required measures for monitoring of the responses to practices at the point of care as well as the care processes, based on identified evidence for practice and care processes.

- *References* – a list of all resources and materials that were used to support the development of the policy.
- *Addendums* – additional information which supports the application of the policy. Examples: sedation scale used; requirements for pre-procedure assessment; list of approved medications for moderate/deep sedation with dosing, clearance, and contraindications; education/competency curriculum; list of areas where moderate/ deep sedation can occur; process for new site approval for procedural sedation.

When a draft of the policy is completed, the document is to be reviewed by key stakeholders for feedback and input. This step will assist the flow through the administrative approval process. To assist the movement of the policy through this phase, an approval plan and an itemized timeline are helpful to ensure all key stakeholders and committees are captured. Concurrently, the oversight committee develops a communication and education plan regarding the policy and practice expectations. This can be accomplished in a number of ways. However, the methods are to be diverse and robust, with the information easily accessible and concise. In-service training may be required, along with ongoing informational reinforcements to make sure all involved professionals are made aware of the policy and care standards to establish continuity of practice for patient safety.

Quality and Risk-Management Considerations

The policy sets the framework for the standard of care for practice. However, it is the presence of a strong quality and risk-management structure that ensures the practices outlined in the policy are appropriately and consistently applied at the point of care (Figure 7.1). This structure has risk management focusing on the minimization of risk for adverse patient outcomes, and quality acting as a mechanism for the improvement of practice and operational processes. The work is collaborative between the two departments and including the committee's leadership and membership. Therefore, every procedural sedation program must have both components in place. The principles of quality and risk must be valued by the interprofessional team, to guarantee that the program structure is functional and effective.

Though most sedation procedures occur without an adverse event or breach in care standards, there are occasions when these events do happen. It is at these times when these structures help to identify the cause and strengthen the care processes and ensure safety.

Professional Liability: Negligence/Malpractice

Risk management mitigates the potential legal risks associated with procedural sedation to promote safety and minimize risk of injury. Negligence and malpractice standards may not be well known and can create confusion for each individual professional and the team. A basic understanding of these terms is needed by the healthcare professional to identify those situations when applicable and to reinforce the safety of practice.

Negligence

Negligence is "conduct which falls below the standard established by law for the protection of others against unreasonable risk of harm" [1]. Medical negligence, in a legal sense, is the failure to act in accordance with the accepted standards of the healthcare practice or as sometimes stated, a breach of the standard of care.

Malpractice

A malpractice case is a type of tort, which is a civil wrong committed by one person against another that can be adjudicated in a court of law. There are four required elements that a plaintiff (the person who brings a case against another person) must prove to substantiate malpractice. The first is a duty that must be owed to the injured person. That duty then must be breached, and that breach must be the cause of an injury. Lastly, there must be damages from the injury [1].

Duty

A duty is established when the healthcare provider develops a relationship with the patient. The duty the healthcare provider owes the patient is to treat the patient within accepted healthcare standards. The provider is then held to the standard of those clinicians with similar education and training in a similar clinical situation.

Breach of Duty

A duty is breached when the provider does not act according to the accepted healthcare standards. This may be a specific act that fails to meet the accepted standard of care, or a failure to act when a particular action is appropriate. Expert testimony is required to discern what the accepted medical and healthcare standard is and why the act (or failure to act) failed to meet that standard.

Causation

The action(s) that did not meet the standard(s) must be shown to have caused an injury. This may be the most difficult element for a plaintiff to prove. Often, it is difficult to separate a known complication from an action that would constitute a breach of duty. Expert testimony is required to establish causation.

Damages

The patient must suffer a form of damage from the injury to establish a case. Damage may take the form of economic damages (financial losses such as medical expenses, lost wages, or other economic harm) and/or non-economic damages (physical suffering, emotional distress, and loss of enjoyment of relationship with significant other and/or family). Some states have caps on non-economic damages. Some states may permit punitive damages on top of economic and non-economic damages when it can be shown that the clinician acted with willful recklessness, gross negligence, malice, or deceit.

Each element needs to be proved by a preponderance of the evidence. A preponderance of the evidence means it is more likely than not that the element has been proved, mathematically speaking a 51% chance. Therefore, as an example of a successful case, the plaintiff is required to establish that the patient was under the care of the provider (*duty*), the provider responsible for the administration of procedural sedation did not act according to the standard of care (*breach*), the failure to act according to the standard of care was directly responsible for the patient's injury (*cause*), and the patient's injury was the cause of some sort of economic or noneconomic harm (*damage*).

In addition, the courts may look to state statutes and regulations when evaluating the breach element. Should it be shown that the clinician defendant was in violation of an applicable statute or regulation, the court may find either that the plaintiff automatically proved this element, or that the violation of the statute or regulation is strong evidence of proof of a breach of the standard of care. As state boards promulgate regulation in the area of procedural sedation, it is wise to review your state regulations to assure all regulatory compliance requirements are met when administering procedural sedation. The courts will also give great weight to the adopted policies on procedural sedation of state boards.

As noted earlier, the most difficult element to prove in a healthcare malpractice case is typically causation. In almost all healthcare malpractice cases, expert opinion is needed to state the standard of care and to prove causation. Expert opinion is required because the subject matter is not within the common knowledge of the average juror. The expert should be an expert in the particular subspecialty at issue in the lawsuit. They do not need to practice in that arena, but must be familiar with it. As applicable to procedural sedation, the clinician expert would not necessarily have to be an anesthesiologist, but would typically have to be familiar with procedural sedation practices, policies, and procedures. The expert would have to show that the clinician's failure to meet the standard of care directly harmed the patient.

Mitigating the Risk of Malpractice Lawsuit: Documentation

Since it is often difficult to distinguish a complication of care from a tortious act, the best defense to a claim of malpractice is good documentation that maps the medical decision making of the care. It has often been said, "If it was not documented, it did not occur." Even the absence of relevant findings should be documented. Failure to document the absent findings may indicate that the clinician failed to elucidate the findings.

A key documentation requirement is the informed consent prior to the procedure. Since the patient must consent to the administration of procedural sedation, the clinician performing the procedure or a member of the procedural team must have a conversation with the patient noting the risks and benefits of procedural sedation (or with the patient's representative, for patients lacking decisional capacity). The patient or representative must sign an informed consent form documenting the conversation. A note in the medical record detailing the conversation and the patient's or representative's understanding of the conversation is equally important. The consent process permits the clinician to understand and manage the patient's expectations, and to individualize the plan of care. A patient who has unreasonable expectations about the success of a procedure may be more likely to initiate a lawsuit should a complication of care occur. Having an open and frank conversation with the patient, addressing all material complications and their likelihood, may dissuade the patient from litigation. Documenting that conversation protects the clinician from allegations that the patient did not understand the nature of the procedure and the likelihood of complications.

Another key documentation requirement is a history and physical documented prior to the procedure. During the procedure, the patient's response to the sedation must be documented and, post procedure, the patient's status must be documented, including that all discharge criteria are met before the patient leaves the facility or is transferred to another care giver. These are also a necessary requirement from a regulatory perspective.

Regulatory Agencies

In the United States, several regulatory bodies have promulgated regulations or developed guide-lines regarding the administration of procedural sedation, both at state and federal levels [2]. The major regulatory bodies include the State Boards of Medicine and Nursing, the CMS (federal government agencies), and TJC (a healthcare facility accreditation organization). Other agencies also accredit ambulatory procedural facilities, such as t he Accreditation Association for Ambulatory Health Care and American Association for Accreditation of Ambulatory Surgery Facilities.

State Boards

State professional boards are charged with licensing and regulating healthcare professionals including physicians, dentists, nurses, pharmacists, and, in some states, anesthesia assistants practicing within hospitals and at other standalone locations such as clinics and professional offices. State legislatures pass statutes that authorize the state boards to promulgate regulation enforceable upon professionals licensed by that board. Boards of medicine and dentistry may provide guidance for developing a policy, in collaboration with the anesthesia department, citing the evidence used to develop the sedation policy; identifying clinicians administering procedural sedation and the necessary credentialing requirements, medications, patient selection, and equipment; and establishing appropriate patient assessment and monitoring frequency [3]. Boards also may establish appropriate resource allocation for sedation procedures, ongoing education requirements for competence, and requirements for anesthetic care performed in the office setting.

Each state's board of dentistry has a statute and/or regulation on the administration of sedation and/or anesthesia in various dental settings. The regulation typically encompasses local anesthesia to general anesthesia and includes all levels of sedation. Many, but not all, boards of medicine have statutes, regulations, or policies on procedural sedation. Board of medicine regulations on procedural sedation are often included in regulations on office-based surgery (Table 7.1).

The Centers for Medicare and Medicaid Services

The CMS promulgate regulations that are enforceable upon hospitals. The CMS also mandates hospital compliance with all applicable state laws [4]. The Condition of Participation 482.52 states, "If the hospital furnishes anesthesia services, they must be provided in a well-organized manner under the direction of a qualified doctor of medicine or osteopathy. The service is responsible for all anesthesia administered in the hospital." Within a facility, the anesthesia service is responsible for all anesthesia administered, including procedural sedation administered by both anesthesia and non-anesthesia providers, including physicians, dentists, certified registered nurse anesthetists, and anesthesiologist assistants (if permissible by state law).

The CMS also requires appropriate anesthesia care throughout the process [4]. The pre-anesthesia process requires a patient assessment within 48 hours before the administration of anesthesia. Intraoperatively, the responsible clinician is required to monitor the patient and document the key elements that are outlined. Postoperatively, the CMS does not require an evaluation. However, it is stated that appropriate postoperative anesthesia evaluation is required. Therefore, current practice dictates that the patient

Table 7.1 State by state rules, regulations, and policies on procedural sedation

State	Medical board law, regulation, or policy	Dental board law, regulation, or policy
AL	Chapters 540- X-10-.06 and 540-X-10-.07	Chapter 9, Sect. 39-9-63 et al.
AK	None	12 AAC 28.600–12 AAC 28.640
AZ	Article 7; R4–16–701 et al.	Article 13; R4–11–1301
AR	Medical Board Regulation 35	Dental Board Regulation, Article XIII
CA	CA Business and Professional Code Division 2, Ch. 5, Art. 11.5 Surgery in certain outpatient settings	CA Business and Professional Code 1647–1647.9 and 1647.10 –1647.26
CO	Medical Board Policy 40-12, Office Based Surgery and Anesthesia	Dental Board Regulation, Rule XIV – Anesthesia
CT	CGSA Sect. 19a-490m, Sect. 19a-493b & Sect. 19a-691	Administration and Use of Anesthesia and Conscious Sedation in Dentistry. Sect. 20-123b
DE	None	Title 24 DE Administrative Code, 7.0 Anesthesia Regulations
Wash DC	None	District of Columbia Municipal Regulation, Ch. 42, Sect. 4212: Requirements for the Administration of Anesthesia
FL	Rule 64B8–9 Standard of Care for Office Surgery	Rule 64B5–14 Anesthesia
GA	GA Medical Board Office Based Anesthesia and Surgery Guidelines	Statute: Title 43, Ch. 11, Sect 21. Regulation: Chapter 150-13 Sedation Permits
HI	HI Administrative Rules, Title 11, Ch. 96–6	HI Administrative Rules, Title 16, Ch. 79, Subch. 8
ID	None	19.01.01 – Rules of the Idaho State Board of Dentistry, Sect 060 Moderate Sedation.

Table 7.1 *(cont.)*

State	Medical board law, regulation, or policy	Dental board law, regulation, or policy
IL	IL Medical Practice Act of 1987, Sect. 1285.340 – Anesthesia Services in an Office Setting	IL Dental Practice Act, Sect. 1220, subpart E – Anesthesia Permits.
IN	Title 844, Article 5, Rule 5	Title 828 IAC 3-1 et. al.
IA	None	IAC 650, Ch. 29.
KS	KAR 100-25-3	KSA 65–1444 & KAR 71–5
KY	KY Board of Medicine Opinion	201 KAR 8:550
LA	Title 46, Part XLV, Ch. 73	LRS 37:793 & Title 46, Part XXIII, Ch. 15.
ME	None	Title 32, Sect 1089 & 02-313, Ch. 14
MD	None	Title 10, Subtitle 44, Ch. 12
MA	Board Endorsed Office-based Surgery Guidelines	234 CMR 3.00
MI	None	Dentistry General Rules, Part 6
MN	None	MN Administrative Rules, Ch. 3100.3600
MS	Board Regulation, Title 30, Part 2635, Ch. 2 – Office Based Surgery	Board Regulation 29 – Administration of Anesthesia
MO	None	20 CSR 2110–4
MT	None	Rule 24, Ch. 138, Subch. 32
NE	NE Board Opinion on Propofol Use	172 NAC 56-008 and 56-009
NV	NRS 449.435 et al.	Nev Admin Code Ch. 631.2211 et al.
NH	None	NH Den Part 304
NJ	NJAC Title 13, Ch. 35, Subchpt 4A	NJAC Title 13, Ch. 30, Subchpt 8.1A, 8.2, and 8.20
NM	None	NMAC Title 16, Ch. 5, Sect. 16, Part 15
NY	NY Public Health Law Sect 230-d	NY State Regulations of the Commissioner Part 61.10
NC	NC Medical Board Position Statement on Office Based Procedures	NCAC Title 21, Subch. 16Q
ND	None	ND Administrative Code 20-02-01-05
OH	OAC Ch. 4731-25	OAC Ch. 4715-5-05 et al.
OK	OK Medical Board Guidelines on Office Based Surgery	OAC Title 195, Ch. 20
OR	OAR 847-017-0000 et al.	OAR 818-026-0000 et al.

Table 7.1 (cont.)

State	Medical board law, regulation, or policy	Dental board law, regulation, or policy
PA	None	PA Code Title 49, Ch. 33, Sect 33.331 et al.
RI	R23–17-PASC	R5–31.1-DHA
SC	Board of Medical Examiners Regulation 81–96	Dental Sedation Act Section 40-15-400
SD	None	SD Code 20:43:09
TN	Rule of TN Board of Medical Examiners Ch. 0880-02-.21	Rule of the TN Board of Dentistry Ch. 0460-02-.07
TX	TAC Title 22, Part 9, Ch. 192	TAC Title 22, Part 5, Ch. 110
UT	None	Dentist Practice Act Rule R156–69–601
VT	None	VT Board of Dental Examiners Administrative Rules, Part 5
VA	VAC 85-20-310 et. al.	VAC 60-21-290 et. al.
WA	WAC 246-919-520	WAC 246–817-701 et.al.
WV	None	WV Code Section 30-4A
WI	WAC 124.20 (3) (b)	WAC DE Ch. 11
WY	WY Dept of Health, Rules and Regulations for Hospital Licensure, Ch. 12, Sect. 10b	Board of Dental Examiners Rules and Regulations, Ch. 5

receiving procedural sedation be monitored and evaluated before, during, and after the procedure by trained practitioners with appropriate documentation to provide evidence of compliance.

The CMS authorizes anesthesia professionals (anesthesiologists, nurse anesthetists, and anesthesiologist assistants) or other qualified non-anesthesiologist physicians (as well as dentists, oral surgeons, or podiatrists who are qualified to administer anesthesia under state law) to administer deep sedation [3]. Registered nurses, advanced practice registered nurses, or physician assistants may not administer deep sedation per the CMS. The 2010 ASA statement on granting privileges for deep sedation to non-anesthesiologist sedation practitioners was created to "assist healthcare facilities in developing a program" for the delineation of procedure-specific clinical privileges for non-anesthesiologist physicians to administer or supervise the administration of sedative and analgesic drugs to establish a level of deep sedation [5]. The statement outlines recommendations for education, training, licensure, performance evaluation, and performance improvement.

In contrast, mild to moderate sedation usually can be administered safely by non-anesthesia practitioners who have had specialized training, as outlined in the ASA statement on granting privileges for administration of moderate sedation to practitioners who are not anesthesia professionals [6]. Knowledge of the pharmacologic profiles of sedation agents is necessary to maximize the likelihood that the intended level of sedation is targeted accurately [7]. If cardiorespiratory compromise occurs, the non-anesthesia practitioners should possess the skills necessary to "rescue" a patient whose level of sedation is deeper than planned, and return the patient to the intended level. Therefore, one person must be available whose only responsibility is to monitor the patient, identify cardiorespiratory compromise, and institute bag-mask ventilation and cardiopulmonary resuscitation if necessary. Backup emergency services, including protocols for summoning emergency medical services, must be established and maintained [7].

The Joint Commission

TJC is an independent, not-for-profit organization. It accredits and certifies more than 18,000 healthcare organizations and programs in the United States. TJC is the "auditor" for the CMS and aligns their care standards with the CMS's conditions of participation, which makes it easier to track compliance. Currently TJC standards for sedation and anesthesia care apply when the administration of analgesia or sedative medication to an individual, in any setting, for any purpose, by any route, induces a partial or total loss of sensation for the purpose of conducting an operative or other procedure [7]. The definitions of four levels of sedation and anesthesia include the following:

1. Minimal sedation (anxiolysis) is a drug-induced state during which patients respond normally to verbal commands. Although cognitive function and coordination may be impaired, ventilatory and cardiovascular functions are unaffected.
2. Moderate sedation/analgesia ("conscious sedation") is a drug-induced depression of consciousness during which patients respond purposefully to verbal commands, either alone or accompanied by light tactile stimulation. Reflex withdrawal from a painful stimulus is not considered a purposeful response. No interventions are required to maintain a patent airway, and spontaneous ventilation is adequate. Cardiovascular function is usually maintained.
3. Deep sedation/analgesia is a drug-induced depression of consciousness during which patients cannot be easily aroused, but respond purposefully following repeated or painful stimulation. The ability to independently maintain ventilatory function may be impaired. Patients may require assistance in maintaining a patent airway, and spontaneous ventilation may be inadequate. Cardiovascular function is usually maintained.
4. Anesthesia consists of general anesthesia and spinal or major regional anesthesia. It does not include local anesthesia. General anesthesia is a drug-induced loss of consciousness during which patients are not arousable, even by painful stimulation. The ability to independently maintain ventilatory function is often impaired. Patients often require assistance in maintaining a patent airway, and positive-pressure ventilation may be required because of depressed spontaneous ventilation or drug-induced depression of neuromuscular function. Cardiovascular function may be impaired.

These definitions are based upon the ASA practice guidelines for sedation and analgesia by non-anesthesiologists, and are generally accepted by most organizations.

These definitions are used for a number of TJC standards related to procedural sedation that address clinician credentials and patient assessment, monitoring, and treatment before, during, and after the administration of procedural sedation (Table 7.2).

Table 7.2 Summary of TJC standards for procedural sedation

Standard number	Standard	Requirement	Compliance
PC.03.01.01	Procedural sedation must be administered by a qualified provider	Plan for procedures requiring procedural sedation	Personnel credentialed, sufficient personnel available, nurse supervising perioperative care, appropriate equipment available to administer medications/blood, resuscitation equipment available
PC.03.01.03	Patients must be assessed prior to sedation/procedure Provider must discuss risks/options with the patient/family prior to sedation/procedure Provider must reassess the patient immediately before sedation is initiated	Provide patient with care prior to the administration of sedation	Pre-procedure assessment conducted and reassessment performed just prior to sedation administration, evidence of post- procedure patient needs planning, pre-procedure education complete and based on plan of care, and clinician responsible for patient concurs with sedation plan
PC.03.01.05	Mandatory monitoring of the patient's oxygenation, ventilation, and circulation during sedation	Monitor patient during the administration of procedural sedation	Documentation of evidence for continuous monitoring of patients during the procedure including oxygenation, ventilation and circulation measures
PC.03.01.07	Post-sedation assessment in the recovery area is necessary before the patient is discharged A qualified provider must discharge the patient from the post-sedation recovery area, or discharge must be based on established criteria	Provide care after the administration of procedural sedation	Assessment of the patient's physiological status, mental status, and pain is complete immediately post procedure and then at determined frequencies, discharge is conducted by a qualified provider based on established criteria, and outpatients are discharged with a responsible individual

Table 7.2 (*cont.*)

Standard number	Standard	Requirement	Compliance
RC.02.01.03	Documentation of the use of procedural sedation	Healthcare record documents the use of procedural sedation	Documentation contains provisional diagnosis, pre-procedure history and physical examination, administration of sedation with patient's response, a procedure note, patient discharged by a qualified unanticipated events/complications followed by how they were managed

Recognizing the risks involved with sedation and analgesia, TJC mandates that sedation practices throughout the institution be monitored and evaluated by the department of anesthesia.

The Joint Commission Sedation and Analgesia Standards

There are additional TJC standards that apply to procedural sedation events located within the Universal Protocol for preventing wrong-site, wrong-procedure, and wrong-person surgeries or procedures (UP.01.01.01–UP.01.03.01) [7]. This protocol applies to all surgical and non-surgical invasive procedures, and is required to reinforce the need for teamwork to ensure and protect patient safety. The protocol specifies three standards: pre-procedure verification, site marking, and a time-out immediately before the procedure.

- First, the *pre-procedure verification* is an ongoing process to obtain and confirm information to ensure all relevant documents, equipment, and information are known and present. The organization, within the policy, should dictate the frequency and location for this process. It may need to occur more than once prior to the procedure, and it is best if the patient can be involved.
- *Site marking* is the second component of the Universal Protocol, and is required to prevent wrong-site procedures. This standard is most successful when a consistent site-marking process is developed within the organization's policy. The markings should be used when the procedure is to be done on those areas that have various sides, limbs, or spine or organ levels. Site marking is not required when the provider doing the procedure is *continuously* with the patient until the procedure is performed.
- A *time-out* or *safety pause* is to be conducted just prior to the procedure to ensure the identification of the patient, and to check for the correct site, ensure all equipment and implants are present, and the correct procedure is being performed. It is ideal
- to conduct the time-out before sedation is administered to the patient, so that the patient can be involved. A member of the procedure team initiates the time-out, which includes active communication and verification from all members of the team. The procedure is not started until all members confirm the information. A standardized process is required throughout the organization.

There are other associated TJC standards which apply generally to a number of other care events that might occur in connection with procedural sedation. These standards, MS.06.01.03, MM.03.01.03, RC.02.01.01, and PI.01.01.01, are denoted within the body of the sedation and analgesia standards and should be evaluated to ensure compliance. The standards for the administration of procedural sedation continue to evolve. The ASA amended the standards for basic anesthetic monitoring, effective December 13, 2020 [8]. Moderate or deep sedation adequacy of ventilation shall be evaluated by continual observation of qualitative clinical signs and monitoring for the presence of exhaled carbon dioxide unless precluded or invalidated by the nature of the patient, procedure, or equipment. Patients administered moderate or deep sedation must have their expired carbon dioxide monitored by capnography.

Ambulatory surgical and procedural facilities may also be accredited by either or both the Accreditation Association for Ambulatory Health Care and/or American Association for Accreditation of Ambulatory Surgery Facilities. Their procedural sedation standards are similar to CMS and TJC standards, but should be reviewed for variations.

The foregoing statutes, regulations, and standards function together to provide a framework for both the individual clinician and the practice site. The regulations and standards demonstrate a strong public interest in providing safe and effective care of the patient undergoing a procedure. The boards regulate the individual clinicians and their office-based practice. CMS and TJC regulate procedural sedation practice in the institutional setting. They each have regulations and standards that govern the clinician, the practice site, and the quality of the program. When TJC surveys a facility, it is also with the eyes of CMS, since CMS deems TJC to be the enforcer of their own conditions of participation. Therefore, if an institution passed a TJC survey and was fully accredited by TJC, that institution is deemed an accredited CMS organization and is permitted to participate in Medicare and Medicaid programs.

Practice-Systems Improvement

The purpose of the quality improvement program is to ensure best practice at the point of care through the review and evaluation of key care processes and patient outcomes, along with the oversight committee, to provide a systems approach to safe, consistent practice. It is through these interrelated dynamics that the standards of care and the mission of the policy are actualized, and consistency of care is assured.

Monitoring Practice and Operational Processes

A data collection system is required to be built into the sedation processes at the departmental and healthcare provider level to capture all key regulatory standards and any other identified important care processes impacting practice at the point of care. The oversight committee is accountable for data collection and for the evaluation of the results at regular intervals. The evaluation is conducted to ensure the understanding and actualization of the policy and to monitor patient outcomes. Depending on the resources available at an institution or facility, the structure of this system may vary. However, the priority is for all areas performing procedural sedation to complete a select volume of random case reviews monthly or, better, concurrently. TJC requires the percentage of records audited to be based upon the number of procedures performed within that area. The best way to track and organize the data for review and analysis is for the data to be electronically entered at the point of care to a database, allowing immediate access to the oversight committee, risk management, and quality improvement leadership. The results are then presented at the oversight committee meeting for discussion and development of an action plan, if needed. This information loop is important as a means of providing in-the-moment feedback to the oversight committee as well as reinforcing the collaboration with risk and quality departments. This type of structure ensures that any potential areas of risk can be addressed or practice improvement initiatives enacted. Figure 7.2 depicts an example of a procedural sedation monitoring tool.

Outcome and Process Measures

The monitoring tool is a collection of process and patient outcome measures. The tool design reflects all mandatory regulatory requirements that need to be measured as well as any identified processes the oversight committee wants to follow. The incorporation of these measures into the procedure's documentation format is an excellent method to ensure actualization of the required care processes. The tool should be reviewed on a yearly basis and revised as needed by the oversight committee.

Quality metrics are required to be monitored to ensure excellence in practice, patient safety and better outcomes. Both process and outcomes measures need to be monitored to reflect the quality of the program [9]. However, process measures may vary depending on the organization's current practice for procedural sedation and TJC requirements.

TJC has a number of measures that may overlap with the AQI's recommendations. However, there are differences, and the standards should be reviewed including required data to support compliance [10, 11]. This review is important to verify the information is collected via another data collection process, and, if not, evaluated to be added to the procedural sedation tool. In addition to the regulatory measurement requirements, the oversight committee may add additional measures to target specific care processes of interest.

Patient Satisfaction

With a patient-centered focus for care, the patient and family cannot be excluded from having an input into the evaluation of the quality and satisfaction of the care. A number of factors influence the patient's perception and evaluation of care, such as comfort, control over sedation, adverse side effects experienced, and the occurrence of adverse events [12]. To account for the patient's perspective, patient satisfaction is suggested to be included in the outcome measures to be reviewed, evaluated, and included in the report with the other clinical and process measures.

Patient Safety Reporting

A safety reporting system, paper or electronic, is an additional tool required to reinforce a culture of safety and provide a direct source of feedback regarding practice by the practitioners at the point of care. The expectation and responsibility to complete the safety reports is for *all* members of the team when a concern regarding care standards or outcomes are in question. These reports are reviewed by both risk and quality

PROCEDURAL SEDATION AUDIT

MRN: Type of sedation   ☐ Deep sedation
Patient Name   ☐ Moderate sedation
Auditor Name
Pod / Area
Procedure Date:

Was PS administered in an outpatient area ?   ☐ Yes   ☐ No

    If yes, patient discharged with designated adult   ☐ Yes   ☐ No

LIP credentials   ☐ Verified   ☐ Not credentialed   ☐ Unable to locate

All sections of pre-sedation assessment completed   ☐ Yes   ☐ No

Consent for sedation signed   ☐ Yes   ☐ No

NPO status confirmed   ☐ Yes   ☐ No

Anesthesia consult obtained   ☐ Yes   ☐ No

Safety pause process completed (time out)   ☐ Yes   ☐ No

Prior to Procedure

○ Yes	○ No	Vital Signs
○ Yes	○ No	Sedation Level
○ Yes	○ No	Pain Level

During Procedure (at least every 5 minutes)

○ Yes	○ No	Vital Signs
○ Yes	○ No	Sedation Level
○ Yes	○ No	Pain Level

Post Procedure (every 10 mins for first 30 mins; then every 15 mins until post sedation score is greater/equal to 8)

○ Yes	○ No	Vital Signs
○ Yes	○ No	Sedation Level
○ Yes	○ No	Pain Level

COMPLICATIONS

☐ Acute coronary syndrome

☐ Adverse drug reaction

☐ Aspiration

☐ Cardiac/Respiratory Arrest

☐ Death

☐ Greater than 5 minutes of mask/bag ventilation

☐ Inability to complete the procedure as planned

☐ Intubation required

☐ Medications used other than those approved

☐ Unplanned hospital admission

☐ Unplanned transfer to ICU

☐ Use of reversal agent

Figure 7.2 Procedural sedation audit reporting form. Courtesy of Vineeta Vaidya, Brigham and Women's Hospital.

management to bring forth practice issues or gaps in care for resolution. An important aspect in creating a successful reporting system is an understanding that the report will be used in a non-punitive fashion, and the information will lend itself to the correction of the causation of the event or a change in the system to prevent further occurrences [13]. The system should also have a feedback loop to the reporting authors as to the follow-up and outcome of the event. Once these components are well established, the goal of robust use by differing practitioners will be achieved and encouraged.

For procedural sedation, any complication that may occur from the pre-procedure phase through recovery must be documented within the patient safety reporting system as well as any breach in policy, or concern regarding the processes surrounding the procedure. These reports are closely monitored by local leadership, risk, and quality management depending on the organization or facility reporting structure. Trending of care events or process issues is conducted, with an immediate response to any adverse event occurrences.

Responding to Risk or Potential Risk Events

The response to potential risk or actual risk events is a collaborative effort by local-level leadership, risk and quality managers, and facility's senior leadership, with the oversight committee acting as the final review for recommendations. The correct tone of the response is essential to ensure psychological safety for the healthcare professional involved and to bolster the culture of safety within the organization. Therefore, the evaluation of the events should be not only from the healthcare professional's contributions to the event, but also an assessment of the contributing factors of the organization. This approach recognizes all the contributing factors to the risk event to ensure a comprehensive action plan to reduce patient harm. The early identification of such events through the active monitoring of practice creates the ability to respond proactively and immediately when needed (Box 7.2). Though the immediacy of a response varies, depending on the severity of the event, the process for the review remains the same, to make certain all possible causation is addressed and not overlooked [13].

Risk and quality management are involved to varying degrees with most responses, working closely with local leadership and other expert practitioners. This activity of review, analysis, and evaluation is the cornerstone to developing and ensuring a clinically excellent and safe sedation program. It provides an opportunity to make sure all policy and procedure steps are followed, ultimately resulting in a reevaluation of practice and care process points. This activity should never be short-changed, and it should be a regular item on the oversight committee's agenda.

The initial communication of an event or concern can occur in various ways depending on the severity of the situation and the hospital structure. For a severe event, local-level leadership notifies risk and quality immediately. A thorough and credible investigation is initiated to gather additional facts and information, including discussions with the practitioners involved. In other situations, risk, quality, or care providers may identify an event or a trend in practice. At that point, leadership is contacted to report on the situation and to support further inquiry. The investigation phase is very important, since it establishes the "What, How, and Why?" of the incident to clearly articulate the issues [13]. A standardized analysis to review an incident should be used to capture all possible areas of causation or influencing factors to identify improvement

Box 7.2 Elements to reduce risk

The director of the anesthesia services assures that all clinicians providing anesthesia, including procedural sedation, in all settings, are doing so in a safe and compliant manner

Each clinician involved in the administration of procedural sedation is competent to do so, and all records are up to date

Each procedural sedation area has required equipment immediately available for the safe administration of the sedating agent, as well as for resuscitation of the patient from oversedation and/ or respiratory depression

A strong informed consent process is established

Pre-procedure assessment is complete and detailed, especially airway, to identify any risk and possible need for anesthesia consultation

Patient monitoring is conducted pre-procedure through recovery

Discharge criteria are established and documented

A process is created to approve sites where procedural sedation is performed

A systematic data collection process is developed at the departmental and physician level to assess compliance with policy and evaluate practice

Table 7.3 Event follow-up framework

Main factors	Contributory factors
Institutional	Economic pressures, regulatory requirements, hospital mission/priorities
Organizational	Financial priorities, structure, policies, standards, safety culture
Work environment	Staffing, skill mix, workload, shift patterns, design, equipment availability and maintenance, support
Team factors	Communication, supervision, team culture
Individual	Knowledge, skills, competence, health
Task factors	Task design, availability and use of protocols, test results, accuracy and availability of patient notes
Patient factors	Complexity and seriousness, language, communication, personality, special factors

Modified with permission from Vincent et al. [13].

areas. One such framework is proposed by Vincent and colleagues [13] (Table 7.3). The event should be reviewed by all those involved as well as interested committee forums that can add to the strength of the overall action plan. Examples of such are morbidity and mortality rounds, medical and nursing departmental practice committees, and quality forums.

The oversight committee chair is notified as well, and the incident is reviewed at the next committee meeting to review the findings from the investigation with all stakeholders in attendance for analysis and resolution, including development of corrective actions as needed. The action plans are carried out and the final findings are documented and reported up through the organization of the facility's committee structure. The oversight committee is responsible for closing the loop, making certain the action plan is completed, and continuing to monitor to verify sustainability of the change as appropriate.

Reportable Events

There are specific events which require a report to one or more regulatory agencies. These sentinel events may require a root-cause analysis to identify causation and an action plan for correction. TJC requires a review of a sentinel event by the institution, and leaves it to each institution whether to report it to TJC. Some state agencies may require a report of a sentinel event. Some procedural-based sentinel events that may involve the administration of procedural sedation include [7]:

- unanticipated death or major permanent loss of function not related to the natural course of the patient's illness or underlying condition
- death or major permanent loss of function associated with a medication error
- patient death or serious injury associated with the use of contaminated drugs, devices, or biologics provided by the healthcare setting
- hemolytic transfusion reaction involving administration of blood or blood products having major blood group incompatibilities
- procedure on the wrong patient or wrong body part
- death resulting from nosocomial infection
- intraoperative or immediately postoperative/post-procedure death in an ASA Class 1 patient
- unintended retention of a foreign object in a patient after the procedure

State regulatory agencies such as the professional boards and departments of public health may also require specific reporting. For example, the Massachusetts Department of Public Health (DPH) requires reporting of all serious reportable events (SREs). These are those on a list of events compiled by the National Quality Forum [14, 15]. In addition, states may require an institution to report the SRE to the patient's third-party insurer and the patient. Further, Massachusetts requires the facility to perform a preventability analysis of each SRE. Should the event be found to be preventable, the institution cannot bill out any charges for care that flow from the event. In a vertically integrated care organization, should the patient be discharged to the care of a sister institution within the organization, the sister institution may not bill for care associated with the event as well. The state agency may also require reporting of other events not captured by SRE reporting requirements. Some states may require reporting to multiple agencies. Reports submitted to a state agency may be available for public review.

Each state will have different review and reporting requirements. The trend in the states is toward more disclosure of adverse events. A review of your own state's regulations will be required to be compliant with your own reporting requirements.

By using a two-pronged, risk and quality, approach in evaluating patient outcomes and care processes, improvement can be identified resulting in changes to treatment algorithms, care processes, and environmental issues. Any change in the procedural process must be evaluated after implementation to ensure the change created an improvement in the process, enhancing the safety of the patient care environment.

Summary

A successful procedural sedation program is built with a collaborative team of experts who clearly articulate the goal and standards of care through an institutional policy. This policy is based upon national and state recognized practice requirements and guidelines, which lay the foundation for patient safety and clinical excellence. A robust risk and quality structure built within the program ensures best practice at the point of care. It is through this framework that procedural sedation program excellence is attained and the policy is actualized beyond the written text.

References

1. American Law Institute. Restatement of the law, third. Torts: medical malpractice. www.ali.org/publications/show/torts-medical-malpractice

2. Benzoni, T, Cascella, M. *Procedural Sedation*. Treasure Island, FL: StatPearls Publishing, 2023. www.ncbi.nlm.nih.gov/books/NBK551685

3. American Society of Anesthesiologists. Statement on granting privileges for deep sedation to non-anesthesiologist sedation practitioners. www.asahq.org/standards-and-practice-parameters/statement-on-granting-privileges-for-deep-sedation-to-non-anesthesiologist-physicians

4. Centers for Medicare and Medicaid Services. Conditions of participation: regulations at 42 CFR 482. www.govinfo.gov/app/details/CFR-2011-title42-vol5/CFR-2011-title42-vol5-sec482-52

5. American Society of Anesthesiologists. Statement on granting privileges for administration of moderate sedation to practitioners who are not anesthesia professionals. www.asahq.org/standards-and-practice-parameters/statement-on-granting-privileges-for-administration-of-moderate-sedation-to-practitioners-who-are-not-anesthesia-professionals

6. Metzner J, Domino KB. Procedural sedation by nonanesthesia providers. In Urman R, Gross W, Philip BK, eds., *Anesthesia Outside of the Operating Room*. Oxford: Oxford University Press, 2011, 49–61.

7. Metzner J, Domino KB. Provision of care, treatment and services standards, record of care, and improving organizational performance. In *Comprehensive Accreditation Manual for Hospitals*. Oakbrook Terrace, IL: The Joint Commission, 2011.

8. American Society of Anesthesiologists. Standards for basic anesthetic monitoring. www.asahq.org/standards-and-practice-parameters/standards-for-basic-anesthetic-monitoring

9. Anesthesia Quality Institute. Quality metrics for procedural sedation. www.aqihq.org/files/Procedural_Sedation_Metrics.pdf

10. The Joint Commission. Who we are. www.jointcommission.org/who-we-are

11. The Joint Commission. Sedation and anesthesia - understanding the assessment requirements, April 11, 2016, last updated January 19, 2023. www.jointcommission.org/standards/standard-faqs/ambulatory/provision-of-care-treatment-and-services-pc/000001645

12. Mahajan RP. Critical incident reporting and learning. *Br J Anaesth* 2010;105:69–75.

13. Vincent C, Taylor-Adams S, Stanhope N. Framework for analysing risk and safety in clinical medicine. *BMJ* 1998;316:1154–7.

14. Massachusetts Department of Public Health regulation 105 CMR 130.332, Serious reportable events.

15. Massachusetts Department of Public Health regulation 105 CMR 130.331, Serious incident and accident reports. Massachusetts Board of Registration in Medicine. Policy 94-04. Patient Care Assessment Guidelines for Intravenous Conscious Sedation.

Additional Reading

Caperelli-White L, Urman RD. Developing a moderate sedation policy: essential elements and evidence-based considerations. *AORN J.* 2014 Mar;99(3):416–30. doi: 10.1016/j.aorn.2013.09.015.

Karamnov S, Sarkisian N, Grammer R, Gross WL, Urman RD. Analysis of adverse events associated with adult moderate procedural sedation outside the operating room. *J Patient Saf.* 2017;13(3):111–21.

Pisansky AJ, Beutler SS, Urman RD. Education and training for nonanesthesia providers performing deep sedation. *Curr Opin Anaesthesiol.* 2016;29(4):499–505. doi: 10.1097/ACO.0000000000000342.

Ranum D, Ma H, Shapiro FE, Chang B, Urman RD. Analysis of patient injury based on anesthesiology closed claims data from a major malpractice insurer. *J Healthc Risk Manag.* 2014;34(2):31–42.

Nursing Considerations for Sedation

Laurie Demeule and Lisa Govoni

Introduction

Historically, nurses have participated in every aspect of patient care related to moderate sedation as allowed by their state of practice and institutional policy. The current standard requires the presence of two qualified professionals when administering moderate sedation. The role of the nurse and their scope of practice has become more defined as an increasing number of procedures are performed in outpatient settings and same-day surgical centers on an older population with increased complexity. Many professional nursing organizations have statements regarding moderate sedation including the American Nurses Association, American Association of Critical Care Nurses, and Association of Operating Room Nurses. In fact, the American Association of Moderate Sedation Nurses (AAMSN),was founded in 2008 to ensure patient safety by developing a curriculum for certification of non-anesthetist registered nurses (RNs) that promotes adherence to the American Nurses Association (ANA), American Association of Nurse Anesthetists (AANA) and American Society of Anesthesiologists (ASA) standards and guidelines for registered nurses who practice moderate sedation and are not certified registered nurse anesthetists [1]. The AAMSN provides a network of support and development that upholds high professional standards and quality care across all practice settings, including private practices, through its collaboration with other professional organizations. In this chapter, the focus will be on the training and responsibilities of nurses functioning as the monitor while caring for patients receiving moderate/procedural sedation.

Training

All patients should be provided the same level and quality of care. In an effort to ensure this, credentialing organizations have mandated standards. The Joint Commission's (TJC) Provisions of Care (PC) 03.01.01: "The hospital plans operative or other high-risk procedures, including those that require the administration of moderate or deep sedation or anesthesia," Element of Performance (EP) 5 along with the corresponding Centers for Medicare and Medicaid Services (CMS) Medicare Requirement (482.23) note that an RN supervises perioperative nursing care. The ASA mandates that regardless of the location where procedural sedation is being provided, all patients should receive comparable levels of care by qualified professionals. In most institutions the standard is that there is a minimum of two qualified professionals attending to the patient: the "operator" and the "monitor." The role of the nurse is to act as a "monitor." The monitor can be defined as a licensed and credentialed healthcare professional (physician, dentist, physician assistant, nurse practitioner, or RN) who will monitor appropriate physiologic parameters as well as the patient's response to the drugs administered and the procedure itself.

According to the ASA statement on granting privileges for administration of moderate sedation to practitioners who are not anesthesia professionals, formal training provides competency in both safe administration of sedatives and analgesics used to establish a level of moderate sedation and the rescue of patients who exhibit adverse physiologic consequences of a deeper-than-intended level of sedation [2]. This training must encompass [2]:

1. Practice guidelines for sedation and analgesia by non-anesthesiologists.
2. Components of informed consent, pre-procedure counseling including risks, benefits, and alternatives pertaining to moderate sedation.
3. The continuum of depth of sedation with definitions of levels of sedation/analgesia.
4. Skills for assessing appropriateness and risks involved in sedation including potential for aspiration and airway management complications. Skills for evaluation of the patient's medical history to evaluate risks and comorbidities. Physical examination should be completed by operator and monitor.
5. The pharmacology and safe administration of sedatives and analgesics used to achieve a level of moderate sedation as well as their appropriate antagonists.
6. The benefits and risks of supplemental oxygen.
7. Airway management with face mask and self-inflating bag–valve mask device.
8. Monitoring and documentation of patient's physiologic parameters including, but not limited to, blood pressure, respiratory rate, oxygen saturation by pulse oximetry, ECG monitoring, depth of sedation, and capnography.
9. Continuous use of appropriately set audible alarms on all physiologic parameters.
10. Documentation of administered drugs and fluids during the pre-, intra-, and post-procedure phases, including the patient's hemodynamic status and level of sedation.
11. Competency in cardiopulmonary resuscitation required for the monitor and certification equivalent to Advanced Cardiac Life Support for the operator as well as recognition of common complications that can occur, and appropriate intervention by both team members.

These educational requirements must be consistent across the institution. In addition to this initial education, a formal re-credentialing process must be in place. Evaluation and documentation of competence occurs on a periodic basis according to each institution's guidelines.

Nurses may obtain certification specific to moderate sedation through the AAMSN. The Certified Sedation Registered Nurse (CSRN) is one who has studied an advanced curriculum in sedation, whose scope of practice includes but is not limited to:

1. Administration of moderate sedation medications by non-anesthetist RNs as allowed by state laws, institutional policy, procedures, and protocol.

2. The orders and medications necessary to achieve moderate sedation selected by the qualified anesthesia provider or attending physician.
3. Guidelines for patient monitoring, drug administration, and protocols for dealing with potential complications or emergency situations available specific to accepted standards of anesthesia practice.
4. The RN managing the care of the patient receiving moderate sedation shall have no other responsibilities that would leave the patient unattended or compromise continuous monitoring.
5. The RN managing the care of patients receiving moderate sedation is able to:
   a. Demonstrate the acquired anatomy, physiology, pharmacology, cardiac arrhythmia recognition, and complications related to moderate sedation and medications.
   b. Assess total patient care requirements and physiologic parameters.
   c. Understand the process of oxygen delivery and respiratory physiology as well demonstrate proficiency in utilization of oxygen delivery devices.
   d. Anticipate and recognize potential complications related to moderate sedation.
   e. Evidence skill set necessary to assess, diagnose, and intervene in the event of complication or undesired outcome.
   f. Demonstrate skill in airway management and resuscitation.
   g. Understand legal ramifications associated with administering moderate sedation and/or monitoring patients receiving moderate sedation, including the nurse's responsibility and liability in the event of an untoward reaction or life-threatening complication.
6. Maintain competency consistent with ASA and AAMSN guidelines as defined by institution of practice [1].

Nursing Responsibilities

Although the nurse's sole responsibility is the care of the patient receiving moderate sedation during the associated procedure, the nurse is also involved in many aspects of pre- and post-procedure care and documentation.

Pre-procedure Responsibilities

Equipment

All necessary equipment must be present and in working order. Examples of such equipment include:

- oxygen – a source and means for providing supplemental oxygen
- an airway and a self-inflating oxygen delivery system capable of delivering 100% oxygen
- a source of suction with Yankauer-type suction catheters
- a pulse oximeter with audible alarms
- a cardiac monitor with audible alarms
- a blood pressure device and stethoscope
- capnography
- an emergency cart and defibrillator

- pharmaceutical agents to be used for the procedure, and their reversal agents
- liter bags of 0.9% normal saline or lactated Ringer's solution

Documentation

It is usually the responsibility of the operator or individual who is performing the procedure to obtain the informed consent for procedural sedation documentation, perform the pre-procedure assessment, and document the plan. However, it is the responsibility of the monitor/nurse to review this documentation and ensure that it is present and complete.

It is the role of the nurse to validate that the following aspects of care are addressed and documented prior to the procedure:

1. Informed consent – which includes risk, benefits, and alternatives. This needs to be accomplished before any procedural sedation drugs are given.
2. Pre-procedure evaluation including review of allergies, body mass index, physical examination, and medical history review, which evaluates the potential for risks and comorbidities. The examination should include a thorough airway assessment to aid in the recognition of potential difficult airway management. The ASA classification of physical status and the classification system have been described elsewhere in this book. (See Chapters 3 and 4.)
3. Review of pre-procedure labs or tests.
4. Oxygen requirements and ability to tolerate supplemental oxygen.
5. Educational needs of patient and significant others regarding the pre-, intra-, and post-procedure aspects and what to anticipate.
6. Verify the ability of the patient to tolerate positioning required for the procedure and recovery phase.
7. Ensure that a functioning intravenous (IV) line is available throughout the procedure until discharge.
8. Ensure that the patient is able to communicate with the monitor and report any problems associated with the procedure immediately.
9. Confirm the appropriateness and availability of a designated adult escort transportation.
10. Coordinate post-procedure recovery and arrangements for transfer or discharge home.

Note: It is the responsibility of the care team members to identify those patients who, based on the information obtained in the aforesaid documents, are deemed at higher risk for complications, and consider an anesthesia consult in high-risk situations.

Patient Education

Patient education is an important nursing responsibility. As the monitor during procedural sedation, the nurse is in constant communication with the patient. Through continuously monitoring the nurse ensures patient safety while the proceduralist is performing the procedure. The procedure should be thoroughly explained before any drugs are given to the patient. Prior to the procedure, the nurse should describe any sensations that the patient might feel – such as burning, pulling, and pressure. Agree on a method of communication for patients to let you know if and when they need something, perhaps by holding up a finger or making eye contact. Instruct them to let you know if they experience any problems. Although individual response to sedation varies greatly, instruct the patient that they may not remember details of the procedure. Reassure the patient they will be continuously monitored during the procedure.

Patients should be made aware of what will happen post procedure and during discharge. They should also be aware that a "responsible adult" should be available to accompany them home when the recovery from the procedure is complete. This is in accordance with TJC regulation 03.01.03, which states: "Patients who have received sedation or anesthesia as outpatients are discharged in the company of an individual who accepts responsibility for the patient" [2].

Immediate Pre-Procedure Responsibilities

Immediately prior to the procedure and the administration of the sedation, the nurse/monitor should verify correct identification of the patient per institution's standards. Using two patient identifiers meets TJC's National Patient Safety Goal 1. Obtain and document baseline vital signs: heart rate and rhythm, blood pressure, respiratory rate, oxygen saturation, temperature, level of consciousness, and level on a reliable and validated sedation and pain scale (Box 8.1). Patient allergies should be reviewed along with confirmation of NPO status (Table 8.1). All required monitoring equipment must be in place with audible alarms enabled. Review orders for sedation analgesia include benzodiazepines, opioids, and other appropriate drugs, including reversal agents and that they are readily available. Confirm patent IV access with fluids administered as ordered. Verify patient is tolerating the position and discuss with patient any last-minute concerns.

Before starting the procedure, all team members team must participate in a time-out or safety pause that adheres to TJC Universal Protocol regulation [3].

Intra-procedure Responsibilities

During this period, the nurse's primary responsibilities are to deliver moderate sedation medications and to assess and monitor patient responses to the therapy. The most common complications are respiratory depression and airway obstruction. Other common complications that can occur are cardiac arrhythmias and hemodynamic

---

Box 8.1 Depth of Sedation Scale*

Score term description
AWAKE = Awake/alert – 0
MIN = Minimally sedated: tired/sleepy, appropriate response to verbal conversation and/ or sounds – 1
MOD = Moderately sedated: somnolent/sleeping, easily arousable with light tactile stimulation – 2
DEEP = Deeply sedated: deep sleep, arousable only with significant physical stimulation – 3
GEN = Unarousable – 4

* Consistent with the American Society of Anesthesiologists 'Continuum of depth of sedation: definitions of general anesthesia and levels of sedation/analgesia' guideline. Available at www.asahq .org/standards-and-practice-parameters/statement-on-continuum-of-depth-of-sedation-definition-of-general-anesthesia-and-levels-of-sedation-analgesia

Table 8.1 American Society of Anesthesiologists (ASA) pre-procedure fasting guidelines [4]

Ingested material	Minimum fasting period^a
Clear liquids^b	2 h
Breast milk	4 h
Infant formula	6 h
Non-human milk^c	6 h
Light meal^d	6 h

These recommendations apply to healthy patients who are undergoing elective procedures. They are not intended for women in labor. Following the guidelines does not guarantee a complete gastric emptying has taken place.
^{a} The fasting periods apply to all ages.
^{b} Examples of clear liquids include water, fruit juices without pulp, carbonated beverages, clear tea, and black coffee.
^{c} Since nonhuman milk is similar to solids in gastric emptying time, the amount ingested must be considered when determining an appropriate fasting period.
^{d} A light meal typically consists of toast and clear liquids. Meals that include fried or fatty foods or meat may prolong gastric emptying time. Both the amount and type of foods ingested must be considered when determining an appropriate fasting period.

instability. According to the ASA's practice guidelines, the following information should be assessed and documented at a minimum of every 5 minutes:

- vital signs – blood pressure, heart rate and rhythm, respiratory rate, oxygen saturation
- medications given – drug, dose, route, and time
- oxygen delivery – amount and the means of delivery
- airway assessment – checking of head position and patency of the airway
- presence of capnography waveform
- level of sedation on approved scale
- level of pain on approved scale
- any observations that occur during procedure (e.g., complaints of pain, treatment of hypotension with IV fluids, and snoring)

One of the most important things the nurse can do to prevent complications is to avoid overmedication. Intravenous sedative and analgesic drugs should be given in small, incremental doses that are titrated to the desired level of sedation and analgesia. Enough time between doses must be allowed for the effect of the drug to take place. A thorough knowledge of each individual drug's usual dose, its mechanism of action, and its onset and duration of action is imperative. The treatment of respiratory complications can usually be relieved by stimulating the patient, delivering oxygen, repositioning airway with chin tilt or jaw thrust, suctioning any upper airway secretions, and withholding further medications until the issue is resolved. Temporary assistance with breathing may be necessary with a bag–valve mask device. If respiratory depression continues, a reversal agent should be considered.

Hemodynamic instability may be resolved with administration of IV fluids, raising the patient's legs, and/or withholding further medications. The operator should be made aware of any complications and a decision to abort the procedure should be made if all efforts to treat complications have failed. In most cases, the judicious administration of the reversal agent remedies the situation.

Medications

The goals of moderate sedation are analgesia, sedation, and amnesia. These are usually accomplished with a combination of opioids and benzodiazepines. The ASA defines moderate sedation as "a drug-induced depression of consciousness during which patients respond purposely to verbal commands, either alone or accompanied by light tactile stimulation. No interventions are required to maintain a patent airway, and spontaneous ventilation is adequate. Cardiovascular function is usually maintained" [2]. One must remember that while this is the intended response, individuals may react differently. The nurse must adhere to the institution's monitoring guidelines.

Procedural sedation is typically accomplished through IV drugs, but oral doses may be appropriate in some situations. The most common combination of drugs used is midazolam and fentanyl. However, no single regimen is ideal for all situations. Your institution may use other combinations for atypical patient populations or for deep sedation. The reader is referred Chapter 2 for a description of medications and their reversal agents. It is important to remember that administering these medications for procedural sedation should not be undertaken without full knowledge of this pharmacology. It is also important to be aware of specific institutional and state board of nursing guidelines regarding the administration of procedural sedation medications.

Post-procedure: Recovery and Discharge

Since most of the medications used in procedural sedation are not immediately metabolized, it is important to establish a post-procedure monitoring routine. The Joint Commission states that the patient receiving sedation or anesthesia must be assessed in a post-sedation recovery area before discharge. Furthermore, a qualified licensed independent practitioner must discharge the patient from the recovery area or from the hospital. In the absence of the aforesaid practitioner, patients are discharged according to criteria approved by clinical leaders. The ASA agrees that continued observation, monitoring, and predetermined discharge criteria decrease the likelihood of adverse outcomes for both moderate and deep sedation. They recommend that patients are observed in an appropriately staffed and equipped area until they are near their baseline level of consciousness and no longer at increased risk for cardiopulmonary depression. If the patient must be moved from the area where the procedure has taken place, the recovery area must have available the same monitoring and resuscitative equipment. Both the operator and the monitor must stay with the patient until they can spontaneously protect their airway and their vital signs are stable. At the conclusion of the procedure, the patient must be monitored for a specified period of time. The duration and frequency of monitoring is subject to institutional and practice standards. Many facilities will monitor the patient every 5–10 minutes for *at least 30 minutes* after the last medication is administered. Monitoring continues at this frequency until the patient reaches baseline. Parameters monitored should be the same as those observed during the procedure. If the patient received a reversal agent during the procedure, the monitoring period is generally extended to at least 2 hours after the reversal agent was administered. This is because once the reversal agent has worn off, respiratory depression can reoccur.

When this standardized time period has passed and the patient is at baseline, they must meet objective discharge criteria. This is true both for the patient being discharged to home and for the patient being transferred within the institution to a less intensively monitored level of care. One of the first sets of objective discharge criteria used was the Aldrete scoring system first published in 1970 [5]. This system scored the patient in five parameters: activity, respiration, oxygenation, circulation, and consciousness (see Chapter 4, Table 4.2). Since that time, many institutions have modified this scale, based on post-sedation advances. Each of the six criteria listed here receives anywhere from 0 to 2 points based on their absence or presence. A total of 8 points must be achieved for discharge. Any patient who receives a score of 7 or less must be reevaluated by a physician before discharge can occur. Within the inpatient setting, patients can be transferred back to their previous unit once they have met the discharge criteria. The nurse who has recovered the patient will provide a complete report to the receiving nurse. This hand-off communication should include, but not be limited to:

- patient name
- diagnosis
- procedure performed
- review of vital signs, oxygen saturation, pain and sedation levels
- sedation medications administered, total dose, and antagonist, if used
- fluid balance
- complications and their treatment

Those patients who will be discharged to home need to receive both verbal and written discharge instructions. It is very important that both the patient and the accompanying adult are present to receive the instructions. The patients may still be experiencing some degree of amnesia and may not remember everything they have been told. Most discharge instructions include specific limitations or requirements associated with the procedure that has been completed. For example, with a colonoscopy, patients will be advised that they may experience abdominal distention or flatus from air that was placed in the gastrointestinal tract. Any activity or diet restrictions should also be addressed. There are certain restrictions that stem from the use of the procedural sedation medications themselves. Post-procedural sedation discharge instructions should include the following statements, which pertain to the next 12 hours:

- Do not drive an automobile.
- Do not drink any alcoholic beverages.
- Do not make any important decisions.
- Do not do anything that requires mental concentration.

Patients should be instructed to contact the healthcare provider listed on the form if they experience problems or have questions. The name and telephone number should be clearly listed. After the information has been discussed and all questions are answered, both the patient and a witness should sign. They should receive a copy, and a copy should go into the patient's medical record. On a rare occasion, despite everyone's best efforts, the patient may decide to travel home without a responsible adult to accompany them.

This is not recommended, and the patient should be dissuaded. If, however, they insist, they should be required to sign an "against medical advice" form.

Summary

The nurse plays a vital role in administering and monitoring procedural sedation. Receiving specialized training, certification, and adhering to strict institutional standards will help to ensure patient safety.

Acknowledgments

The authors wish to acknowledge Ellen K. Bergeron and Jennifer Kales, the authors of the previous version of this chapter in the second edition of this textbook.

References

1. American Association of Moderate Sedation Nurses. Certified sedation registered nurse (CSRN) scope of practice. https://aamsn.org

2. American Society of Anesthesiologists (ASA). Statement on granting privileges for administration of moderate sedation to practitioners who are not anesthesia professionals. www.asahq.org/standards-and-practice-parameters/statement-on-granting-privileges-for-administration-of-moderate-sedation-to-practitioners-who-are-not-anesthesia-professionals

3. Joint Commission. *Comprehensive Accreditation Manual for Hospitals*. Oakbrook Terrace, IL: Joint Commission, 2016. https://store.jcrinc.com/2024-comprehensive-accreditation-manuals

4. American Society of Anesthesiologists Committee. Practice guidelines for preoperative fasting and the use of pharmacologic agents to reduce the risk of pulmonary aspiration: application to healthy patients undergoing elective procedures: an updated report by the American Society of Anesthesiologists Committee on Standards and Practice Parameters. *Anesthesiology*. 2017;126(3):376–93. doi.org/10.1097/ALN.0000000000001452

5. Aldrete JA, Kroulik D. A postanesthetic recovery score. Anesth Analg 1970;49: 924–34.

Additional Reading

Antonelli MT, Seaver D, Urman RD. Procedural sedation and implications for quality and risk management. *J Healthc Risk Manag*. 2013;33(2): 3–10. doi: 10.1002/jhrm.21121. PMID: 24078203.

Caperelli-White L, Urman RD. Developing a moderate sedation policy: essential elements and evidence-based considerations. *AORN J*. 2014;99(3):416–30. doi: 10.1016/j. aorn.2013.09.015. PMID: 24581648.

Davis AG. *A Nursing Guide to Adult Moderate Sedation*. Create Space Independent Publishing Platform, 2014.

Gorski L, Hadaway L, Hagle M, et al., eds. *Policies and Procedures for Infusion Therapy*, 5th ed. Norwood, MA: Infusion Nurses Society, 2016.

O'Donnell J, Bragg K, Sell S. Procedural sedation: safely navigating the twilight zone. *Nursing* 2003;33(4):36–44.

Pisansky AJ, Beutler SS, Urman RD. Education and training for nonanesthesia providers performing deep sedation. *Curr Opin Anaesthesiol*. 2016 Aug;29(4):499–505. doi: 10.1097/ACO.0000000000000342. PMID: 27054416

Voynarovska M, Cohen LB. The role of the endoscopy nurse or assistant in endoscopic sedation. *Gastrointest Endosc Clin N Am*. 2008;18:695–705.

Physician Assistants and Nurse Practitioners

Chelsi J. Flanagan, Anish P. Saikumar, Allie Shea, Jennifer Kales, and Heather Trafton

Introduction

Nurse practitioners (NPs) and physician assistants (PAs) are trained healthcare professionals who strive to deliver high-quality healthcare and are providers that aim to take care of their patients in an effective, caring, and efficient manner. As of November 2022, there are about 355,000 NPs and 132,940 PAs providing healthcare services to patients across the United States [1].

NPs are licensed practitioners who work in ambulatory, acute and long-term care facilities as primary care or specialty providers [2]. Their scope of practice varies but is primarily determined by their education and training, national certification, state law, and institutional policy. As such, NPs located in certain states can practice and bill independently without the oversight of a physician. In a graduate NP program, the primary focus is on the development of clinical and professional skills and expertise that is necessary for comprehensive primary and specialty care by providing theoretical and evidence-based clinical knowledge and learning experiences [3].

PAs are also nationally certified and state-licensed healthcare professionals who practice medicine as part of a team under the supervision of physicians. They also can provide a broad range of medical and surgical services to diverse populations in both rural and urban settings. As part of their responsibilities, PAs conduct physical examinations, diagnose, and treat illnesses, order tests, and interpret their results, provide counseling regarding preventative healthcare, assist in surgery, and prescribe medications [4]. There are four parameters that define the scope of practice for a PA: state law, institutional policy, education and experience and physician delegation. The PA education and training is derived from that of physicians – rigorous coursework in medicine is followed by more than 2,000 hours of supervised clinical practice in a diverse healthcare institutions and medical practices.

The utilization of NPs and PAs has steadily increased – the United States Bureau of Labor Statistics has projected that the number of PA jobs will increase by 28% between

2021 and 2031, which is much faster than the average for all occupations [5]. Additionally, the Patient Protection and Affordable Care Act of 2010 included several provisions that encourage the continued utilization of NPs and PAs in healthcare settings, specifically including the provision of financial support for PA training and establishment of NP-led clinics. NPs and PAs are also playing a prominent role in academic medical centers. These centers are hiring NPs and PAs to improve healthcare accessibility, increase patient throughput, improve continuity of care, reduce length of stay, and fill the void caused by workforce shortages created by restrictions placed on resident physician work hours.

Regulatory Considerations

The Centers for Medicare and Medicaid Systems (CMS), Medicare Conditions of Participation (CoP), the Joint Commission (TJC), state boards, private payer policies, established institutional policies, medical staff bylaws are all examples of entities that govern the way NPs and PAs can practice. Unfortunately, the language used within the respective policies relayed from the various groups can be contradictory and/or interpreted differently by different institutions. The following sections provide clarification on each of the entities' policies regarding the administration of moderate sedation by NPs and PAs and highlight the nuances of such language.

The Centers for Medicare and Medicaid Systems and The Joint Commission

According to CMS and TJC regulations, NPs and PAs are allowed to administer moderate sedation, but are not allowed to administer deep sedation. Deep sedation is classified as a form of anesthesia that requires specific medical training that is not obtained by NPs and PAs. Interpretive guidelines for the anesthesia services condition of participation (Section 42 CFR 482.52) of the CMS Manual System outlines the requirements an organization must meet if it provides "anesthesia services" [6]. These guidelines outline what types of services are considered to be anesthesia services and defines which individuals may provide such services. Minimal and moderate sedation are classified as analgesia, not anesthesia – therefore the guidelines covering who may administer these two types of sedation are not dictated by the guidelines of the CMS Manual System. This important distinction between anesthesia and analgesia is the reason why NPs and PAs are granted permission to administer minimal and moderate sedation but cannot administer deep sedation.

These guidelines have a significant impact on NP and PA practice; they require that each organization's anesthesia department be responsible for developing policies and procedures that dictate the provision of all categories of "anesthesia services." These policies and procedures include addressing whether specific clinical situations involve anesthesia versus analgesia and specifying the minimum qualifications for each category of practitioner who is permitted to provide anesthesia services. TJC anesthesia care standards do not define specifically who can administer sedation but instead require that the individuals who are permitted to administer sedation are able to rescue patients at whatever level of sedation or anesthesia achieved, intentionally or unintentionally [7].

Determination of the capability of individuals to perform rescue efforts is left up to each organization. It is not always possible to predict how a patient will respond to sedation, and as such the level of sedation has the potential to become deeper than originally intended. The CMS defines "rescue" from a deeper level of sedation as the correction of adverse physiologic consequences of the deeper-than-intended level of sedation that returns the patient to the originally intended level of sedation. Rescue in this situation requires that the provider administering the sedation can fulfill this responsibility – this needs advanced training in advanced life support, airway management, and/or courses developed by an institution specifically for this purpose. Rescue in moderate sedation requires that the provider has the ability to manage a compromised airway or hypoventilation; training for this scenario can be successfully completed by both NPs and PAs. In fact, NPs and PAs often receive this type of instruction when training to provide other types of care aside from anesthesia.

The TJC language in relation to sedation and throughout their policies includes the term "licensed practitioner" (LP), which creates confusion because PAs are not defined as LPs. In response to this obscurity, TJC has added the following addendum to the definition of LP: "When standards reference the term licensed practitioner, this language is not to be construed to limit the authority of a licensed practitioner to delegate tasks to other qualified healthcare personnel (for example, physician assistants and advanced practice registered nurses) to the extent authorized by state law or a state's regulatory mechanism or federal guidelines and organizational policy" [8].

State Laws and Regulations

Individual states can also regulate anesthesia practices; their regulations can be more restrictive than federal laws and CMS and TJC policies. Certified Registered Nurse Anesthetists (CRNAs) and anesthesia assistances (AAs) are professionals who administer anesthesia and there has been a large increase in these professionals over the past 10 years. Because of this boom in CRNAs and AAs, there is now a need for states to review their laws and determine the types of professionals allowed to practice within their state, the scopes of practice of those professionals and whether they require professional registration or licensure. These decisions have prompted statue and regulation language changes to include a definition of what constitutes anesthesia.

The manner in which individual states define anesthesia determines whether the different levels of sedation are included or excluded from anesthesia regulations. The specific definition of anesthesia in some states has led to the prohibition of NPs and PAs from administering any kind of sedation. Consequently, many NPs and PAs that practice in procedural areas where sedation is required have lost their ability to provide those services.

The PA laws generally state that physicians can delegate any legal task for which the PA is appropriately trained to complete. The issue arises when the task that the physician would like to delegate is a task that is prohibited in other sections of state law, those outside of the ones defining physician and PA practice in relation to anesthesia and sedation. When a discrepancy exists within the language, it must be determined which law takes precedence. In these cases, the state regulatory body governing medical and PA practice may provide guidance and help make this determination.

Institutional Policies and Privileging

The scope of sedative-related practices an NP or PA can administer is limited to local anesthetics, minimal sedation, and moderate sedation. Both the TJC and CMC mandate institutions that employ non-anesthesiologists for the use of moderate sedation to implement policies that regulate these practitioners. These policies must include criteria that determine the extent of anesthesia services a practitioner can provide including the type and complexity of procedures they may perform. In addition, a set of procedures must be maintained to determine which individuals are qualified and the policies must address any necessary supervision requirements. For PAs, the law generally allows a supervising physician to delegate tasks they determine a PA to be competent in. Consequently, if a PA is privileged to administer moderate sedation, the supervising physician should have equivalent privileges. NPs however are afforded more flexibility as certain states permit them to practice independently. In these states, the administration of analgesics by NPs does not require physician oversight, and therefore privileging is solely determined by the training criteria outlined by respective institutions. Conversely, in states where NPs practice with a collaborating physician, the scope of practice is governed by the institution and the collaborating physician must supervise the NP regularly for case review.

Credentialing, Privileging, and Education

The TJC policies require that privileging is competency driven with defined criteria to meet and maintain competency. TJC does not stipulate that the administration of moderate sedation be a separately defined privilege, and it may be encompassed within procedure-based privileges. However, institutions may require their own set of privileges that are specific to moderate sedation practices. The privileging process should specify the required training for practitioners, and ASA guidelines recommend formal training in (1) the safe administration of sedative and analgesic drugs used for moderate sedation, (2) the use of reversal agents for opioids and benzodiazepines, (3) monitoring of patients' physiologic parameters and (4) recognition of abnormalities in monitored variables that require intervention by the non-anesthesiologist sedation practitioner or anesthesiologist.

Testing of core competency may include a knowledge-based examination that assesses a practitioner's understanding of concepts including moderate sedation practice guidelines, pediatric-specific training, pharmacology of sedatives and their dosing, airway management, sedation complications, monitoring of physiologic variables, understanding of alarms of physiologic monitoring equipment, appropriate documentation, and advanced cardiovascular life support skills. Credentialing and privileging should remain an ongoing process with routine audits and internal reviews to assess continued competency. Ultimately, the educational requirements for NPs and PAs administering moderate sedation should be at minimum equivalent to those of a non-anesthesia physician and should cover all the components outlined in Chapter 6.

Clinical Practice

Before the administration of moderate sedation, a pre-procedure patient evaluation must occur. The evaluation includes a history and physical, a review of any previous sedation-related adverse effects, and an airway assessment. Of note, the Association of periOperative Registered Nurses (AORN) recommends that nurses should consult the supervising licensed independent practitioner or anesthesia professional when a patient presents with a presumed ASA classification of III or higher [9].

After initiation of moderate sedation, AORN recommends the practitioner should remain with the patient to provide continual monitoring and should have unrestricted access to the patient. There should be no competing responsibilities that could distract them from monitoring and assessing the patient. All practitioners should have the ability to manage complications during moderate sedation and the ability to activate the appropriate emergency response team for that practice area.

Summary

With appropriate training, NPs and PAs can increase the accessibility of analgesic services through the administration of local anesthetics and moderate sedation. By clarifying the guidelines from regulatory bodies such as CMS, CoP, and TJC we can better illustrate and define the specific niche these practitioners have. In doing so, we intend to highlight the vital contribution NPs and PAs play in improving sedation-related patient care.

References

1. AANP National Nurse Practitioner Database, 2022. (accessed March 3, 2023)

2. American Academy of Nurse Practitioners. Quality of nurse practitioner practice. Fact sheet. www .aanp.org/about/all-about-nps/np-fact-sheet

3. American Academy of Nurse Practitioners. Nurse practitioner curriculum. www.aanp.org/advocacy/ advocacy-resource/position-statements/ nurse-practitioner-curriculum

4. American Academy of Physicians. AAPA Annual Survey Report. www.aapa.org

5. Bureau of Labor Statistics, US Department of Labor. Occupational Outlook Handbook: physician assistants. www.bls.gov/ooh/healthcare/physician-assistants.htm (accessed March 3, 2023)

6. Centers for Medicare and Medicaid Systems. CMS Manual System: Revised Appendix A, Interpretive Guidelines for Hospitals, December 2011. www.cms.gov/ Regulations-and-Guidance/Guidance/ Transmittals/downloads/R74SOMA.pdf (accessed May 2016)

7. The Joint Commission. Sedation and anesthesia - rescue requirements: Is the availability of an on demand "cardio-respiratory code team" acceptable in lieu of the person who is permitted to administer moderate or deep sedation being able to perform the rescues required by the sedation and anesthesia standards? www.jointcommission.org/ standards/standard-faqs/ambulatory/ provision-of-care-treatment-and-services-pc/000001646

8. The Joint Commission. Revisions to eliminate term "licensed independent practitioner". www.jointcommission .org/-/media/tjc/documents/standards/ prepublications/effective-2023/lip_hap_ glossary_prepub.pdf

9. Williams, K. "Guidelines in Practice: Moderate Sedation and Analgesia." AORN J. 2022;115(6): 553–64. https://doi .org/10.1002/aorn.13690

High-risk Patients: Sedation Considerations in Coexisting Disease

Alan D. Kaye, Henry Liu, Elyse M. Cornett, and Charles J. Fox III

Introduction

Certain patient populations requiring sedation for procedures present the clinician with challenging decisions regarding their care and management. Some underlying medical disease states, airway abnormalities, or extremes of age require cautious pre-procedural assessment and planning when sedation is required to minimize the incidence of morbidity or mortality. It should be noted that some of these higher-risk patients should only be sedated by trained anesthesia providers. The following commonly encountered conditions are considered high risk and are associated with a higher rate of complications: old age, obesity, chronic obstructive pulmonary disease, coronary artery disease, and chronic renal failure. This chapter discusses important features of these higher-risk patients and practice management when sedation is required. In all cases, appropriate monitoring, prudent selection and dosing of sedative agents, and careful assessment are important to ensure the best outcome for these higher-risk patients.

The Elderly

The elderly population (e.g., 65 years of age or older) is a rapidly growing segment of our society. The Census Bureau predicts that by 2030, 1 in 5 Americans (71 million) will be older than 65. Currently, we have 36 million Americans who are older than 65. Although those individuals considered elderly are at higher risk for complications, the more accurate predictor of outcome may be the patient's physiologic age. This may be determined more clearly during a pre-procedure evaluation. For example, a 65-year-old patient who is wheelchair-bound may be considered higher risk than an 85-year-old marathon runner. Careful pre- procedure evaluation of the patient's coexisting diseases and medications, and a thorough physical examination, are the initial steps in risk stratification for these patients. Knowledge of the physiologic changes associated with aging is important when trying to determine a medication plan for sedation (Table 10.1).

Table 10.1 Physiologic differences and sedation considerations in the elderly population

System	Physiologic differences	Sedation considerations
Cardiovascular	Reduced tissue elasticity in arteries and veins Ventricular hypertrophy Reduced cardiac output Reduced arterial oxygenation Deterioration of the cardiac conduction system	Increased oxygen consumption Inability of the body to adjust to hemodynamic changes Higher likelihood of arrhythmias Slower cardiorespiratory response to hypercarbia and hypoxia
Body composition	Higher proportion of body fat Less intracellular fluid	Expanded distribution volume for pharmacologic agents Higher risk of oversedation with water-soluble drugs Slower recovery period for lipid-soluble drugs
Pulmonary	Decreased respiratory drive Less lung capacity Diminished response to hypoxemia or hypercarbia Increased work of breathing due to loss of chest wall elasticity	Decreased ability for the body to compensate for respiratory depression caused by sedative agents Higher incidence of transient apnea
Neurologic	Loss of neuronal density Reduced levels of neurotransmitters	Increased sensitivity to CNS-depressant drugs Higher incidence of confusion and delirium with sedation
Renal	Reduced blood flow to the kidneys Decreased glomerular filtration rate	Increased risk of renal insufficiency Longer duration of action for some anesthetics and adjuvant drugs
Hepatic	Reduced blood flow to the liver Less liver enzyme activity	Increased duration of action for lipid-soluble drugs Altered metabolism of drugs
Airway	Diminished gag reflex Chronic microaspirations Loss of teeth and use of dentures Arthritis of the neck	Increases risk of aspiration Difficulty in mask ventilation Difficulty performing head-tilt, jaw-thrust maneuver of airway

Cardiovascular System

A large portion of the elderly report participation in strenuous and frequent athletic activities, so the patient's self-reported list of daily activities and exercise tolerance provides the best initial assessment of cardiac function. This can be more accurately expressed in metabolic equivalent levels (METs). Patients achieving a level of four METs or higher have a significantly decreased risk of complications. If the patient has a limited exercise tolerance, chemical stress testing, stress echocardiography, or cardiac catheterization should be considered to explore possible etiologies and degree of cardiovascular disease before proceeding with sedation.

Elderly patients experience a reduction in exercise tolerance (maximally obtainable cardiac output, heart rate, and stroke volume) and progressive loss of vascular elasticity. This loss of elasticity commonly leads to a compensatory left ventricular hypertrophy and hypertension. Chronic elevation of blood pressure leads to decreased baroreceptor sensitivity. If this process continues, the development of congestive heart failure is common. Lastly, it should be recognized that the elderly have an increased incidence of coronary artery disease, heart failure, and valvular heart disease. Because of this, the elderly have an increased risk of mortality and major adverse cardiovascular events within 30 days after surgery. Physicians are experiencing an increase in the request of assessment of perioperative cardiac risks of non-cardiac surgery for this population [1, 2].

An important concept for many elderly patients, along with those with decreased cardiac function, is the principle of delayed response to an intravenous (IV) sedative agent related to a slower circulatory time. This means that IV medications can take a longer time to circulate to the brain and provide sedative effects. Further, the majority of medications used for sedation produce a vasodilatory effect, while a smaller percentage also depress cardiac function. Typical patients with chronic hypertension have overly constricted arterioles and consequently a reduction in intravascular volume. Long-standing hypertension, valvular disease, or coronary artery disease may result in depression of ventricular function. Depending upon the type and dose of medication administered and level of sedation achieved, these patients can experience clinically significant hemodynamic changes, including drops in blood pressure. An excellent example is seen in the response to propofol, which in any population can cause significant hypotension.

Respiratory System

The respiratory system undergoes numerous changes related to aging. The upper airway protective reflexes (coughing and swallowing) are diminished in the elderly by the reduction in nerve endings of irritant receptors. This potentially results in chronic alveolar inflammation and loss of alveolar surface area from constant microaspirations. Thus, elderly patients can potentially aspirate with no or low levels of sedation, so the clinician must constantly assess the patient's level of consciousness and aggressively seek to eliminate risks for aspiration.

The elderly lose chest wall elasticity and respiratory muscle mass and see an increase in turbulent flow in airway passages as they narrow. Because of these changes, the elderly experience reductions in forced vital capacity and forced expiratory volume at 1 second, and increased air trapping, closing capacity, and respiratory residual volume. The summation of these changes is a reduction in arterial oxygenation and an increase in the work of breathing, and this is reflected in the increased incidence of shortness of breath that elderly people experience when performing their daily activities. Mean arterial oxygenation tension averages 70 mmHg at age 80, which is significantly decreased from the oxygen tension of 95 mmHg at age 20. Additionally, the elderly have a decreased responsiveness to hypercapnia and hypoxemia. Therefore, these patients are at increased risk for considerable respiratory depression when receiving sedation medications. With the epidemic of smokers worldwide, an elderly patient can easily have damaged lungs, which are discussed later in this chapter.

Hepatic and Renal Systems

Hepatic and renal changes seen in the elderly primarily reflect a reduction in cardiac output. This reduction decreases hepatic and renal blood flow, dramatically affecting their metabolic capabilities. Also, in the liver there is a reduction in protein synthesis. These two changes in liver physiology decrease drug metabolism and mandate decreased dosing with sedation medications. The reduction in renal blood flow decreases the glomerular filtration rate and prolongs the elimination half-life of drugs cleared by the kidneys. Additionally, renal parenchymal atrophy results in a 50% reduction in glomeruli by age 80, and the kidneys reduce their ability to conserve free water and concentrate urine changes as we age.

Chronic kidney disease (CKD) can cause further complications. Drugs that are normally excreted by the kidney can accumulate and become toxic in a patient with CKD. This can be further complicated in an elderly patient who has decreased kidney function or is on a variety of drugs to support kidney function. Demerol should be avoided in patients with CKD or renal disease as the active metabolite, normeperidine, can accumulate and cause seizures [3]. Morphine is glucoronidated to an active morphine 6-glucuronide, which has significant analgesic effects, and therefore should not be given to patients with renal failure.

Central Nervous System

Aging causes multiple changes in the central nervous system. By age 80, there is a 30% reduction in brain mass and a concomitant decrease in serotonin, dopamine, and acetylcholine receptors. The incidence of diseases such as Parkinson's and Alzheimer's increases as one ages. For example, 3% of people aged 66 have symptoms of Parkinson's, and by age 85 that number increases to 50%. Delirium, a disturbance of consciousness that limits one's ability to focus or shift attention, affects 10–15% of elderly hospitalized patients. Patients with a history of preexisting cognitive dysfunction experience delirium and cognitive dysfunction more frequently post procedure. Postoperative cognitive disorder (POCD) is a concern in the elderly and may persist for weeks after the surgery. However, there is limited evidence of POCD after 6 months post surgery [4]. Because of this, an understanding of the patient's baseline cognitive function should be established before sedation medications are administered.

Temperature Regulation

The ability to regulate body temperature is diminished in elderly patients. Shivering does not occur until a much lower temperature is reached, and the ability to vasoconstrict or conserve heat is impaired in this population. These factors, together with a decreased ability to generate body heat (lower metabolic rate), increase the time needed to recover from hypothermia and can dramatically increase the time required to metabolize and clear sedation medications. Complications of perioperative hypothermia include coagulopathy, prolonged recovery, shivering, and thermal discomfort [5]. Forced-air warming of the patient, along with warming IV solutions and warming the procedure room, can help prevent hypothermia in these patients.

In neonates, temperature is an important physiologic outcome measure and it can be significantly altered by the operating room conditions. There is a dose-dependent increase in mortality with decreasing body temperature and an increase in the likelihood for severe respiratory distress. Fetal temperature is affected by maternal temperature; therefore, mitigating maternal temperature can help control the temperature of the neonate [6].

Obesity

The rate of obesity in the United States has increased dramatically in the last decade. In 1990, the incidence of adult obesity was less than 15%; by 2000, that percentage had increased to 27%. Some estimate that over 67% of our adult population is either overweight or obese. Annually, obesity is responsible for more than 300,000 premature deaths and more than $100 billion of related costs. The rate of obesity now affects 17% of children between the ages of 2 and 19. This rate has tripled in the last two decades [7].

The calculation of overweight, obese, or morbidily obese is based on a patient's body mass index (BMI). The BMI is calculated using the patient's height and weight: BMI = [weight (kg)]/[height (m)]^2 or BMI = [weight (lb)]/[height (inches)]^2 A BMI > 25 is considered overweight while a BMI > 30 is considered obese. An individual with a BMI > 40 is considered morbidly obese.

These patients present a multitude of challenges for the clinician (Box 10.1). Special gowns, operating room tables, monitoring equipment, stretchers, and wheelchairs are needed to properly care for these individuals. They also have anatomical, organ-system, and pharmacokinetic changes that add complexity to their care. A subset of these patients has advanced anatomical and physiologic changes, resulting in diseases such as obstructive sleep apnea, coronary artery disease, and pulmonary hypertension, which may warrant sedation by trained anesthesia providers. In this regard, special care for obese and morbidly obese patients in the prone position with moderate and deep sedation always requires experienced anesthesia personnel providing careful titration of sedative drugs (typically lower doses and over a longer period of time) and standard American Society of Anesthesiologists (ASA) monitors, including quantitative end-tidal carbon dioxide to assess appropriate real-time ventilation. Obese patients that are hypoventilating or apneic can rapidly desaturate and this can result in a catastrophic

---

Box 10.1   Health consequences of severe obesity

High blood pressure
Diabetes
Heart disease
Joint and bone problems
Sleep apnea
Decreased self-esteem
Decreased mobility/daily function
Decreased longevity
Higher incidence of nerve injury under sedation

outcome without proper monitoring of oxygenation and ventilation. Finally, newer anti-diabetic medication/weight loss drugs such as glucagon-like peptide-1 (GLP-1) receptor agonists (e.g., semaglutide, dulaglutide, exenatide, liraglutide, etc.) reduce gastric emptying and, therefore, can theoretically increase the risk of aspiration of gastric contents under sedation. These agents mimic the action of the human incretin GLP-1 increasing the secretion of insulin and improving glycemic control. To date, the ASA has not provided any recommendations on managing patients taking these drugs and therefore consideration of the increased risk of aspiration must be contemplated in providing a safe sedation plan for these patients. There is a trend to use these GLP-1 agonists drugs in younger and healthier patients who are less obese or not diabetics, for weight-loss purposes. Therefore, patient evaluation preoperatively requires identification of this class of medications and a careful plan to address the delayed gastric-emptying effects. These medications most likely will be held in the future, prior to sedation, once recommendations, guidelines, or best practice consensus on the subject is completed in the future by the ASA.

Pulmonary and Airway Systems

Many critical changes happen to both the pulmonary system and the airway in people who are obese (Box 10.2).

The extra weight added to the thoracic cage and abdominal cavity restricts thoracic wall and diaphragmatic movement. This process progresses to a restrictive lung disease (Figure 10.1), initially reducing the functional residual capacity and expiratory reserve volume. The functional residual capacity serves as the oxygen "storage tank," and this is reduced exponentially with increasing BMI (Figure 10.2). As BMI continues to increase, airway closure ensues when the functional residual capacity equals the closing capacity. Morbid obesity causes a reduction in the vital capacity and total lung capacity, and the added weight reduces chest wall compliance and increases airway resistance. These changes are accentuated by medications that cause respiratory depression when the obese patient is sedated in the supine position. Also, obese individuals have increases in both oxygen consumption, which can be double or triple that of lean patients, and carbon dioxide production. Therefore, the rate of desaturation is much faster in the obese patient (Figure 10.2).

Obstructive sleep apnea (OSA) is present in 5% of obese patients; it increases postoperative complication rates, increases the need for intensive care intervention, and prolongs hospital stays. This condition is associated with serious health consequences, such as stroke and a number of cardiovascular conditions – hypertension, coronary artery disease, and atrial fibrillation.

With sleep apnea, breathing stops and starts as one sleeps. These individuals have redundant adipose and soft tissue that narrows the airway. Pharyngeal patency and prevention of airway collapse are dependent on the action of pharyngeal muscle tone.

Box 10.2 Pulmonary and respiratory changes in the obese patient

Increased oxygen consumption due to the metabolic activity of fat
Increased energy expenditure in breathing due to increased chest and abdomen wall mass
Faster desaturation in obese patients
Airway changes that can make ventilation difficult

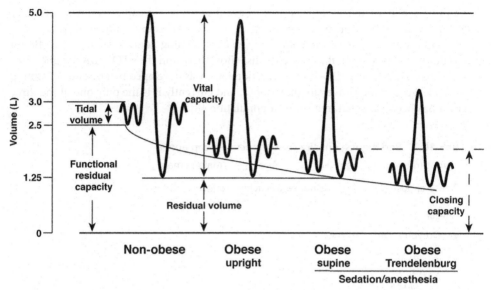

Figure 10.1 Pulmonary mechanics as a function of weight and position. Adapted from Baker and Yagiela [7].

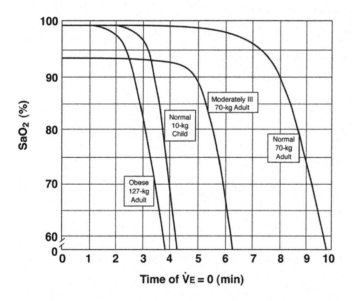

Figure 10.2 Rate of desaturation with apnea as a function of weight. Adapted from Practice Guidelines for the Perioperative Management of Patients with Obstructive Sleep Apnea: A Report by the American Society of Anesthesiologists Task Force on Perioperative Management of Patients with Obstructive Sleep Apnea. Anesthesiology 2006; 104:1081–93 doi: https://doi.org/10.1097/00000542-200605000-00026

This tone is decreased during sleep or sedation, resulting in airway obstruction. As the disease advances, some patients will develop obesity hypoventilation syndrome, which can progress into Pickwickian syndrome. This syndrome is characterized by gross obesity, somnolence, periodic breathing (when awake), hypercapnea, hypoxemia, polycythemia, and pulmonary hypertension. Patients with OSA are considered high risk for obstruction when sedated and should be approached cautiously by the clinician. Because these patients are usually sedated by anesthesiologists or nurse anesthetists, they should be screened pre-procedurally by the sedation service to avoid potential mishaps. Failure to recognize OSA preoperatively is one of the major causes of post-procedural complications.

Presently, there are three commonly used screening tools for OSA: the Berlin questionnaire (Box 10.3), the ASA checklist (Box 10.4), and the STOP–BANG question-naire (Box 10.5). The STOP–BANG questionnaire was developed by Dr. Frances Chung and colleagues at the University of Toronto, and currently it is the only one of the three which has been validated in a surgical population [8].

Box 10.3 Berlin questionnaire for obstructive sleep apnea

Height (m) _____ Weight (kg) _____ Age _____ Male/Female _____

Please choose the correct response to each question

Category 1

- Do you snore?

    . (a) Yes
    . (b) No
    . (c) Don't know

If you snore:

- Your snoring is:

    . (a) Slightly louder than breathing
    . (b) As loud as talking
    . (c) Louder than talking
    . (d) Very loud – can be heard in adjacent rooms

- How often do you snore?

    . (a) Nearly every day
    . (b) 3–4 times a week
    . (c) 1–2 times a week
    . (d) 1–2 times a month
    . (e) Never or nearly never

- Has your snoring ever bothered other people?

    . (a) Yes
    . (b) No
    . (c) Don't know

- Has anyone noticed that you quit breathing during your sleep?

    . (a) Nearly every day
    . (b) 3–4 times a week
    . (c) 1–2 times a week
    . (d) 1–2 times a month
    . (e) Never or nearly never

Category 2

- How often do you feel tired or fatigued after your sleep?

    . (a) Nearly every day
    . (b) 3–4 times a week
    . (c) 1–2 times a week

Box 10.3 (*cont.*)

- (d) 1–2 times a month
- (e) Never or nearly never

- During your waking time, do you feel tired, fatigued, or not up to par?

  - (a) Nearly every day
  - (b) 3–4 times a week
  - (c) 1–2 times a week
  - (d) 1–2 times a month
  - (e) Never or nearly never

- Have you ever nodded off or fallen asleep while driving a vehicle?

  - (a) Yes
  - (b) No If yes:

- How often does this occur?

  - (a) Nearly every day
  - (b) 3–4 times a week
  - (c) 1–2 times a week
  - (d) 1–2 times a month
  - (e) Never or nearly never

Category 3

- Do you have high blood pressure?

  - Yes
  - No
  - Don't know

Categories and scoring

Category 1: items 1, 2, 3, 4, 5

> Item 1: if "yes," assign 1 point
> Item 2: if "c" or "d" is the response, assign 1 point
> Item 3: if "a" or "b" is the response, assign 1 point
> Item 4: if "a" is the response, assign 1 point
> Item 5: if "a" or "b" is the response, assign 2 points
> Add points. Category 1 is positive if the total score is 2 or more points

Category 2: items 6, 7, 8 (item 9 should be noted separately)

> Item 6: if "a" or "b" is the response, assign 1 point
> Item 7: if "a" or "b" is the response, assign 1 point
> Item 8: if "a" is the response, assign 1 point
> Add points. Category 2 is positive if the total score is 2 or more points

Category 3 is positive if the answer to item 10 is "yes" or if the BMI of the patient is greater than 30 kg/m^2 (BMI must be calculated. BMI is defined as weight [kg] divided by height [m] squared, i.e., kg/m^2)

High risk: if there are two or more categories where the score is positive
Low risk: if there is only 1 or no categories where the score is positive
Additional question: item 9 should be noted separately

Adapted from Chung et al. [8].

Box 10.4 American Society of Anesthesiologists (ASA) checklist for obstructive sleep apnea

Category 1: predisposing physical characteristics

- BMI: 35 kg/m^2
- Neck circumference: 43 cm/17 inches (men) or 40 cm/16 inches (women)
- Craniofacial abnormalities affecting the airway
- Anatomical nasal obstruction
- Tonsils nearly touching or touching the midline

Category 2: history of apparent airway obstruction during sleep

Two or more of the following are present (if patient lives alone or sleep is not observed by another person, then only one of the following need be present)

- Snoring (loud enough to be heard through closed door)
- Frequent snoring
- Observed pauses in breathing during sleep
- Awakens from sleep with choking sensation
- Frequent arousals from sleep

Category 3: somnolence

One or more of the following is present

- Frequent somnolence or fatigue despite adequate "sleep"
- Falls asleep easily in a non-stimulating environment (e.g., watching TV, reading, riding in or driving a car) despite adequate "sleep"
- Parent or teacher comments that child appears sleepy during the day, is easily distracted, is overly aggressive, or has difficulty concentrating[a]
- Child often difficult to arouse at usual awakening time[a]

Scoring

- If two or more items in category 1 are positive, category 1 is positive
- If two or more items in category 2 are positive, category 2 is positive
- If one or more items in category 3 are positive, category 3 is positive

High risk of OSA: two or more categories scored as positive
Low risk of OSA: only one or no category scored as positive

Adapted from Gross et al. [9].
[a] Items in brackets refer to pediatric patients.

Cardiovascular System

There are many changes in the cardiovascular system of obese people (Box 10.6). Systemic hypertension, ischemic heart disease, and congestive heart failure are common cardiovascular issues found in the obese patient. Mild to moderate systemic hypertension is found in approximately 50–60% of the obese population. Obesity-induced hypertension is commonly associated with hypervolemia (increased extracellular fluid volume)

Box 10.5 STOP–BANG screening for obstructive sleep apnea

STOP

S (snore)	Have you been told that you snore?	Yes/No
T (tired)	Are you often tired during the day?	Yes/No
O (obstruction)	Do you know if you stop breathing or has anyone witnessed you stop breathing while you are asleep?	
P (pressure)	Do you have high blood pressure or on medication to control high blood pressure?	

Yes/No

If you answered yes to two or more questions on the STOP portion you are at risk for obstructive sleep apnea
To find out if you are at moderate to severe risk of obstructive sleep apnea, complete the BANG questions below

BANG

B (BMI)	Is your body mass index greater than 28?	Yes/No
A (age)	Are you 50 years old or older?	Yes/No
N (neck)	Are you a male with a neck circumference greater than 17 inches, or a female with a neck circumference greater than 16 inches?	
G (gender)	Are you a male?	Yes/No

Yes/No

The more questions you answer yes to on the BANG portion, the greater your risk of having moderate to severe obstructive sleep apnea
$\geq$ 3 yes answers: high risk for OSA
$<$ 3 yes answers: low risk for OSA

Adapted from Chung et al. [8].

Box 10.6 Cardiovascular changes in the obese patient

Hypertension, congestive heart failure, and pulmonary hypertension are more likely in these patients, adding to the challenge of managing safe anesthesia delivery
Framingham study demonstrated direct link between blood pressure and weight

↑ blood volume with obesity
↑ stroke volume with obesity
↑ cardiac output with obesity

↑ Pulmonary wedge pressures

pulmonary hypertension
especially when aggravated by perioperative hypoxic vasoconstriction in the lung

Moderate hypertension is seen in 50%
Risk of ischemic heart disease is doubled in the obese patient

and increased cardiac output. Cardiac output increases approximately 0.1 L/minute for each kilogram of weight gained related to fat tissue. Over time, this increase in systemic hypertension and cardiac output can result in cardiomegaly [9].

Obesity is an independent risk factor for the development of heart disease. Ischemic heart disease is commonly found in patients with a central distribution of fat. Lastly, these individuals are at higher risk for diabetes mellitus and hypercholesterolemia, which are significant risk factors for the development of ischemic heart disease.

Concentric left ventricular hypertrophy can develop over time in patients with systemic hypertension. This increase in ventricular mass eventually causes a decrease in ventricular compliance. In obese patients, coupled with hypervolemia, this increases the risk of congestive heart failure and the development of obesity-induced cardiomyopathy.

Gastrointestinal System

Obesity invokes changes in the gastrointestinal system over time. Although many believe that the increased intra-abdominal pressure, higher rate of hiatal hernias, and increased rate of gastroesophageal reflux exists in this population and leads to an increased risk for aspiration pneumonitis, it is not true. The obese population, without symptoms of gastroesophageal reflux, experiences the same gradient between the stomach and esophagus as the non-obese population. However, gastric emptying in this population may be increased when compared to the non-obese patient. The high incidence of diabetes in the obese population will affect how most providers administer sedation. Given that all diabetic patients have a degree of gastroparesis and therefore a risk of aspiration, nothing by mouth (NPO) status should be carefully evaluated when sedation is planned. It is typical, although not uniform, practice to intravenously administer an histamine-2 blocker such as famotidine and a drug that will increase gastric emptying such as metoclopramide.

The changes invoked by obesity commonly invade the hepatobiliary section of the gastrointestinal system. Fatty infiltration of the liver and the development of gallbladder and biliary tract disease are the most common culprits in obese patients. This may influence the pharmacokinetics (distribution, binding, and elimination) of sedation medications. The volume of distribution is increased because of the hypervolemia and increased cardiac output experienced by obese patients. If liver disease exists, reductions in protein binding can occur, but the overall effects are variable. The elimination of medications can be slowed, especially in obese patients with congestive heart failure. It is not a surprise that providing sedation to this group of patients results in higher morbidity and mortality (Box 10.7).

Box 10.7   Sedation issues with overweight patients

Increased risk of complications
Difficulty with maintaining and recovering the airway
Increased risk of positioning injuries
Increased comorbidities (e.g., diabetes, coronary artery disease, obstructive sleep apnea)

Chronic Obstructive Pulmonary Disease

Chronic obstructive pulmonary disease (COPD) is a common pulmonary disorder that affects millions of people worldwide, and is frequently found in patients with chronic bronchitis or emphysema. It is characterized as a progressive inflammatory process and/or parenchymal destruction of small airways resulting in increased resistance to expiratory gas flow. Patients with COPD need a prolonged period of time for lung emptying. The process may be fixed or variable (reversible with medications), and some patients have features of both.

Because of increased airway resistance and/or parenchymal destruction, patients with COPD have an inefficient gas exchange. The muscles of respiration must generate a significantly greater negative pressure to overcome the increased airway resistance and over time become dysfunctional. This dysfunction ultimately leads to hypoxemia and hypercapnia. Chronic hypercarbia resets the central receptor, thus blunting the ventilatory response to carbon dioxide. Most sedation medications compromise this response and, in the patient with COPD, can result in severe respiratory depression and significant complications if the patient is oversedated. Lastly, most procedures are performed in the supine position, which impairs chest wall muscle function, further reducing functional residual capacity and oxygenation.

Patients with COPD should have a thorough pre-procedural evaluation to ensure that any reversible component to their disease (e.g., bronchospasm, infection) is maximally treated with appropriate drugs (e.g., bronchodilators, antibiotics, or corticosteroids) before proceeding. Bronchodilators should be administered before initiation of sedation, and supplemental oxygen and airway management equipment must be readily available. Sedation medication should be slowly titrated in smaller doses and used sparingly. If possible, local anesthetics should be used in combination with sedation medication to reduce dosing of the latter.

Common procedural complications in this patient population include hypoventilation (hypoxemia and hypercapnia) and bronchospasm. Bronchospasm manifests as wheezing, and it is commonly caused by an exacerbation of the patient's COPD, but an anaphylactoid reaction to a sedation medication should be ruled out.

Coronary Artery Disease

Patients with coronary artery disease present a multitude of challenges for the clinician. Prevalence of coronary artery disease in American adults is 6.2% [10]. This disease presents with various symptoms or conditions, and regardless of the indicator (chest pain, exercise intolerance, hypertension, congestive heart failure, or valvular heart disease), the patient presenting with any of them should be explored meticulously before receiving sedation. There are several issues in these patients that should be cleared up before proceeding.

Frequently, patients presenting for sedation have a history of angina. In the pre-procedure evaluation, the clinician needs to identify if the condition is stable or unstable. Unstable angina is characterized by a change in frequency, intensity, or duration from the usual pattern of angina or if it does not recede with rest or the use of angina medication. Any angina patient classified as unstable should be evaluated by a cardiologist before proceeding with sedation.

Exercise tolerance is a central element of any pre-procedure evaluation. This serves as a rough estimate of the patient's left ventricular ejection fraction and correlates with the heart's ability to function during stressful events. Since patients with coronary artery disease struggle with both oversedation and undersedation, this serves as a useful predictive guide. Anesthesiologists commonly ask patients if they can climb two flights of stairs without chest pain or shortness of breath. This approximates four METs and is the amount of cardiac reserve needed by a patient when starting or concluding an anesthetic for surgery.

Striking the balance between adequate sedation and maximal cardiac functioning can be difficult. Patients with known coronary artery disease who become oversedated experience cardiac complications related to hypotension and/or hypoxemia. On the other hand, the undersedated patient experiences an increase in anxiety and pain, which stimulates the release of catecholamines, and increases the demands on the heart. Because of this, all cardiac medications, especially beta-blockers and statins, should be taken on the day of the procedure. Oxygen is always advised for these patients, and the MONA (morphine, oxygen, nitroglycerin, and aspirin) protocol should serve as an initial treatment plan if cardiac ischemia occurs.

Chronic Renal Failure

Chronic renal failure is a progressive permanent loss of renal function, and it is caused by a multitude of diseases. Hypertension and diabetes mellitus are the two leading causes. These patients ultimately lose significant renal function and require dialysis or transplantation. The manifestations of chronic renal failure are summarized in Box 10.8.

When these patients present for their pre-procedure evaluation, a thorough medication list, post-dialysis labs, and exploration of other comorbidities should be undertaken before proceeding with the case. All antihypertensive medication should be taken on the day that the procedure is to be performed, and because many of these patients are diabetics there should be a mechanism in place for glucose management. Ideally these patients should undergo dialysis within 24 hours of the planned procedure. Knowledge of the pre- and post- dialysis weight will help the clinician better understand the fluid status of the individual. Lastly, the post-dialysis potassium level should not exceed 5.5 mEq/L.

Medication used for sedation should be titrated in slowly, carefully watching hemodynamic response to the medication. These patients are commonly hypertensive and have a decreased intravascular volume or they may respond as if they were hypovolemic because of the central nervous system effects of the antihypertensive medication when combined with the sedation medication. Because of this, they should always be treated as if they were hypovolemic.

Box 10.8 Manifestations of chronic renal failure

Electrolyte imbalance: Hyperkalemia, hypermagnesemia, hypocalcemia
Metabolic acidosis
Unpredictable intravascular fluid status
Anemia: Increased cardiac output, and oxyhemoglobin dissociation curve shifted to the right
Uremic coagulopathies: Platelet dysfunction
Neurologic changes: Encephalopathy
Cardiovascular changes: Systemic hypertension, congestive heart failure, attenuated sympathetic nervous system activity due to antihypertensive drugs

Many pharmacokinetic changes occur in these patients. Hypoalbuminemia and acidosis are usually present, and this can increase the free drug availability of medications that are highly protein-bound. Benzodiazepine dosing should therefore be reduced in this patient population. Most post-dialysis patients have a decreased volume of distribution, and therefore reduced dosing requirements.

Certain sedation medications should be avoided or used very cautiously in patients with chronic renal failure. Meperidine should be avoided because it produces a metabolite, normeperidine, which accumulates in these patients, increasing the risk of seizures. Also, morphine produces a neurotoxic metabolite that is nondialyzable, so it should be avoided in this patient population. Fentanyl is an attractive option, because it produces no active metabolites, but it should be slowly titrated to avoid complications.

Summary

Certain patient populations provide challenging clinical situations for the sedation provider. Patients with cardiovascular disease, COPD, chronic renal failure, obesity, or advanced age are considered high risk and possess a higher rate of procedural complications. Because of this, these higher-risk patients in particular should have a thorough pre-procedural assessment, appropriate ASA standard monitoring (including ventilation with quantitative end-tidal carbon dioxide), careful and potentially decreased sedative dosing considerations, and an overall prudent and safe sedation plan before proceeding, in order to minimize morbidity and mortality. In particular, these patients may require additional personnel, including the presence of an anesthesiologist throughout the procedure to ensure the best outcome possible for these higher-risk patients.

References

1. Hansen PW, Gislason GH, Jørgensen ME, et al. Influence of age on perioperative major adverse cardiovascular events and mortality risks in elective non-cardiac surgery. *Eur J Intern Med.* 2016; S0953–6205(16):30164–9.

2. Gualandro DM, Calderaro D, Yu PC, Caramelli B. Acute myocardial infarction after noncardiac surgery. *Arq Bras Cardiol.* 2012;99(5):1060–7.

3. Tawfic QA, Bellingham G. Postoperative pain management in patients with chronic kidney disease. *J Anaesthesiol Clin Pharmacol* 2015; 31(1):6–13.

4. Ancelin M-L, de Roquefeuil G, Scali J, et al. Long-term post-operative cognitive decline in the elderly: the effects of anesthesia type, apolipoprotein E genotype, and clinical antecedents. *J Alzheimers Dis* 2010; 22(Suppl 3): 105–13.

5. Sessler DI. Perioperative thermoregulation and heat balance. *Lancet* 2016;387(10038):2655–64.

6. Perlman J, Kjaer K. Neonatal and maternal temperature regulation during and after delivery. *Anesth Analg* 2016; 123(1):168–72.

7. Baker S, Yagiela JA. Obesity: a complicating factor for sedation in children. *Pediatr Dent* 2006;28(6):487–93.

8. Chung F, Yegneswaran B, Liao P, et al. STOP questionnaire: a tool to screen patients for obstructive sleep apnea. *Anesthesiology* May 2008;108(5):812–21.

9. Gross JB, Bachenberg KL, Benumof JL, et al., and American Society of Anesthesiologists Task Force on Perioperative Management. Practice guidelines for the perioperative management of patients with obstructive sleep apnea: a report by the American Society of Anesthesiologists Task Force on Perioperative Management of patients

with obstructive sleep apnea. *Anesthesiology*. 2006;104(5):1081–93; quiz 1117–18.

10. Duncan D, Wijeysundera DN. Preoperative cardiac evaluation and management of the patient undergoing major vascular surgery. *Int Anesthesiol Clin*. 2016;54(2):1–32.

Additional Reading

Adams JP, Murphy PG. Obesity in anaesthesia and intensive care. *Br J Anaesth*. 2000;85:91–108.

Chambers EJ, Germain M, Brown E, eds. *Supportive Care for the Renal Patient*. New York, NY: Oxford University Press, 2004.

Hevesi Z. Geriatric disorders. In Hines R, Marschall K, eds., *Anesthesia and Co-Existing Diseases*, 5th ed. Philadelphia, PA: Churchill Livingstone, 2008: 639–49.

Kalarickal P, Fox C, Tsai J, Kaye AD. Perioperative statin use: an update. *Anesthesiol Clin*. 2010;28:739–51.

Maddali MM. Chronic obstructive pulmonary disease: perioperative management. *Middle East J Anesthesiol*. 2008;19:1219–40.

Martin ML, Lennox PH. Sedation and analgesia in the interventional radiology department. *J Vasc Interv Radiol*. 2003;14:1119–28.

Murphy EJ. Acute pain management pharmacology for the patient with patient undergoing major vascular surgery. *Int Anesthesiol Clin*. 2016;54(2):1–32.

Murphy EJ. Acute pain management pharmacology for the patient with concurrent renal or hepatic disease. *Anaesth Intensive Care*. 2005;33:311–22.

Older P, Hall A, Hader R. Cardiopulmonary exercise testing as a screening test for perioperative management of major surgery in the elderly. *Chest*. 1999;116: 355–62.

Tillquist MN, Gabriel RA, Dutton RP, Urman RD. Incidence and risk factors for early postoperative reintubations. *J Clin Anesth*. 2016;31:80–9. doi: 10.1016/j.jclinane.2015.12.038

Vaughan S, McConachie I, Imasogie N. The elderly patient. In McConachie I, ed. *Anesthesia for the High Risk Patient*, 2nd ed. Cambridge: Cambridge University Press, 2009, 225–40.

Respiratory Compromise in Moderate and Deep Sedation

Ashish K. Khanna and Fredrik Olsen

Introduction

Sedation and anesthesia are common triggers of respiratory compromise, which often manifests as depression of respiratory drive, airway occlusion, and resultant hypoxemia and hypercarbia. The respiratory compromise cascade (Figure 11.1) can be understood as a set of states through which a patient moves from respiratory insufficiency toward respiratory failure and, ultimately, respiratory arrest. While the movement of a patient through the cascade is not linear, the effect of increasing momentum with progression to

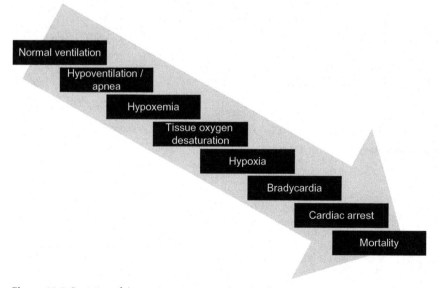

Figure 11.1 Depiction of the respiratory compromise cascade.

each phase occurs. Therefore, the later the patient is recognized in the cascade, the more serious the interventions to restore normal gas exchange become.

The potential to halt patient progression through the cascade and return patients to a healthy state is depicted by the decreasing incidence of complications as we move down the cascade (see Table 11.1). The majority of respiratory complications are thus transient and many do not cause lasting patient injury or harm [1]. In cases of hypoxemia, simple

Table 11.1 Incidence of patient safety endpoints on the respiratory compromise cascade during moderate and deep sedation

Definition of respiratory compromise	Incidence in clinical trials when using standard of care	Incidence in retrospective studies
Mild desaturation, < 90%	Beitz 2012: 19.79% Friedrich-Rust 2014: 32.33% Mehta 2016: 54.5% Qadeer 2009: 68.55% Klare 2016: 44.35% Zongming 2014: 19.5%	Bellolio 2016: 2.30% Campbell 2006: 1.4% Cravero 2009: 1.54% Green 2015: 2% non-trauma; 1% trauma Kamat 2015: 1.48% McGrane 2011: 1.40%
Severe desaturation, < 85%	Beitz 2012: 7.75% Friedrich-Rust 2014: 8.27% Klare 2016: 26.09% Mehta 2016: 17.57% Qadeer 2009: 30.65% Zongming 2014: 7.8%	
Bradycardia	Beitz 2012: 8.29% Friedrich-Rust 2014: 1.5% Klare 2016: 9.57% Mehta 2016: 7.66% Zongming 2014: 8.36%	Bellolio 2016: 1.41% Green 2015: 3% non-trauma; 2% trauma
Hypotension	Beitz 2012: 4.01% Campbell 2016: 1.4% Friedrich-Rust 2014: 16.54% Klare 2016: 10.43% Mehta 2016: 8.11% Qadeer 2009: 4.84% Zongming 2014: 3.9%	Campbell 2006: 1.3% Green 2015: 16% non-trauma; 20% trauma McGrane 2011: 2.33%
Bag–mask ventilation required	Beitz 2012: 0.27% Campbell 2016: 0.6% Friedrich-Rust 2014: 3.34% Klare 2016: 0.87% Slagelse 2013: 1.08% Zongming 2014: 0.84%	McGrane 2011: 0.93% Sayfo 2012: 1.55%

Randomized, controlled trials: Beitz 2012 [18]; Campbell 2016 [19]; Friedrich-Rust 2014 [20]; Klare 2016 [21]; Mehta 2016 [22]; Slagelse 2013 [17]; Qadeer 2009 [23]; Zongming 2014 [24]. Retrospective studies: Bellolio 2016 [25]; Campbell 2006 [26]; Cravero 2009 [27]; Green 2015 [28]; Kamat 2015 [29]; McGrane 2011 [30]; Sayfo 2012 [31].

airway maneuvers such as a chin lift can reopen the airway and prevent patient harm. Progression to hypoxia may be corrected via supplemental oxygen, although care is required to ensure that this does not artificially mask an ongoing ventilatory problem [2, 3]. The next stop on the respiratory compromise cascade, respiratory arrest, is one of the most common causes of a code blue event in the hospital setting [3]. The progression from respiratory failure to arrest has two major causes [4]:

- Type I respiratory failure: Respiratory arrest that follows from a ventilation–perfusion mismatch and impaired alveolar oxygen diffusion.
- Type II respiratory failure: Alveolar hypoventilation, which results in retained alveolar carbon dioxide and respiratory arrest. This pathway is of particular pertinence to the sedation team because it is linked to both opiates and disordered breathing [5].

Clinical Significance of Respiratory Compromise in Sedation

Medications used in procedural sedation have key characteristics to ensure patient amnesia, somnolence, and analgesia. Almost all these medications have the potential alone or in combination to cause respiratory compromise. Indeed, respiratory complications are the most common form of adverse event during procedural sedation [6, 7]. Respiratory complications are most often associated with oversedation and/or an adverse patient response to medication [6, 8, 9]. In addition to patient safety, respiratory compromise events have economic impact [10]. The Agency for Healthcare Research and Quality reported in 2010 that respiratory compromise was one of the most frequent conditions contributing to increasing hospital costs for Medicare-covered admissions [11]. It was associated with nearly 386,000 inpatient stays and a cost of $7.7 billion in 2007. Two reviews of US closed claims reported that inadequate oxygenation/ventilation was the most frequent event resulting in a claim related to sedation outside of the operating room [12, 13]. The direct cost of respiratory complications and their potential to evolve into expensive legal proceedings has been estimated to be a major factor in the overall cost of sedation outside of the operating room [14, 15].

Because of the complex and broad spectrum of sedation providers and patients, consensus uniform reporting of safety events during these cases varies considerably. For example, in clinical trials using moderate sedation, the definition of mild oxygen desaturation varies from an oxygen level of < 95%, through < 93%, to the more frequently reported < 90% for at least 10 seconds [16, 17]. The application of different end-point definitions makes comparison between studies and settings difficult. When consistently defined and reported, complications during sedation are more common than many would anticipate (Table 11.1). Clinical trials comparing standard of care monitoring with capnography monitoring during moderate sedation report that mild desaturation < 90% occurs in one in five patients, severe desaturation < 85% occurs in one in five patients, while bag mask ventilation is likely to be required at least once per every 333 sedations using moderate or deep sedation. Retrospective studies report consistently lower complication rates but are likely hampered by limitations to end-point definitions and reporting. These studies may indicate the rate of more clinically significant events that could be entered into reporting systems as efforts are made to standardize patient safety and risk assessment worldwide. Although many may consider mild oxygen desaturation to be of minor clinical importance, several recent studies have suggested that mild desaturation can have an impact on post-surgical outcomes [7]. If we consider a mild oxygen desaturation event as one of the first steps on the respiratory compromise cascade, its clinical importance increases. If a patient's oxygenation level is prevented from falling below 90%, the potential for progression to more serious complications may be averted (Figure 11.1).

Risk Factors for Respiratory Compromise in Sedation

For an individual patient, the risk of respiratory compromise may be much lower or higher than indicated by analysis of general trends and incidence rates. It is impossible to accurately quantify risk for each individual patient, but through consideration of risk factors, informative stratification can be achieved. Risk factors for respiratory compromise fall under three main headings: procedure profile, patient characteristics, and area of care (Table 11.2). There are clearly procedures and settings in which patient safety is more at risk; in no case, though, is a procedure using sedation 100% safe.

Beyond patient risk factors, sedation is not binary but a continuum, with different levels of sedation associated with different levels of patient consciousness. As consciousness cannot be easily quantified, the levels of sedation targeted and achieved are subjectively measured. In line with standard practice, while under moderate sedation, a patient's ability to independently maintain ventilatory function, to be able to breathe on his or her own accord, should not be compromised. In contrast, deep sedation can result in ventilatory function being impaired and necessitating ventilatory assistance. Partly due to the subjective nature of sedation levels, the movement of a patient into a deeper sedated state than planned is possible and can have potentially serious consequences.

Studies indicate that the risk of oversedation during procedural sedation can be substantial. Sayfo and colleagues reported 91.2% of patients receiving propofol with a target of moderate sedation for implantable cardioverter-defibrillator procedures reached deep sedation [31]. High rates of oversedation were also reported by Erden

Table 11.2 Risk factors associated with respiratory compromise

Level of risk adjustment	Procedure	Patient	Area of care
Strong	Choice of sedative [29, 30] Oversedation Inadequate monitoring [1] Procedure length	ASA status > 2 [14] Respiratory disease [14, 29] Obesity [31]	
Moderate	Patient positioning [32] Route of sedative administration [14]	Increased age [14, 32] Trauma [25] Concomitant medication	Nurse to patient ratio [29] Level of risk education [14]

et al., who used propofol 0.5 mg/kg plus ketamine 0.25 mg/kg during interventional radiology procedures. In this study, 57.8% of patients reached a Ramsay sedation level greater than 4, although a level 2–3 was targeted [32]. Other reported rates for oversedation are much lower, in the range of 0.02%, and so its incidence is likely dependent on many factors such as procedure length and the sedative given [33]. The sedation team should be aware of patient and procedural risk factors for over-sedation and use appropriate monitoring to minimize the risks for respiratory compromise [34, 35].

Prevention and Treatment of Respiratory Compromise

Prevention

In planning for a patient's care during procedural sedation, all members of the sedation and procedural team must keep patient safety at the forefront of their thinking. It is important to undertake a thorough risk assessment to identify patients at higher risk of respiratory compromise and other sedation-related and procedure-related complications. A simple but informative risk score is the American Society of Anesthesiologists (ASA) Physical Status Classification, which has six classes. Although designed for surgery requiring general anesthesia, the ASA classification can be applied to both moderate and deep sedation. Any patient in Class 3 or above is considered to be at higher risk of respiratory complications, and additional care should be taken with these patients to ensure that the procedure is completed safely [35, 36].

Other characteristics to consider before undertaking the procedure are:

- NPO (nothing by mouth) status
- airway anatomy
- presence of obstructive sleep apnea
- overweight and obesity
- smoking, drug and/or alcohol abuse
- older age, > 70 years
- any history of failed sedation or aborted procedures
- past medical, surgical, and anesthetic history

Ongoing education of the sedation team on the dangers of sedation and pharmacological attributes of sedatives and analgesics in use is of paramount importance [35, 37, 38]. Care should also be taken if the patient uses concomitant medication that can also increase the risk of respiratory compromise, for example compounds such as promethazine and diphenhydramine, and a list of such drugs should be maintained and made available to the sedation team.

Identification

Patient monitoring is the standard of care during procedural sedation, and at a minimum should include pulse oximetry and visual assessment by a dedicated member of the sedation team. For moderate sedation the use of capnography is indicated unless it is not possible due to the nature of the procedure or patient [35,

36]. A protocol for monitoring and the frequency of monitoring should be set by the institution to balance procedure efficacy, cost, and most importantly, patient safety. The early stages of respiratory compromise present most commonly as airway obstruction, and either obstructive or central (sedation-mediated) apnea. Compared with minimal requirements in monitoring (pulse oximetry and visual assessment), the addition of continuous monitoring of patient ventilation using capnography has been shown to reduce the incidence of complications along the respiratory compromise cascade [23]. Providers who fail to monitor airway patency and ventilation with continuous capnography risk being presented with a desaturation event caused by obstructive or central apnea. Indeed, patients who are apneic can maintain saturations > 90% for over a minute. Therefore, a desaturation due to airway obstruction or apnea may represent a patient in whom ventilation has been compromised for some time. The resulting respiratory acidosis and hypercapnia can set the stage metabolically for rapid progression through the respiratory compromise cascade. This is one of the reasons why visual assessment of patient respiration must be used in conjunction with pulse oximetry monitoring. Visual assessment must consider:

- *patient depth of sedation*, using tools such as the Ramsay Sedation Scale: a Ramsay score of 2 is usually considered optimal for moderate sedation
- *respiratory rate*: to assess adequacy of ventilation and to identify possible apnea (no breath for 15 seconds)
- *air entry on auscultation*: to assess adequacy of ventilation
- *heart rate*: to evaluate potential bradycardia or tachycardia
- *patient appearance*: may allow for assessment of general well-being, with loss of color and clammy skin potential indicators of problems

Treatment

It is impossible to prevent every potential episode of respiratory compromise and so every sedation team must be prepared when the time comes to respond to a patient. In fact, most paradigms in current sedation care focus on rescue over prevention. It is outside of standard practice for any sedation to be performed without having reversal agents and an airway recovery kit at hand. Appropriate monitoring and early identification of patient compromise should negate the use of these interventions in the majority of cases. The intervention required is patient and case dependent, but in general the more severe the respiratory complication, the more complex the rescue intervention (Table 11.3) and the greater the disruption to the planned procedure.

First and foremost, the arterial oxygen saturation must be normalized as quickly as possible. In some cases, when airway obstruction is the cause, a simple chin-lift or other airway maneuver may be sufficient to rescue the patient. Other situations require more involvement to increase the oxygen saturation. A common option is the use of supplemental oxygen, though the patency of the patient's airway must first be confirmed. In more severe compromise, intubation and/or bag–mask ventilation may be required to stabilize the patient and allow time for an appropriate rescue response. In cases of severe or increasing respiratory compromise, timely involvement of an anesthesiologist may be the best course of action.

Table 11.3 Guideline recommendations for interventions by respiratory complication

End point	Intervention options if mild–moderate	Intervention options if severe
Oxygen desaturation	Airway repositioning Vigorous tactile stimulation Supplemental or increased oxygen delivery	Intubation Oral or nasal airway Bag–mask ventilation
Apnea	Vigorous tactile stimulation Airway repositioning (if obstructive apnea)	Intubation Bag–mask ventilation Reversal agents
Airway obstruction	Airway repositioning Suctioning	Intubation Additional sedation agents Administration of neuromuscular blockade drugs
Bradycardia	Vigorous tactile stimulation Airway repositioning Suctioning Supplemental or increased oxygen delivery	Intubation Bag-mask with assisted ventilation Chest compressions
Hypotension		Intravenous fluids Appropriate medication Chest compressions

Summary

While respiratory compromise can occur at any level of sedation, it is clear that deeper levels present higher risk. Inadvertent oversedation and the movement of patients into deeper planes of sedation is relatively common and the identification of such events should be a target of patient periprocedural monitoring. With effective monitoring and a well-trained sedation team, the incidence and risk of respiratory compromise progressing to respiratory failure and respiratory arrest can be reduced. In the event that a patient develops respiratory compromise, working quickly to ensure airway patency, oxygen delivery, and adequate ventilation are the cornerstones of team-rescue action. Once the patient is stabilized, the sedative dose and patient risk factors should be reviewed to minimize the risk of recurrent respiratory compromise.

References

1. Cook T, MacDougall-Davis S. Complications and failure of airway management. *Br J Anaesth*. 2012;109 (Suppl 1):i68–85.

2. Lynn LA, Curry JP. Patterns of unexpected in-hospital deaths: a root cause analysis. *Patient Saf Surg*. 2011;5(1):3.

3. Lamberti JP. Respiratory monitoring in general care units. *Respir Care*. 2020;65(6):870–81.

4. Prasad S, O'Neill S. Respiratory failure. *Surgery (Oxford)*. 2021;39(10):654–9.

5. Khanna A, Saager L, Bergese SD, et al. Opioid-induced respiratory depression increases hospital costs and length of stay in patients recovering on the general

care floor. *BMC Anesthesiol.* 2021;21(1):88.

6. Jones PM, Cherry RA, Allen BN, et al. Association between handover of anesthesia care and adverse postoperative outcomes among patients undergoing major surgery. *JAMA.* 2018;319(2):143.

7. van Schaik EPC, Blankman P, Van Klei WA, et al. Hypoxemia during procedural sedation in adult patients: a retrospective observational study. *Can J Anesth.* 2021;68(9):1349–57.

8. Stone AB, Brovman EY, Greenberg P, Urman RD. A medicolegal analysis of malpractice claims involving anesthesiologists in the gastrointestinal endoscopy suite (2007–2016). *J Clin Anesth.* 2018;48:15–20.

9. Yeh T, Beutler SS, Urman RD. What we can learn from nonoperating room anesthesia registries: analysis of clinical outcomes and closed claims data. *Curr Opin Anesthesiol.* 2020;33(4):527–32.

10. McGrath SP, McGovern KM, Perreard IM, et al. Inpatient respiratory arrest associated with sedative and analgesic medications: impact of continuous monitoring on patient mortality and severe morbidity. *J Patient Saf.* 2021;17(8):557–61.

11. Wier LM, Henke R, Friedman B. Diagnostic groups with rapidly increasing costs, by payer, 2001–2007. In *Healthcare Cost and Utilization Project (HCUP) Statistical Briefs*. Rockville, MD: Agency for Healthcare Research and Quality (US), 2006, Feb. Statistical Brief 91.

12. Robbertze R, Posner KL, Domino KB. Closed claims review of anesthesia for procedures outside the operating room. *Curr Opin Anesthesiol.* 2006;19(4):436–42.

13. Metzner J, Posner KL, Domino KB. The risk and safety of anesthesia at remote locations: the US closed claims analysis. *Curr Opin Anesthesiol.* 2009;22(4):502–8.

14. Urman RD, Moucharite M, Flynn C, Nuryyeva E, Ray CE. Impact of respiratory compromise in inpatient interventional radiology procedures with moderate sedation in the United States. *Radiology.* 2019;292(3):702–10.

15. Saunders R, Erslon M, Vargo J. Modeling the costs and benefits of capnography monitoring during procedural sedation for gastrointestinal endoscopy. Endosc Int Open. 2016;4(03):E340–51.

16. Ishikawa M, Sakamoto A. Postoperative desaturation and bradypnea after general anesthesia in non-ICU patients: a retrospective evaluation. *J Clin Monit Comput.* 2020 Feb;34(1):81–7.

17. Slagelse C, Vilmann P, Hornslet P, Jørgensen HL, Horsted TI. The role of capnography in endoscopy patients undergoing nurse-administered propofol sedation: a randomized study. *Scand J Gastroenterol.* 2013;48(10):1222–30.

18. Beitz A, Riphaus A, Meining A, et al. Capnographic monitoring reduces the incidence of arterial oxygen desaturation and hypoxemia during propofol sedation for colonoscopy: a randomized, controlled study (ColoCap Study). *Am J Gastroenterol.* 2012;107(8):1205–12.

19. Campbell SG, Magee KD, Zed PJ, et al. End-tidal capnometry during emergency department procedural sedation and analgesia: a randomized, controlled study. *World J Emerg Med.* 2016;7(1):13–8.

20. Friedrich-Rust M, Welte M, Welte C, et al. Capnographic monitoring of propofol-based sedation during colonoscopy. *Endoscopy.* 2014;46(3):236–44.

21. Klare P, Reiter J, Meining A, et al. Capnographic monitoring of midazolam and propofol sedation during ERCP: a randomized controlled study (EndoBreath Study). *Endoscopy.* 2016;48(1):42–50.

22. Mehta PP, Kochhar G, Albeldawi M, et al. Capnographic monitoring in routine EGD and colonoscopy with moderate sedation: a prospective, randomized, controlled trial. *Am J Gastroenterol.* 2016;111(3):395.

23. Qadeer MA, Vargo JJ, Dumot JA, et al. Capnographic monitoring of respiratory activity improves safety of sedation for

endoscopic cholangiopancreatography and ultrasonography. *Gastroenterology.* 2009;136(5):1568–76; quiz 1819–20.

24. Zongming J, Zhonghua C, Xiangming F. Sidestream capnographic monitoring reduces the incidence of arterial oxygen desaturation during propofol ambulatory anesthesia for surgical abortion. *Med Sci Monit.* 2014;20:2336–42.

25. Bellolio MF, Gilani WI, Barrionuevo P, et al. Incidence of adverse events in adults undergoing procedural sedation in the emergency department: a systematic review and meta-analysis. *Acad Emerg Med.* 2016;23(2):119–34.

26. Campbell SG, Magee KD, Kovacs GJ, et al. Procedural sedation and analgesia in a Canadian adult tertiary care emergency department: a case series. *Can J Emerg Med.* 2006 Mar;8(2):85–93.

27. Cravero JP, Beach ML, Blike GT, et al. The incidence and nature of adverse events during pediatric sedation/anesthesia with propofol for procedures outside the operating room: a report from the Pediatric Sedation Research Consortium. *Anesth Analg.* 2009;108(3):795.

28. Green RS, Butler MB, Campbell SG, Erdogan M. Adverse events and outcomes of procedural sedation and analgesia in major trauma patients. *J Emerg Trauma Shock.* 2015;8(4):210–5.

29. Kamat PP, McCracken CE, Gillespie SE, et al. Pediatric critical care physician-administered procedural sedation using propofol: a report from the Pediatric Sedation Research Consortium database. *Pediatr Crit Care Med.* 2015;16(1):11.

30. McGrane O, Hopkins G, Nielson A, Kang C. Procedural sedation with propofol: a retrospective review of the experiences of an emergency medicine residency program 2005 to 2010. *Am J Emerg Med.* 2012;30(5):706–11.

31. Sayfo S, Vakil KP, Alqaqa'a A, et al. A retrospective analysis of proceduralist-directed, nurse-administered propofol sedation for implantable cardioverter–defibrillator procedures. *Heart Rhythm.* 2012;9(3):342–6.

32. Erden IA, Pamuk AG, Akinci SB, Koseoglu A, Aypar U. Comparison of two ketamine–propofol dosing regimens for sedation during interventional radiology procedures. *Minerva Anestesiol.* 2009;76(4):260–5.

33. Karamnov S, Sarkisian N, Grammer R, Gross WL, Urman RD. Analysis of adverse events associated with adult moderate procedural sedation outside the operating room. *J Patient Saf.* 2017;13(3):111–21.

34. Martin JG, Bercu ZL, Becker L, et al. Modifying institutional guidelines reduces the likelihood of oversedation during interventional procedures. *J Am Coll Radiol.* 2018;15(8):1185–7.

35. Hinkelbein J, Lamperti M, Akeson J, et al. European Society of Anaesthesiology and European Board of Anaesthesiology guidelines for procedural sedation and analgesia in adults. *Eur J Anaesthesiol.* 2018;35(1):6–24.

36. Practice guidelines for moderate procedural sedation and analgesia 2018: a report by the American Society of Anesthesiologists Task Force on Moderate Procedural Sedation and Analgesia, the American Association of Oral and Maxillofacial Surgeons, American College of Radiology, American Dental Association, American Society of Dentist Anesthesiologists, and Society of Interventional Radiology. *Anesthesiology.* 2018;128(3):437–79.

37. Jarzyna D, Jungquist CR, Pasero C, et al. American Society for Pain Management Nursing guidelines on monitoring for opioid-induced sedation and respiratory depression. *Pain Manag Nurs.* 2011;12(3):118–145.e10.

38. Tran TT, Beutler SS, Urman RD. Moderate and deep sedation training and pharmacology for nonanesthesiologists: recommendations for effective practice. *Curr Opin Anesthesiol.* 2019;32(4):457–63.

Management of Complications of Moderate and Deep Sedation

Saninuj Nini Malayaman, Elyse M. Cornett, Alan D. Kaye, and Henry Liu

Introduction

Intravenous pharmacologic sedation is often chosen for surgical and nonsurgical procedures and is administered by an anesthesiologist, nurse anesthetist, or other trained professional. Sedation is described as a continuum, encompassing minimal, moderate, and deep sedation that can be categorized according to the patient's level of consciousness (Figure 12.1). This categorization is subjective and the different levels of sedation can be achieved through changes in medication choice and dosage. There exist overlapping zones between levels of sedation. In clinical practice, deep sedation and general anesthesia share many of the same features in terms of patient awareness, lack of responsiveness, and risk of airway compromise.

Sedation, as opposed to general anesthesia, may be requested for reasons of surgeon preference, patient preference, cost, and availability of resources. For patients undergoing diagnostic and therapeutic procedures, intravenous sedation can be a positive experience by reducing anxiety, pain, and discomfort. Further benefits include decreasing stress on the cardiovascular system.

Importantly, intravenous sedation can potentially cause complications. Clinicians requesting and administering sedation should be aware of these possible complications and be prepared to manage changes in the patient's hemodynamic and respiratory status. In many respects, moderate and deep sedations can be more challenging for anesthesia providers than general anesthesia with endotracheal intubation. There are several factors

Minimal Sedation	Moderate Sedation	Deep Sedation	General Anesthesia
Awake	Asleep, Easy to awaken	Asleep, Difficult to awaken	Unconscious

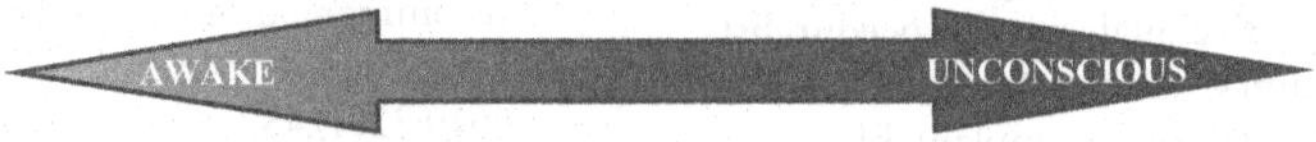

AWAKE　　　　　　　　　　　　　　　　UNCONSCIOUS

Figure 12.1 The sedation continuum.

that make sedation challenging: (1) sedation procedures are frequently requested for sites away from operating rooms with likely limitation of anesthesia supplies, equipment, and personnel; (2) procedure room layouts may place anesthesia machines and sedation providers at a great distance from the patient; (3) airway obstruction is likely since the airway is not provided an open path via an endotracheal tube or held open with a laryngeal mask airway. Boynes et al. reported that in dental procedures airway obstruction occurred in 18 out of 286 patients, and nausea/vomiting in 12 out of 286 patients, although no severe complications occurred [1].

Sedation Scoring Scales

Scoring systems have been developed to assess the patient's depth of sedation; these include the Richmond Agitation–Sedation Scale (RASS), Sedation Agitation Scale (SAS) and the Inova Health System Sedation Scale (ISS) [2] (Table 12.1). The RASS and SAS each assess agitation in addition to consciousness. Sedation scoring scales are logical, easily administered, and readily recalled evaluation systems with inter-rater reliability. Scoring systems, with levels for awake states, are used for ventilated, non-ventilated, sedated, and non-sedated adult patients in both medical and surgical intensive care units (ICUs) [3] as opposed to patients undergoing procedural sedation.

Because procedural sedation often involves hypnotic medications in addition to analgesic medication, the ISS, which does not include awake states, may be a more practical scale to assess level of sedation [4]. In the ISS, levels 1 and 2 appear equivalent to minimal sedation, levels 3 and 4 are equivalent to moderate sedation, level 5 corresponds best to deep sedation, and level 6 is general anesthesia.

Preoperative Risk Assessment

Prevention of complications starts with a thorough pre-procedural patient assessment. Knowledge of a patient's coexisting diseases gives the clinician insight into possible medications or equipment that may be necessary and to plan for successful management of potential complications. Further details of some of the patient-related risk factors discussed in the following subsections can be found in Chapter 10.

Table 12.1 Inova Health System Sedation Scale (ISS)

Level	Description
1	Alert
2	Occasionally drowsy
3	Dozing intermittently
4	Asleep, easy to waken
5	Difficult to awaken
6	Unresponsive

Source: Nisbet and Mooney-Cotter [2].

Patient-Related Factors

Age

Advanced age is a factor for developing complications for patients receiving intravenous sedation. Closing capacity, the volume in the lungs at which respiratory bronchioles begin to collapse, becomes equal to functional residual capacity (FRC) at the age of 66. Older edentulous patients have a higher probability of having loose oropharyngeal tissue, which potentially narrows or obstructs the airway when in the supine position.

The elderly experience metabolic changes such as reduction in first-pass metabolism that can lead to increased bioavailability of sedation medications which predisposes older patients to sedative, hypnotic, and analgesic complications. Older patients also tend to have more coexisting medical conditions often with related declines in renal function [5]. A prudent approach to sedation of elderly patients is to decrease the initial dose and monitor closely during incremental dosing. Additionally, the clinician should attempt to minimize the use of multiple sedatives, because of potential synergistic effects.

A study of endoscopic retrograde cholangiopancreatography performed under propofol sedation in 450 patients (126 patients $\geq$ 65 years of age, 324 patients < 65 years, with a higher incidence of comorbid conditions in those $\geq$ 65 years, $p < 0.001$) reported anesthetic complications in 6% of patients, but found no statistical significance among American Society of Anesthesiologists (ASA) groups ($p = 0.7$) or age groups ($p = 0.1$). No procedure-related mortality was documented. The authors concluded that deep intravenous propofol sedation is safe in elderly patients and has a low anesthetic complication rate [6]. Another study of procedural sedations in elderly patients in the emergency department found no statistically significant difference in complication rates for patients 65 years or older, although there was a significant decrease in mean sedation dosing with increased age and ASA score [7].

In pediatric patients, airway obstruction and respiratory depression are the most common complications, with children aged 1–5 years at greatest risk [8]. For pediatric patients with reactive airway disease (asthma), bronchodilator therapy should be continued until the procedure commences. Airway irritants and histamine-releasing agents should be avoided if at all possible. The patient's neurologic status should be evaluated before surgery, and any intracranial pressure-increasing medication should be avoided if the patient has preexisting increased intracranial pressure. In most cases, pediatric patients are not ideal candidates for sedation in clinical practice; a significant number of procedures in pediatric patients will be done under general anesthesia (see chapters 23 and 24).

Body Weight

Obesity, defined as body mass index (BMI) equal or greater than 30 kg/m^2, increases the risk for moderate and deep sedation, including both ventilatory and circulatory risks. Clinically severe obesity, also known as morbid obesity, with a BMI equal or greater than 40, confers the greatest challenges for mask ventilation and oxygen saturation as well as initiation, maintenance, and recovery from sedation. A consultation with an anesthesiologist is highly recommended for patients with severe obesity.

A higher BMI is associated with a higher risk for procedural sedation. Obese patients usually have a short, thick neck and a large tongue. A bulk of soft tissue and large tongue can cause supraglottic obstruction during sedation. Patients with clinically severe obesity have associated physiological changes including decreased total lung capacity, decreased arterial oxygen pressure (PaO$_2$), increased arterial carbon dioxide pressure (PaCO$_2$), and increased oxygen consumption. Additionally, patients that have undergone bariatric surgery may require higher sedative doses than those without a history of bariatric surgery [9, 10].

Obese patients have a larger amount of adipose mass and an increase in lean body weight. Increased fat mass leads to an increase in volume of distribution for lipophilic medications such as propofol. Although a greater dose of propofol may be needed to achieve the desired level of sedation, it is advisable to start with a low dose of sedative or anxiolytic mediations and proceed to titrate these medications slowly. For most medications used for sedation, dosing in obese patients should be calculated for lean body weight as opposed to total body weight. Realistic goals of sedation should be discussed and patients should be informed that light sedation might be necessary for their safety. Communication with the patient is key to providing a satisfactory sedation experience [10].

NPO Status

Fasting, nil/nulla per os (NPO), guidelines are a subject of much debate. The goal of preoperative fasting is to decrease gastric content and reduce risk of pulmonary aspiration. Current guidelines are applied to all healthy patients, with the exception of patients in labor, undergoing elective procedures under sedation, regional, and general anesthesia [11]. These recommendations allow clear fluid up to 2 hours and milk and some solids up to 6 hours preoperatively; in practice, prolonged fasting beyond these time periods often occurs. Given the low incidence of pulmonary aspiration in elective procedures, prolonged fasting – which can occur in afternoon cases, when patients are told to have nothing after midnight – should be avoided [12]. If a patient has a full stomach and is a high risk for aspiration, sedation should be avoided, and the scheduled procedure should be done under general anesthesia with a secured airway.

Airway Anatomy

The following anatomic features predispose patients to a high risk of difficult ventilation with a face mask or tracheal intubation:

- micrognathia: mandibular hypoplasia, lower jaw is undersized
- retrognathia: mandible displaced posteriorly
- prognathia: protruding upper jaw
- macroglossia: large tongue
- protruding teeth
- high arched palate
- glossoptosis: downward displacement of the tongue
- deviated trachea
- short, thick, and firm neck

One or more of these features should be anticipated in a patient with syndromes including: Beckwith Wiedemann, Trisomy 21, Pierre Robin, Treacher Collins, Goldenhar, Alpert, Klippel Feil, and Hallermann–Streiff–François.

Pregnancy

Pregnancy is accompanied by airway changes due to edema of soft tissue mucosa of the upper respiratory tract. This swelling can lead to difficulties in ventilation and increased risk of difficult endotracheal intubation. The gravid uterus and consequent increased abdominal pressure during pregnancy pushes upwards against the diaphragm leading to decreased FRC by 20% and increased oxygen demand by 20%. If sedative medications are given, the provider should be aware that the pregnant patient will have a faster time to desaturation and should be prepared to administer supplemental oxygen [13, 14].

Pregnant patients have increased risk of aspiration due to reduced lower esophageal sphincter tone and increased gastric volume. Pharmacologic prophylaxis, such as a histamine-2 (H_2)-receptor blocker and metoclopramide, may be used to decrease the aspiration risk. Benzodiazepine medication can be used to decrease anxiety. Regional anesthesia is recommended to avoid airway management. All pregnant patients should be treated as a full stomach and, if a regional anesthetic technique is not used, general anesthesia with rapid sequence induction is mandatory [14].

Medications commonly administered for general anesthesia are safe during pregnancy; however, insufficient evidence exists on the safety of sugammadex in terms of teratogenicity and this should be avoided for neuromuscular blockade reversal. Maternal death, miscarriage, and fetal loss occur at a higher rate in the first trimester; therefore, delaying surgery until the second trimester is recommended when possible [14, 15].

Substance Use Disorder

Providing sedation for a person with an opioid use disorder can be challenging. Understanding the level of sedation required for the particular diagnostic or therapeutic procedure can help guide the amount of anxiolytic and sedation medications administered. These patients usually have developed a high tolerance to sedatives and a low tolerance to pain and discomfort. During the pre-anesthetic evaluation and informed consent process, a discussion about expectations for pain levels in the peri-procedural period will help set realistic goals for pain management.

Acknowledging the increase in deaths due to prescription opioid overdose, various states have established prescription drug monitoring programs (PDMPs) to encourage appropriate opioid prescribing, reduce opioid misuse, and reducing deaths from opioid overdose. These programs have been effective with clinicians expressing greater satisfaction when the PDMP date is accessed via electronic health records integration [16].

Current opioid users are more likely to require postoperative opioid analgesics for routine procedures. However, they are also more likely to receive inappropriate prescriptions [17].

Coexisting Pulmonary Diseases

Any pulmonary disease compromising the oxygen-delivering pathway or oxygenating function will increase the risk of airway complications when a patient undergoes intravenous sedation. The risk increases in parallel with the severity of the underlining pulmonary pathology.

Chronic obstructive pulmonary disease (COPD) patients have a blunted ventilatory response to carbon dioxide, and commonly used sedatives further decrease the ventilatory response to carbon dioxide. These patients also have increased airway reactivity and are at risk for bronchoconstriction and bronchospasm if airway management becomes necessary [18]. When a patient with COPD is scheduled for a procedure with intravenous sedation, consider administering a bronchodilator prior to sedation. The total dose of sedatives should be decreased to avoid events requiring airway manipulation.

Smokers are at increased risk for developing procedural hypoventilation and hypoxemia, especially when they have COPD and decreased pulmonary function. Smokers usually have increased airway secretions and are more prone to coughing, bronchospasm, and laryngospasm.

Obstructive sleep apnea (OSA) is caused by the total or partial collapse of the airway, which can lead to episodes of apnea and hypopnea during sleep. Being overweight is a strong risk factor for OSA, and OSA may increase the risk of cardiopulmonary adverse events during endoscopy [19].

Coexisting Cardiovascular Diseases

Patients with coronary artery disease present risks during sedation in cases of both undersedation and oversedation. Oversedation can lead to cardiac complications as a consequence of hypoxemia and hypotension. Undersedation that does not adequately control pain and anxiety will be accompanied by an increased catecholamine plasma level, pain, hypertension, and tachycardia, which will increase cardiac workload and oxygen demand [20].

Sedation providers need to achieve a balance by providing adequate sedation so that the patient is calm and does not have a high catecholamine level while, at the same time, avoiding oversedation with subsequent hypoventilation- and hypotension-related problems.

Patients with heart failure and a low ejection fraction will have delayed onset of sedation when given medications intravenously. A cautious approach will minimize risk of oversedation. Goals for sedation should include encouraging inotropy and forward flow without hypotension and ischemia. Medications, in classes other than sedatives and hypnotics, may be necessary to maintain blood pressure and control heart rate in these patients.

Coexisting Liver Diseases

The preoperative evaluation of patients with liver disease should focus on a history of alcohol use, which may increase tolerance to benzodiazepines and opioid medications. Gastric emptying may be delayed with an increased risk of aspiration.

During a procedure, hepatic dysfunction may lead to decreased metabolism, elimination, and excretion of multiple sedatives and hypnotics. In advanced liver disease, decreases in blood flow and portosystemic shunting can decrease the clearance of medications. Lower albumin production decreased the amount of plasma binding of mendicants, which leads to greater availability of medication and increased volume of distribution of sedatives and hypnotics. For most sedative and hypnotic medications, reductions in both dosing and frequency should be considered. In the postoperative period, recovery time may be prolonged due to decreased metabolism [21].

Other Coexisting Diseases

Anterior mediastinal mass, post-radiation therapy for cancer in the head and neck, thyroid diseases, and associated tracheomalacia could present serious airway problems during procedures under moderate to deep sedation. Maintaining spontaneous breathing is crucial, and keeping the patient in the beach-chair (also known as sitting or Fowler's) position can help if there are problems maintaining the airway in the supine position. Although some debate has been raised over the necessity of continuous end-tidal capnography for procedural sedation, it remains a useful and essential monitor of changes in ventilation and should be used when feasible for moderate to deep sedation [22].

Procedure-Related Factors

Position

The supine (dorsal decubitus) position, routinely used for most procedures, causes abdominal contents to exert cephalad pressure on the diaphragm and lungs. This position reduces the FRC by almost 30% compared with an upright position. When the patient is in the supine position, the closing lung capacity becomes equal to FRC when the patient reaches their mid-40s.

The lateral position is often used for gastroenterological endoscopic procedures. This induces ventilation/perfusion (V/Q) mismatch and causes a pulmonary shunting phenomenon, which means that deoxygenated blood bypasses the pulmonary oxygenating unit. All these positioning-related factors (decreased FRC, V/Q mismatch, pulmonary shunt) will, in the presence of other coexisting negative conditions, cause intraoperative problems if the patient is sedated.

Special Procedures

During gastroscopy, esophagogastroduodenoscopy, or endoscopic retrograde cholangiopancreatography, gastroenterologists insert a gastroscope through the patient's mouth and to examine the upper part of the gastrointestinal tract. The shared airway and procedural space make airway management a challenging task when the procedure is performed under moderate or deep sedation. It is critically important to identify and prepare for those at high risk of intraoperative issues preoperatively; for example, patients with morbid obesity, full stomach, history of difficult airway, history of difficult monitored anesthesia care, and recent vomiting. For patients at high risk, it is may be safer to proceed with general endotracheal anesthesia and ensure that the airway is secured before the gastroscope is inserted.

Potential Complications and Their Management

Respiratory System Complications

Among all the complications induced by intravenous sedation, respiratory issues are most common. Respiratory complications may manifest a myriad of symptoms including respiratory depression, hypoventilation, hypoxemia, hypercapnia, laryngospasm, bronchospasm, and complete airway obstruction [23]. These are usually caused by oversedation or an untoward response to sedative or hypnotic medications as well as to airway maneuvers. Laryngospasm and bronchospasm often occur in patients with excessive airway secretions and in patients undergoing a procedure that involve stimulation of the airway system.

Hypoventilation and Hypoxemia

Hypoventilation and hypoxemia may be the most common complications for a patient under sedation, especially deeper sedation. There are multiple mechanisms for hypoventilation, such as relaxed laryngeal tissue obstructing the airway and decreased respiratory drive caused by opioids and other sedatives; the pharmacokinetics and pharmacodynamics of the sedative may be altered in critically ill patients, so that a

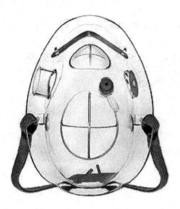

Figure 12.2 A POM Medical Procedural Oxygen Mask (from company website).

sedative that normally does not cause hypoventilation or hypotension may cause cardiopulmonary complications even with reduced medication dosing. Benzodiazepines and opioids are synergistic in their respiratory depressant effects when used in combination. This respiratory depressant effect is dose dependent and can compromise the pulmonary function by inhibiting respiratory drive response to hypoventilation, hypoxemia, and hypercapnia. Benzodiazepines and opioids can also decrease the muscle tone, which will lead to weaker ventilatory efforts, resulting in a V/Q mismatch [23].

Oversedation can be effectively prevented by applying the following strategies:

- Slowly titrate smaller doses of sedatives over an extended period of time to achieve the sedative end point.
- Avoid giving multiple sedatives simultaneously. If you intend to give several sedatives/hypnotics, administer the different medications over an extended period of time.
- Adjust dosage according to the patient's physiologic status. In elderly patients, dehydrated patients, and critically ill patients, the dosage needs to be further reduced.

For procedures such as esophagogastroduodenoscopy, sometimes it is not easy to provide adequate inspired partial oxygen concentration (FiO_2). If the patient is mouth-breathing, a nasal cannula is not the best option and a regular face mask cannot be used because the endoscope has to pass through the mouth. There are two solutions to this problem. A face mask with a specially designed hole for endoscope probe to pass through, such as the POM Medical Procedural Oxygen Mask [24] (Figure 12.2)

Another solution is a high-flow nasal oxygen cannula, such as the Optiflow Nasal Cannula (Figure 12.3) [25], which will provide significantly higher FiO_2 than regular nasal cannula.

Airway Obstruction

Airway obstruction can be caused by a relaxed tongue and oropharynx, closed epiglottis, laryngospasm, bronchospasm, airway mass, airway foreign body, compression, or secretions. The tongue and oropharynx are two very common places where airway obstruction develops. It is the submandibular muscle tone that maintains the patency of the upper airway and indirectly supports the epiglottis. Obesity, older age, and a history of sleep apnea are risk factors for airway obstruction.

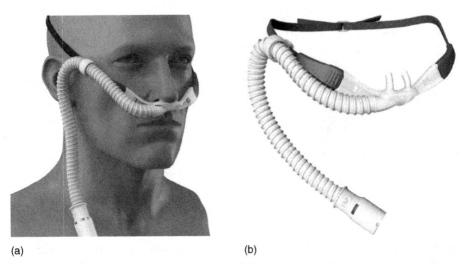

(a)   (b)

Figure 12.3 Optiflow High Oxygen Flow Nasal Cannula (from company website).

Laryngospasm is a form of airway obstruction that occurs when there is tonic contraction of glottic muscles, including the true and false vocal cords. This obstruction may be partial or total. With total obstruction, the vocal cords are stringently closed and no air exchange is possible despite chest wall movement. In partial laryngospasm, the laryngeal opening is narrowed, but some air exchange is possible. The usual precipitants of laryngospasm are vocal cord irritation due to secretions, vomitus, or blood as well as preexisting upper respiratory infection. Mechanical irritations that can occur with oral and nasal airways are potential triggers of laryngospasm. Airway obstruction is recognizable without too much difficulty and can usually be managed with positive airway pressure and suctioning of secretions can be used to decrease laryngeal irritability. Small doses of succinylcholine can be given if initial maneuvers are unsuccessful. Fortunately, laryngospasm is significantly less common in sedation cases than following general anesthesia. However, it has the potential to cause perioperative morbidity and mortality, especially if managed poorly.

Bronchospasm is a lower airway obstruction due to an increase in bronchial smooth muscle tone. Although it is a complication less frequently experienced than laryngospasm, it can lead to morbidity and mortality if left undiagnosed and untreated. Presenting symptoms are directly related to the degree of bronchospasm. Mild bronchospasm involving a small number of bronchioles presents as mild wheezing, only detectable with a stethoscope. Chest tightness, audible wheezing, chest retractions, and accessory muscle usually signify a substantial airway obstruction requiring immediate attention. Risk factors for developing bronchospasm include COPD, histamine release, upper respiratory or pulmonary infection, excessive airway secretions, aspiration, and bronchial irritation from suctioning. Propofol has been reported to induce bronchospasm [26].

Negative-pressure pulmonary edema (NPPE) is a rare pulmonary complication that occurs when the patient spontaneously takes an inspiratory breath against an upper airway obstruction. This results in significant generation of negative intrathoracic pressure, which pulls fluid from the pulmonary capillary bed and into the alveoli, resulting in significant ventilation and perfusion defects. Patients with a history of sleep apnea, laryngospasm, foreign body aspiration, opioid use, or obesity, and young healthy males, are at risk for developing NPPE. Resolution of NPPE can occur without treatment but may require supplemental oxygen and endotracheal intubation with positive pressure ventilation [27].

Complete airway obstruction is a clinical emergency that may arise in several scenarios. If a patient has a history of sleep apnea, neck mass, has undergone radiation therapy for head and neck cancer, or has a chronic large thyroid mass that might have caused an acquired tracheomalacia, sedation providers should be highly alert to the risk of loss of airway patency. If a patient has obstructive airway disease, or a difficult airway plus sedative-induced decreased respiratory drive and muscle relaxation, airway obstruction is likely to occur with sedation. These patients may be better candidates for general anesthesia with endotracheal intubation, with consideration that advanced airway management techniques (e.g., fiberoptic intubation) may be required to secure the airway. It may be too risky to proceed with moderate or deep sedation with the possibility of oversedation and loss of respiratory drive.

In the clinical emergency of complete airway obstruction, sedation providers immediately need to identify whether the patient can be ventilated with a bag-valve mask. If bag-valve-mask ventilation is not possible, immediate establishment of airway patency is necessary, either by endotracheal intubation or with a laryngeal mask airway. If the anesthesia provider is still unable to intubate the patient or ventilate the patient with the laryngeal mask airway, for whatever reason, immediate cricothyrotomy or tracheostomy may be needed.

Several maneuvers can be used to help ventilate a patient with a face mask:

- Insert oral airway and/or nasal trumpet.
- Jaw-thrust: lift the mandibular angle perpendicularly away from the patient's vertical plane while using the thumbs to push open the mouth and apply forward pressure, as shown in Figure 12.4; this maneuver opens up the airway by upward and potentially

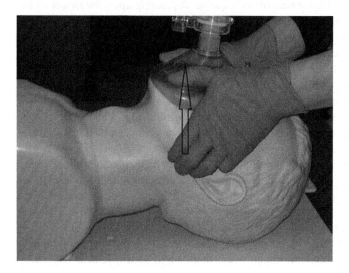

Figure 12.4 Jaw-thrust maneuver: lift the mandibular angle perpendicularly away from the vertical plane and push the mandibular body to open the patient's mouth with both thumbs. Note the direction of the lifting force, as shown by the arrow. Source. Photograph by Henry Liu, MD.

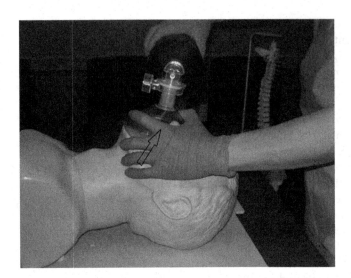

Figure 12.5 The routine chin-lift technique. Note the direction of the lifting force, as shown by the arrow. Source. Photograph by Henry Liu, MD.

forward forces; it is better than chin-lifting, which helps to open the airway by upward and backward forces (Figure 12.5): the backward force may not be beneficial to maintaining the patency of the airway.

- Positioning the patient in a semi-sitting or beach-chair position will help open up the airway, especially in a patient with neck mass, mediastinal mass, thyroid mass, and neck radiation, etc.

On many occasions during intravenous sedation, inadequate ventilation and hypoxemia are caused by a combination of decreased respiratory drive, decreased muscle strength of the respiratory system, and partial airway obstruction.

Pulmonary Aspiration of Gastric Contents

Pulmonary aspiration is the entry of gastric content into the lungs and trachea. Pulmonary aspiration can produce a variety of hazardous sequelae, depending upon the nature of the aspirate, which may include large food fragments (obstructing airway), small particles (causing granulomatous inflammation), gastric acid (causing chemical pneumonitis), and blood and digestive enzymes (causing irritation and chemical reaction) [28].

Signs and symptoms of pulmonary aspiration include rales and rhonchi, wheezing, dyspnea, tachypnea, tachycardia, and oxygen desaturation. Prophylactic strategies include head elevation/reverse Trendelenburg position, cricoid pressure, suctioning the stomach before the procedure, and administering the following medications: non-particulate antacids, H_2-receptor antagonists (cimetidine), and gastrokinetic drugs (metoclopramide).

Patients predisposed to aspiration are those with increased intra-abdominal pressure, poor gastric emptying, or gastroesophageal reflux. Increases in intra-abdominal pressure are commonly seen in pregnant patients, in patients with ascites, and in patients with intra-abdominal masses. Poor gastric emptying is related to mechanical obstruction or poor gastric muscular contraction.

Medications used for sedation have multiple effects that leave patients vulnerable to aspiration. Opioid medications commonly cause nausea and vomiting as a side effect.

Protective reflexes, which guard against aspiration, are obtunded by many of the medications used for sedation.

If the patient has a full stomach and has pyloric stenosis or other gastrointestinal obstruction, suctioning of the stomach can be effective in reducing the gastric volume. This patient should then proceed with general anesthesia with rapid sequence induction and intubation.

Hypoventilation/Hypoxemia Summary

General rules of thumb in managing patients with hypoventilation/hypoxemia during moderate or deep sedation are outlined as follows:

- If the patient has decreased respiratory drive, compromised airway, and decreased pulse oximetry readings, immediately inform the proceduralist to pause the procedure and have you or the proceduralist apply chin-lift and jaw-thrust maneuvers, to attempt to open the airway. If these maneuvers are not effective, insert an oral and/or nasal airway.
- If the patient maintains spontaneous breathing, apply positive airway pressure and assist patient breathing. If the patient has no spontaneous breathing, gentle positive pressure mask ventilation should be started immediately with 100% FiO_2.
- Suspending the procedure or switching to general endotracheal intubation can be a hard decision to make. If the patient is not expected to resume spontaneous breathing quickly, sedation should be converted to general anesthesia with endotracheal intubation or a laryngeal mask airway. If ventilation can be established, the procedure can be resumed.

Cardiovascular System Complications

Typically, minimal sedation has a negligible effect on the cardiovascular system. Moderate and deep sedation may have varying degrees of depressive effects on cardiovascular function, depending on the patient's physiologic status and the dosage of sedative agents administered. Excessive sedative dosages in addition to a large dose of local anesthetics with vasoconstrictors and procedural factors may induce significant cardiovascular changes during sedation, such as hypotension, hypertension, tachycardia, bradycardia, and dysrhythmias.

Hypotension

There are various potential causes of hypotension during sedation. Intravenous sedatives can lower systemic blood pressure, especially when the patient is overdosed with sedative medications [8]. Mechanisms for development of hypotension include decreased sympathetic tone leading to vasodilation, decreased venous return, and direct myocardial-depressant effects. Hypotension can also arise from dehydration, vasovagal response, hemorrhage, sepsis, and anaphylaxis [23]. Patients with preexisting cardiovascular disease may have prescription medications that act synergistically with sedative medications. Patients may also have preexisting depressed ventricular function and less "reserve" so that even small doses of sedative medications cause exaggerated responses. If sedative medications such as benzodiazepines, opioids, and intravenous induction agents are administered simultaneously, they will have synergistic effects, which may present as hypotension. Hypotension during sedation is not rare. It can be managed by intravenous hydration as well as sympathomimetic agents to increase vascular tone.

Hypertension

An elevation in blood pressure is possible during procedural sedation. It usually reflects inadequate intravenous sedation, procedural stimulation, or epinephrine added to local anesthetics. Stress and pain experienced by patients directly results in an increased autonomic response. This increase in catecholamine release is manifested in tachycardia and hypertension. The addition of epinephrine as a vasoconstrictor to local anesthetic is another additional risk factor for hypertension. Epinephrine is often used in dental procedures to prolong duration of local anesthetic action. In patients with preexisting hypertension, some may develop a hypertensive crisis during the procedure, and this will require immediate and controlled reduction of blood pressure. Medications commonly used to treat these perioperative hypertensions include nicardipine, sodium nitroprusside, nitroglycerin, and beta-blockers.

Tachycardia

Just like hypertension, tachycardia is usually caused by undersedation and/or procedural stimulation. An undersedated patient is likely to remain anxious and will very likely develop tachycardia and hypertension, especially if there is pain or discomfort. Tachycardia can also be a reflex response to hypoxia or hypotension, and these should be considered during patient assessment before treatment. Once these possibilities have been attended to, persistent tachycardia may cause the patient to complain of palpitations. In this scenario, intravenous fluids should be administered to support blood pressure to help sustain cardiac output. If the tachycardia continues, a selective beta-1-receptor antagonist such as esmolol can be titrated intravenously to gradually decrease sympathetic stimulation to the heart. Esmolol has a short duration, so if the heart rate drops too precipitously, it should recover within a few minutes.

Syncope

Syncope is one of the most common cardiac complications during sedation [29]. The mechanism for the pathogenesis of syncope is mostly cardiovascular in nature and commonly associated with hypoxemia, hypotension, or other cardiac rhythmic abnormalities. Syncope needs to be recognized immediately when it occurs, to avoid or decrease morbidity and mortality [30].

Other Dysrhythmias

Other dysrhythmias may include premature ventricular contractions, bigeminy, and premature atrial contractions. The majority of these complications are likely to be associated with hypotension and hypoxemia. These cardiac dysrhythmias should be recognized promptly and managed aggressively with appropriate therapeutic interventions.

Gastroenterological Complications

Nausea and Vomiting

Postoperative nausea and vomiting (PONV) is a very common and unpleasant problem for patients with undesirable outcomes such as electrolyte imbalances, increased length of stay in the post-anesthesia care unit, and unplanned admissions. The incidence of PONV is estimated to be 25–30%, while in high-risk groups the incidence is as high as 80%. Certain patient characteristics are associated with a higher risk of intraoperative nausea and vomiting (IONV) and PONV: younger age (< 50 years), female gender, and history of PONV or motion sickness, and non-smoking status. Nausea can also be due to hypotension and disease states affecting the gastrointestinal system or intracranial pressure [29, 30, 31].

The incidence of PONV in patients who received intravenous sedation medications is not clear; it should be lower than after general anesthesia. Opioids used in intravenous sedation can potentially cause IONV and PONV. Prophylaxis for high-risk patients is necessary. Avoidance of inhalational agents including nitrous oxide is recommended. Intravenous dexamethasone and ondansetron (a serotonin-receptor antagonist) are each effective at PONV risk reduction. Transdermal scopolamine patches have been successfully to decrease risk [31].

Constipation

Chronic use of opioids for the purpose of sedating patients in the ICU setting can potentially lead to constipation, although opioids used for procedural sedation are very unlikely to cause this complication. A stool softener or plant-derived laxative (e.g. Senna) can help avoid constipation when opioids are prescribed for post-procedural pain.

Other Complications

Urine Retention

Some opioids used for procedural sedation can potentially cause urine retention. Morphine is most associated with this complication. Urinary catheter placement to drain the bladder may be necessary.

Delirium

Delirium is a state in which the patient has altered consciousness, orientation, memory, perception, and behavior. A patient's reaction to hypoxemia, hypercarbia, and airway obstruction can sometimes mimic delirium, so thorough examination of the patient to rule out life-threatening events is critical. Risk factors for delirium are preoperative (including advanced age, cerebrovascular disease, alcohol or sedative withdrawal, and endocrine and metabolic disorders), intraoperative (the administration of multiple sedatives, anticholinergic agents, barbiturates, and benzodiazepines, as well as hypotension/hypoperfusion, and ophthalmic procedures), and postoperative (hypoxia and sepsis). Delirium can be managed by treating the underlying causes. Haloperidol is sometimes chosen for the patient with delirium. It can be used orally, intramuscularly, or intravenously. Droperidol and chlorpromazine are also used. However, the use of physostigmine for the management of delirium is controversial [32].

Psychogenic Non-epileptic Seizures

Psychogenic non-epileptic seizures can occur in the post-anesthesia recovery unit, although they are rare. They manifest as sudden motor and cognitive disturbances that mimic epileptic seizures and closely resemble shivering. A psychiatric background is common with the presentation of psychogenic non-epileptic seizures. Treatment includes providing the patient with high levels of psychologic support and reassurance. Anesthetic considerations should be limited to short-acting agents [33].

Propofol Infusion Syndrome

The term propofol infusion syndrome was first used by Bray in 1998 to describe a clinical state associated with propofol infusion in children [34]. The syndrome is defined by FDA investigators as metabolic acidosis with or without rhabdomyolysis with progressive myocardial dysfunction [35]. The presentation of this syndrome, also referred to as propofol-related infusion syndrome (PRIS), varies considerably from unexplained lactic acidosis, lipemic serum, and cardiac dysfunction or Brugada-like electrocardiogram changes, to cardiac failure, tachyarrhythmias or heart block, ventricular fibrillation or ventricular tachycardia, rhabdomyolysis (manifesting as elevated creatine kinase and myoglobinuria), hyperkalemia, renal failure, and fatty degeneration of the liver [36].

Risk factors for PRIS include severe head injury, airway infection, young age, large total cumulative dose, high catecholamine and serum glucocorticoid levels, low carbohydrate intake/high fat intake, critical illness, or inborn errors of fatty acid oxidation. Infusion rate and duration of infusion are particularly important risk factors for the development of PRIS. The mortality rate is as high as 83% [34]. It is recommended that infusions of 0.4 mg/kg per hour for longer than 48 hours be avoided. Early PRIS, however, has been shown to develop during high-dose, short-term infusions. Special care should be taken when such patients have factors that may increase the likelihood of development of PRIS (such as mitochondrial disease or fatty acid oxidation defects, young age, critical illness of central nervous system or respiratory origin, exogenous catecholamine or glucocorticoid administration, or inadequate carbohydrate intake). The monitoring of pH, lactate, and creatine kinase is recommended when unusually high doses or long infusion periods are unavoidable. If prolonged or high-dose propofol administration is necessary, supplemental sedatives can be used to decrease the amount of propofol necessary for the desired level of sedation [36]. The lactate-to-pyruvate ratio has been reported as a marker for the diagnosis of PRIS [37]. There is a report of successfully using extracorporeal membrane oxygenation to treat a patient with PRIS [32].

Methemoglobinemia

When benzocaine [38] or prilocaine [39] is used as a local anesthetic agent for some sedated endoscopic or echocardiographic procedures, methemoglobinemia can occur. In contrast to hemoglobin, methemoglobin is unable to bind oxygen. The clinical manifestations include cyanosis, low oxygen saturation reading, and normal arterial PaO_2 values. Kane et al. reported 28,478 patients who underwent transesophageal echocardiography (TEE), all of whom had topical benzocaine to the area for its local anesthetic effects. Nineteen patients (0.07%) developed methemoglobinemia (with a mean methemoglobin level of 32%). Eighteen of these 19 patients were treated with methylene blue [38].

The American Society for Gastrointestinal Endoscopy (ASGE) guidelines for conscious sedation and monitoring during gastrointestinal endoscopy recommend against the routine use of topical pharyngeal anesthetics in most patients [40]. However, pharyngeal anesthesia before upper endoscopy or TEE may improve the conduction of these procedures and also improves patient tolerance and comfort. Therefore, applying local anesthetics may be acceptable under certain conditions, especially if light or no sedation is administered.

Methemoglobinemia can be treated with methylene blue or ascorbic acid. Methylene blue should be avoided in patients with glucose-6-phosphate-dehydrogenase deficiency and those taking selective serotonin reuptake inhibitors.

Paradoxical Sedative Excitement

A state of excitement can occur in some patients as a reaction to sedation with benzodiazepines or propofol. This can affect the performance of the procedure, and sometimes the procedure has to be stopped so that the sedation providers can manage the patient. These paradoxical reactions can include uncooperativeness, excessive talkativeness, violent movement, and emotional release. Certain factors predispose a patient to a paradoxical reaction: young and advanced age, genetic predisposition, alcoholism or drug abuse, psychiatric and/or personality disorders. These reactions are relatively uncommon, occurring in less than 1% of cases [41].

There are reports of using physostigmine to treat these paradoxical reactions. The therapeutic effect occurs by two mechanisms: physostigmine reestablishes central nervous system homeostasis via augmented cholinergic pathways, with the net result being thalamocortical excitation, and a cholinergically mediated increase in cerebral blood flow increases the rate of redistribution of the intravenous sedative agents [42].

Summary

When patients are appropriate candidates for moderate to deep sedation, this level of anesthesia care can provide safety and comfort during procedures. For those patients at high risk for gastric content aspiration, general endotracheal anesthesia is likely a safer choice. For those who are morbidly obese or have a potentially difficult airway, general anesthesia is the better option in order to ensure that the patient's airway is secured.

Patients who are borderline risk for aspiration, or have a borderline difficult airway, pose a dilemma to the sedation provider. Proceeding with intravenous sedation and completing the procedure can be the ideal clinical course. However, this approach runs the risk of intraoperative loss of airway or aspiration. Borderline patients warrant a consultation with an anesthesiologist and strong consideration should be given to endotracheal intubation and general anesthesia, thereby securing the airway and preventing aspiration.

References

1. Boynes SG, Lewis CL, Moore PA, Zovko J, Close J. Complications associated with anesthesia administered for dental treatment. *Gen Dent.* 2010;58(1):e20–5.

2. Nisbet AT, Mooney-Cotter F. Comparison of selected sedation scales for reporting opioid-induced sedation assessment. *Pain Manag Nurs.* 2009;10(3):154–64.

3. Sessler CN, Gosnell MS, Grap MJ, et al. The Richmond Agitation–Sedation Scale: validity and reliability in adult intensive care unit patients. *Am J Respir Crit Care Med.* 2002;166(10):1338–44.

4. Waldmann C. Using and understanding sedation scoring systems. *JICS.* 2010;11(1):15–16.

5. Shi S, Klotz U. Age-related changes in pharmacokinetics. *Curr Drug Metab.* 2011;12(7):601–10.

6. Garcia CJ, Lopez OA, Islam S, et al. Endoscopic retrograde cholangiopancreatography in the

elderly. *Am J Med Sci.* 2016;351(1): 84–90.

7. Weaver CS, Terrell KM, Bassett R, et al. ED procedural sedation of elderly patients: is it safe? *Am J Emerg Med.* 2011;29(5):541–4.

8. Martin ML, Lennox PH. Sedation and analgesia in the interventional radiology department. *J Vasc Interv Radiol.* 2003;14(9):1119–28.

9. Jirapinyo P, Thompson CC. Sedation challenges: obesity and sleep apnea. *Gastrointest Endosc Clin N Am.* 2016;26(3):527–37.

10. Bautista A, Hrushka L, Lenhardt R. Procedural sedation in the morbidly obese: implications, complications, and management. *Int Anesthesiol Clin.* 2020;58(3):41–6.

11. Practice guidelines for preoperative fasting and the use of pharmacologic agents to reduce the risk of pulmonary aspiration: application to healthy patients undergoing elective procedures: an updated report by the American Society of Anesthesiologists Task Force on preoperative fasting and the use of pharmacologic agents to reduce the risk of pulmonary aspiration. *Anesthesiology.* 2017;126:376–93.

12. Friedrich S, Meybohm P, Kranke P. Nulla per os (NPO) guidelines: time to revisit? *Curr Opin Anaesthesiol.* 2020;33(6):740–5.

13. Reitman E, Flood P. Anaesthetic considerations for non-obstetric surgery during pregnancy. *Br J Anaesth.* 2011;107(Suppl 1):i72–8.

14. Vasco Ramirez M, Valencia G CM. Anesthesia for nonobstetric surgery in pregnancy. *Clin Obstet Gynecol.* 2020;63(2):351–63.

15. Heesen M, Klimek M. Nonobstetric anesthesia during pregnancy. *Curr Opin Anaesthesiol.* 2016 June;29(3):297–303.

16. Calcaterra SL, Butler M, Olson K, Blum J. The impact of a PDMP–EHR data integration combined with clinical decision support on opioid and benzodiazepine prescribing across

clinicians in a metropolitan area. *J Addict Med.* 2021;11:10.

17. Waljee JF, Zhong L, Hou H, et al. The use of opioid analgesics following common upper extremity surgical procedures: a national, population-based study. *Plast Reconstr Surg.* 2016;137(2):355e–64e.

18. Chino K, Ganzberg S, Mendoza K. Office-based sedation/general anesthesia for COPD patients, Part II. *Anesth Prog.* 2019;66(1):44–51.

19. Jirapinyo P, Thomson CC. Sedation challenges: obesity and sleep apnea. *Gastrointest Endosc Clin N Am.* 2016; 26(3):527–37.

20. Derry S, Straube S, Moore RA, Hancock H, Collins SL. *Cochrane Database of Systematic Reviews*, vol. 1. Chichester: John Wiley & Sons, Ltd, 1996.

21. Fung BM, Leon DJ, Beck LN, Tabibian JH. Pre-procedural preparation and sedation for gastrointestinal endoscopy in patients with advanced liver disease. *Dig Dis Sci.* 2022;67(7):2739–53.

22. Chawla N, Boateng A, Deshpande R. Procedural sedation in the ICU and emergency department. *Curr Opin Anaesthesiol.* 2017;30(4):507–12.

23. Odom-Forren J, Watson DS. Management of complications. In *Practical Guide to Moderate Sedation/ Anesthesia*, 2nd ed. New York, NY: Mosby, 2005, 71–96.

24. POM Medical procedural oxygen masks: adult male or female procedural oxygen mask - 1001-MF. Available at www .graylinemedical.com/products/pom-medical-procedural-oxygen-masks-adult-male-or-female-procedural-oxygen-mask-1001-mf?variant

25. Fisher and Paykel OptiFlow+ Nasal Cannula for my AIRVO 2 High Flow Systems. Available at www .directhomemedical.com/cart/merchant .mvc?Screen=PROD&Product_ Code=optiflow-nasal-cannula-myairvo-2-fisher-paykel&Store_Code

26. Takahashi S, Uemura A, Nakayama S, Miyabe M, Toyooka H. Bronchospasms and wheezing after induction of

anesthesia with propofol in patients with a history of asthma. *J Anesth.* 2002;16(4):360–1.

27. Bhattacharya M, Kallet RH, Ware LB, Matthay MA. Negative-pressure pulmonary edema. *Chest.* 2016;150(4):927–33.

28. Tasch MD. Pulmonary aspiration. In Atlee JL, ed., *Complications in Anesthesia*, 2nd ed. Philadelphia, PA: Saunders/Elsevier, 2007, 186–8.

29. D'eramo EM, Bookless SJ, Howard JB. Adverse events with outpatient anesthesia in Massachusetts. *J Oral Maxillofac Surg.* 2003;61(7):793–800.

30. Gan TJ, Diemunsch P, Habib AS, et al. Consensus guidelines for the management of postoperative nausea and vomiting. *Anesth Analg.* 2014;118(1):85–113.

31. Stoops S, Kovac A. New insights into the pathophysiology and risk factors for PONV. *Best Pract Res Clin Anaesthesiol.* 2020;34(4):667–79.

32. Guitton C, Gabillet L, Latour P, et al. Propofol infusion syndrome during refractory status epilepticus in a young adult: successful ECMO resuscitation. *Neurocrit Care Aug.* 2011;15(1):139–45.

33. Ramos JA, Brull SJ. Psychogenic non-epileptic seizures in the post-anesthesia recovery unit. *Brazilian J Anesthesiol.* 2016;66(4):426–9.

34. Bray RJ. Propofol infusion syndrome in children. *Paediatr Anaesth.* 1998;8(6):491–9.

35. Wysowski DK, Pollock ML. Reports of death with use of propofol (Diprivan) for nonprocedural (long-term) sedation and literature review. *J Am Soc Anesthesiol.* 2006;105(5):1047–51.

36. Wong JM. Propofol infusion syndrome. *Am J Ther.* 2010;17(5):487–91.

37. Pisapia JM, Wendell LC, Kumar MA, Zager EL, Levine JM. Lactate-to-pyruvate ratio as a marker of propofol infusion syndrome after subarachnoid hemorrhage. *Neurocrit Care Aug.* 2011;15(1):134–8.

38. Kane GC, Hoehn SM, Behrenbeck TR, Mulvagh SL. Benzocaine-induced methemoglobinemia based on the Mayo Clinic experience from 28 478 transesophageal echocardiograms: incidence, outcomes, and predisposing factors. *Arch Intern Med.* 2007; 167(18):1977–82.

39. Adams V, Marley J, McCarroll C. Prilocaine induced methaemoglobinaemia in a medically compromised patient. Was this an inevitable consequence of the dose administered? *Br Dent J.* 2007;203(10):585–7.

40. Waring JP, Baron TH, Hirota WK, et al. American Society for Gastrointestinal Endoscopy, guidelines for conscious sedation and monitoring during gastrointestinal endoscopy. *Gastrointes Endosc.* 2003;58(3):317–22.

41. Mancuso CE, Tanzi MG, Gabay M. Paradoxical reactions to benzodiazepines: literature review and treatment options. *Pharmacotherapy.* 2004;24(9):1177–85.

42. Milam SB, Bennett CR. Physostigmine reversal of drug-induced paradoxical excitement. *Int J Oral Maxillofac Surg.* 1987;16(2):190–3.

Recovery and Discharge After Monitored Anesthesia Care

Christopher Hoffman, Alan D. Kaye, Charles J. Fox III, and Henry Liu

Introduction

Monitored anesthesia care (MAC) has been increasingly utilized in anesthesia services for diagnostic or therapeutic procedures for various non-surgical and surgical procedures in the last several decades [1]. It is also steadily increasing in demand by many different medical specialties: cardiology for cardioversion, defibrillation, transesophageal echocardiography, pacemaker/defibrillator implantation or removal, cardiac catheterization, and other cardiac monitoring devices; gastroenterology for endoscopic examinations, potential biopsies, and other therapeutic interventions; urology for cystoscopy, etc. [1, 2]. MAC has also been gradually applied for more complex procedures in patients receiving endovascular aortic stent placements, transcatheter aortic valve replacements, and even sophisticated procedures like Mitroclip. The aims of MAC for procedures are to enhance patient comfort and cooperation, maintain airway patency and hemodynamic stability, thus facilitating efficient and safe completion of the scheduled procedures.

For most procedures or surgeries, there may be several different anesthetic techniques available. The strategies to alter a patient's consciousness level can be a continuum from giving no medication to full-scale general anesthesia [3]. The patient's preference, safety considerations, the proceduralist's preference, and equipment availability play major roles in the decision process regarding which anesthetic technique is appropriate or best for the patient. While no sedation and conscious sedation with small doses of sedatives, such as intravenous (IV) 1 mg benzodiazepines and/or 25–50 µg fentanyl, are options for motivated patients, many patients and families, and proceduralists, would prefer deeper levels of IV sedations or even general anesthesia for a planned procedure, depending on the duration and complexity of the

Table 13.1 Comparison of MAC and moderate sedation [4]

	MAC	Moderate sedation
Physician service	Yes	Yes
Physician	Anesthesiologist	Any licensed physician
Proceduralist	Different from sedating physician	Same as sedating physician
Peri-procedural anesthesia assessment	Yes	None
Ready to convert to general anesthesia	Yes	No
Provider's focus	MAC anesthesia service	Scheduled procedure
Level of sedation	Continuum from light to general anesthesia	Light to moderate
CPT code	00100-01999	99151– 99157

CPT, Current Procedural Terminology; MAC, monitored anesthesia care.

scheduled procedure. Although MAC is often interchangeably used with conscious/moderate sedation, it is different from moderate sedation based on the definitions; the differences are listed in Table 13.1. Both are physician services that are not equivalent to procedural sedation, because of the different expectations, perspectives, and qualifications of the provider(s). According to the American Society of Anesthesiologists (ASA)'s latest definition of MAC, the MAC provider(s) must be able to support a compromised airway and hemodynamics while simultaneously managing the patient's comfort and monitoring their overall well-being during a diagnostic or therapeutic procedure [3, 4].

Optimal Monitored Anesthesia Care

In some regards, providing safe care for patients undergoing moderate and deep sedation can be more challenging when compared to general anesthesia as the patient is typically breathing on their own and surgical changes throughout the case can significantly create alterations in depth of sedation and anesthesia requirements. The ideal status of a patient undergoing moderate or deep sedation includes [4]:

- maintaining consciousness of the patient
- maintaining patent airway
- retaining protective reflexes (swallow and gag)
- ensuring patient cooperation and response to physical and verbal commands
- avoiding anxiety or panic
- providing adequate pain relief
- maintaining vital signs within normal limits
- recovering patient to pre-procedural status safely and promptly

Risks Related to Monitored Anesthesia Care Service

Anesthesia provider(s) understand the transition of a patient from complete consciousness through various depths of sedation to general anesthesia, is a continuum, not a set of discrete, well-defined stages (see Table 13.2). The patient's response to sedatives, hypnotics, analgesics, and anesthetics varies enormously among patients. Loss of consciousness with the risk of loss of airway reflex protection may occur rapidly and unexpectedly. All of these following risks need to be addressed during and after the procedure [6, 7]:

- depression of respiration, especially with administration of IV opioids and/or induction agents
- depression and/or loss of protective airway reflexes
- loss of airway patency
- depression of the cardiovascular system leading to significant hypotension and lowered cardiac output
- risks inherent in the wide variety of procedures performed under procedural sedation and/or analgesia
- drug interactions or adverse drug reactions, including anaphylaxis and allergic reactions
- unexpectedly high sensitivity to the drugs used for procedural sedation and/or analgesia, which may result in undesired loss of consciousness, and respiratory or cardiovascular depression
- the possibility of requiring deeper sedation or anesthesia to compensate for inadequate analgesia or local anesthesia [7]

One basic element of MAC service is that the provider(s) must be always prepared and qualified to convert MAC to general anesthesia when necessary. And the service

Table 13.2 American Society of Anesthesiologists (ASA) continuum of sedation [5]

	Minimal sedation anxiolysis	Moderate sedation/ analgesia ("conscious sedation ")	Deep sedation/ analgesia	General anesthesia
Responsiveness	Normal response to verbal stimulation	Purposeful* response to verbal or tactile stimulation	Purposeful* response following repeated or painful stimulation	Unarousable even with painful stimulus
Airway	Unaffected	No intervention required	Intervention may be required	Intervention often required
Spontaneous ventilation	Unaffected	Adequate	May be inadequate	Frequently inadequate
Cardiovascular function	Unaffected	Usually maintained	Usually maintained	May be impaired

* Reflex withdrawal from a painful stimulus is *not* considered a purposeful response (pushing away the painful stimulus would be considered purposeful).

provider(s) of a MAC care should be able to rescue a patient's airway from any sedation-induced compromise [4, 7, 8].

Transfer from the Procedure Room to the Post-anesthesia Care Unit

The transport of a patient from the operating room or procedure room after the surgery or procedure is done can be a perilous endeavor. It is often a time when the patient is not as closely monitored and where resources are not immediately available if the patient somehow decompensates. The risk factors inherent to the patient, such as age, body mass index, and other comorbidities, can lead to complications. There are also environmental factors that can increase the likelihood of troublesome patient transportation, such as a longer distance to the recovery unit, to different buildings, small elevators, etc.

Safely transporting a patient to the post-anesthesia care unit (PACU) requires close monitoring of the patient's airway and their respiratory and hemodynamic status. Hypoventilation is a common phenomenon after anesthesia care, and supplemental oxygen is always advisable to prevent hypoxemia. However, vigilance must always be maintained, especially in patients at risk of hypoventilation and hypercarbia, and the patient's mental status should also be closely observed as this can be the main symptom of hypercarbia. Unless there is a contraindication to placing the patient in a seated position, the head of the bed should be elevated to at least 30 degrees to improve the patient's respiratory dynamics. Talking to the patient during transportation is one of the best ways to monitor patient. Placing a hand in front of the patient's nose is an effective way to check patient's breathing during transportation. Once the patient arrives at the PACU, monitors should be immediately reconnected/applied and the patient should be reassessed prior to giving the PACU nurse a care-transfer report.

The following are procedures are recommended:

- The patient is transferred from the procedure room to the PACU by appropriately trained staff, and supervised by an anesthesiologist if necessary.
- Portable monitoring is recommended if any alteration or deterioration of the patient's condition is anticipated or the distance to the PACU makes it reasonable.
- Measures should be taken to avoid hypoxemia, trauma, hypothermia, airway compromise, and disconnection of IV lines, drains, oxygen, etc.
- On arrival at the PACU, the anesthesia staff will give a report to the PACU staff regarding the patient's history, procedure, medications given, fluids given, urine output, blood loss, and any complications or problems encountered during the anesthetic. The anesthesia provider(s) should also give specific verbal and written instructions for postoperative care and make sure patient is stable before leaving the PACU.
- Physiological parameters should be measured and recorded at regular intervals during transferring the patient [3, 7].

Recovery of Patients After Procedural Sedation

All patients who have received MAC service should receive appropriate post-anesthesia management. Postoperative management is also one important element in MAC service [4, 7]. The ASA recommendations include [5, 7]:

1. A PACU or a designated area where basic monitoring equipment equivalent to a PACU is available, for example, a surgical intensive care unit (ICU), shall be available

to receive patients after MAC service. All patients who receive anesthesia care shall be admitted to PACU or its equivalent facility except by specific order(s) of the anesthesiologist responsible for the patient's care.

2. The medical aspects of care in PACU (or equivalent area) shall be governed by policies and procedures which have been reviewed and approved by the department of anesthesiology and the hospital.
3. The design, equipment and staffing level of the PACU shall meet the requirements of the facility's accrediting and licensing bodies.

Postanesthesia Phase Definitions

Most units are separated into a *phase I* recovery area for those patients that are still deeply under the influence of the sedatives and narcotics administered for anesthesia and require close attention, and a *phase II* recovery area where patients are prepared to be discharged home.

Phase I Recovery

This phase focuses on providing care to the patient immediately after procedure/surgery, transitioning the recovering patient to postanesthesia phase II care, the inpatient regular ward setting, or to an ICU setting for continued care. Basic life-sustaining needs of the patient are of the highest priority and constant vigilance is required during this phase. A physician (more often an anesthesiologist) determines whether a patient can bypass phase I recovery in certain situations, which are discussed later in the chapter [4, 7].

Phase II Recovery

This phase focuses on preparing the patient, family, and/or significant other for care in the home, or an extended care environment [4, 7].

PACU Facility and Equipment Requirements

The PACU should be equipped with life-support and patient-monitoring equipment [3, 4, 7, 8]. The following should be readily available:

- vital signs monitor(s) including ECG, pulse oximetry, blood pressure, respiratory rate, and/or end-tidal carbon dioxide
- suction canister, catheter, and wall-source negative pressure
- oxygen supply and suitable devices for the administration of oxygen to a spontaneously breathing patient
- emergency airway equipment
- adequate space to perform resuscitation if necessary
- appropriate lighting
- cardiopulmonary resuscitation cart
- defibrillator
- adequate access throughout the facility to allow the patient to be transported easily and safely

PACU Patient Monitoring and Assessment

A patient who received MAC/procedural sedation should be monitored similarly to a patient who underwent general anesthesia. These parameters essentially include blood pressure, ECG, pulse oximetry, end-tidal carbon dioxide/respiratory rate, temperature, and urine output.

Postanesthetic management of the patient after MAC/procedural sedation for procedures should include periodic assessment and monitoring of mental status, respiratory function, cardiovascular function, neuromuscular function, temperature, pain, nausea and vomiting, fluid assessment, urine output and voiding, and drainage and bleeding [3, 4, 7].

The ASA Task Force on Postanesthetic Care recommendations for assessment and monitoring of post-MAC patients are as follows [3, 7, 8]:

1. Periodic assessment of oxygen saturation, respiratory rate, and airway patency should be carried out when necessary. Particular attention should be given to monitoring oxygenation and ventilation.
2. Close monitoring of heart rate and blood pressure should be done during recovery, and ECG monitoring should always be available in the PACU.
3. Mental status should be periodically assessed during recovery.
4. Body temperature should be checked during recovery.
5. Pain score should be periodically assessed during recovery.
6. Nausea and vomiting should be assessed routinely during recovery.
7. Postoperative hydration status should be assessed in the PACU and managed accordingly. Any procedure involving excessive loss of blood or fluids may require blood transfusion and additional volume replacement.
8. Urine output and urinary voiding should be evaluated on a case-by-case basis for selected patients or selected procedures during recovery.
9. Drainage and bleeding should be assessed during recovery, or prompted by increased drainage or bleeding [3,7,8].

Management of the Post-anesthesia Care Unit

The following considerations are important in the management of the PACU.

1. *Oxygenation and respiration*: Oxygen supplementation via a nasal cannula or face mask may be needed to maintain oxygen saturation (SpO_2) above 90%, and some patients may need 100% non-rebreather to achieve this goal. Some patients with obstructive sleep apnea (OSA) may need special equipment like continuous or bilevel positive airway pressure (CPAP/BiPAP) to maintain their airway patency and oxygenation.
2. *Management of respiratory depression or airway obstruction*: Sometimes an opioid reversal agent (naloxone) is needed to treat respiratory depression if it is related to an overdose of narcotics. Flumazenil, a benzodiazepine antagonist, may also be required. Oral airway, nasal trumpet, CPAP and BiPAP are often used to maintain the airway patency, and emergency airway equipment should be immediately available in the event that a patient requires intubation.
3. *Adequate circulation*: The goal of mean arterial pressure (MAP) and heart rate should be within 20% of the patient's baseline range. Administration of vasopressor(s) either in bolus or continuous infusion may be necessary to treat postoperative hypertension. Beta-blockers or other antihypertensive drugs may be needed to manage postoperative hypertension. Analgesic(s) are often used to provide analgesic effects, thus lowering blood pressure [4, 7].

4. *Maintaining normothermia*: Pharmacologic agents for the treatment of shivering are sometimes needed to reduce the increased oxygen and energy consumption associated with shivering. Meperidine is very effective in the treatment of patient shivering. Magnesium sulfate and tramadol have also been found effective in controlling postoperative shivering [9]. The PACU should also be a comfortable temperature and have warm blankets and warming devices immediately available.

5. *Postoperative nausea and vomiting (PONV)*: The ASA Task Force recommends the following measures for PONV [10]. What is emphasized is the multimodal approach in current anesthetic practice in controlling PONV. Non-pharmacological measures such as acupuncture have been adopted in minimizing PONV. Pharmacological agents for the prophylaxis of PONV include:

- serotonin antiemetics: ondansetron
- tranquilizers/neuroleptics
- antihistamines: diphenhydramine, hydroxyzine, benztropine
- metoclopramide
- scopolamine: should be applied preoperatively and the patient may keep the patch on for up to 72 hours.
- dexamethasone: should be given pre-incision as the onset of action is prolonged.
- small doses of propofol (10–20 mg) may also be used for refractory PONV

6. *Management of post-procedure pain*: Analgesic(s) will likely be needed to control pain. The Centers for Disease Control and Prevention recently published guidelines on minimizing the prescribing of opioids for chronic pain [11]. Although the post-surgical patient is excluded from the guidelines, a multimodal pain regimen is wise to minimize patient dependence on opioids. Multimodal pain therapies should be tailored to the individual patient, but may include: acetaminophen, non-steroidal anti-inflammatory drugs, dexamethasone, local anesthetics, certain antidepressants and anti-epileptic drugs (pregabalin, gabapentin, duloxetine) and regional/neuraxial blocks [12].

Modified Aldrete Score

The original Aldrete score was initially published in 1970. The scoring system has been modified since then (Table 13.3), but a similar version was adopted by the Joint Commission on Accreditation of Health Care Organizations in the United States, as well as in numerous other countries, as the standard by which PACU nurses and anesthesiology staff should complete patient assessments and determine patient readiness for discharge. A score of 9 out of 10 signifies that the patient is ready for discharge [8].

Management based on the modified Aldrete scores includes [11]:

- as a general rule, frequency of assessing patients in PACU as follows:
  - 3 points below baseline: every 5 minutes with constant (1:1) monitoring
  - 2 points below baseline: every 15 minutes with constant monitoring of vital signs
  - 1 point below baseline: every 15–30 minutes with vital signs depending upon patient condition.

- baseline: utilize your facility's protocols for standard post-procedural care.

Table 13.3 Modified Aldrete score

	2	1	0
Consciousness	Fully awake	Arousable on calling	Not responding
Respiration	$SpO_2 > 92\%$ on room air, able to cough	Dyspnea/shallow breathing	Apnea
Circulation/ blood pressure (BP)	BP ±20mmHg pre-op level	BP ±20–50 mmHg pre-op level	BP ±50 mmHg pre-op level
Oxygenation	$SpO_2 > 92\%$ on room air	Needs oxygen to maintain $SpO_2 > 90\%$	$SpO_2 < 90\%$ with supplemental oxygen
Activity/ movement	Able to move four extremities	Able to move two extremities	Unable to move extremity

Adapted from Marshall SI and Chung F [8].

Fast-Tracking Post-Procedural Care

Bypass PACU Recovery Phase I

Some patients can be transferred from the procedure room directly to phase II recovery, thus bypassing phase I recovery and expediting discharge from the hospital or surgical center. Criteria for a post-procedural sedation patient to bypass PACU phase I requires that the patient recovers to a modified Aldrete score of 9 or higher prior to leaving the procedure/operating room. This may only be done at the discretion of the attending anesthesiologist.

Strategies to Reduce PACU Stay

McLaren et al. reported that they achieved a significant decrease in operating room hold rates, improvement in perioperative throughput, improved efficiency, increased team-work between the perioperative team, PACU stay and improved patient family satisfaction, by implementing the education program and using the American Society of PeriAnesthesia Nurses (ASPAN) standards to educate the perioperative staffs. They analyzed the length of stay (LOS) before and after education, and the team decreased the LOS in the phase I PACU by 20%, which resulted in a cost savings of $46,000 over a 3-month period [13].

Transfer from Phase I to Phase II Postanesthesia Care

The criteria for transfer from phase I to phase II postanesthesia care [7, 8] are:
- patient returns to pre-procedural orientation level and/or is awake and alert
- stable vital signs
- patients who had spinal/epidural anesthesia must have full return of sensory and motor function to lower extremities and demonstrate the ability to stand and walk with minimal assistance
- patients can tolerate sitting in an upright position without presentation of orthostatic hypotension

Discharge of Patients Who Received Procedural Sedation

All monitored anesthesia care patients should meet discharge criteria for phase I and phase II recovery.

The discharge criteria of phase II patients to home are as follows [7, 8]:

1. The patient is awake, alert, responds to commands appropriate to age, or returns to pre-procedure mental status.
2. The SpO$_2$ is greater than 95% or returns the pre-procedure baseline on room air for 30 minutes without airway support. Breathing is even and unlabored. The respiratory rate is greater than 10 and less than 30 for adults.
3. The patient is able to sit in an upright position without signs and symptoms of orthostatic hypotension and no active bleeding. The BP is ±20 mmHg of pre-procedure range or within patient's stated normal range.
4. The patient is able to ambulate with minimal assistance or at pre-procedure level.
5. The pain score at rest is less than 4 or at the pre-procedure level at rest and the patient states that there is adequate pain control. No IV opioids or sedatives have been given within 30 minutes, or any intramuscular agents within 1 hour.
6. The patient is not actively vomiting and nausea is mild in severity.
7. The patient is able to void if they had spinal or epidural anesthesia, or contrast media.
8. IV infusion is discontinued unless ordered to the contrary.
9. Arrangements have been confirmed for a responsible adult to accompany the patient home and an individual remains available for the first 24 hours.
10. Discharge medication prescriptions are given to the patient.
11. The patient discharge teaching and written instructions are provided to the patient and/or companion.

The ASA Task Force on Postanesthetic Care has the following recommendations:

1. The ASA Task Force believe routine requirement for urination by the patient before discharge should not be part of a discharge protocol and may only be necessary for selected patients.
2. The requirement of drinking clear fluids should not be part of a discharge protocol and may only be necessary for selected patients This should be determined on a case-by-case basis (e.g., diabetic patients).
3. As part of a recovery room discharge protocol, all patients should be required to have a responsible individual to accompany the patient return home.
4. Patients should be observed until they are no longer at increased risk for cardiorespiratory depression. A mandatory minimum stay should not be required. Discharge criteria should be designed to minimize the risk of central nervous system or cardiorespiratory depression after discharge [3, 4].

Finally, the Postanesthesia Discharge Scoring System (Table 13.4) can be used to decide if discharge is appropriate. A score of 8 or more indicates that the patient is ready to be discharged.

Responsibility for Discharge

A physician is responsible for the discharge of a patient from the PACU [3, 7]:

1. When discharge criteria are used, they must be approved by the department of anesthesiology and the medical staff. They may vary depending upon

Table 13.4 Post-anesthesia Discharge Scoring System (PADSS)

	Patient status	PADSS score
Vital signs	Within 20% of preoperative value	2
	20–40% of preoperative value	1
	> 40% of preoperative valve	0
Nausea and vomiting	Minimal, treated with oral medications	2
	Moderate, treated with parenteral medications	1
	Continues after repeated treatments	0
Ambulation	Steady gait/no dizziness	2
	Ambulates with assistance	1
	Not ambulating/dizziness	0
Pain	Acceptable to patient (oral medications)	2
	Acceptable to patient (parenteral medications)	1
	Pain not controlled/not acceptable to patient	0
Bleeding	Minimal/no dressing changes required	2
	Moderate bleeding	1
	Severe bleeding	0

Adapted from the University of British Columbia College of Physicians and Surgeons, Postanesthesia Care and the National Association of PeriAnesthesia Nurses of Canada [8, 13].

whether the patient is discharged to a hospital room, the ICU, a short-stay unit, or home.

2. In the absence of the physician responsible for the discharge, the PACU nurse shall determine that the patient meets the discharge criteria. The name of the physician accepting responsibility for discharge shall be noted on the record.

Patients with Obstructive Sleep Apnea

Patients with OSA should be managed differently because of their higher risk to develop respiratory depression and hypoxia. The ASPAN standards include a practice recommendation established to describe best nursing practice for managing adult patients with OSA. Based on an extensive literature review, the ASPAN strategic work team members identified several nursing-specific recommendations intended to promote safe care of these patients. The literature review unveiled very little empirical evidence on discharge of the patient with known or suspected OSA from the PACU phase I care, thus they made a vague suggestion for an anticipated "extended PACU stay." Some literature did reveal evidence to support observing outpatients with OSA an average of 3 hours longer than non-OSA patients, anticipating a minimum observation period of 2–6 hours. In case the patient demonstrates sustained desaturations or episodes of apnea, the care team should plan on at least seven additional hours of monitoring for each hypoxemic and/or obstructive event witnessed. The only other "time-based" recommendation for the patient with known or suspected OSA is to assure that the patient maintains oxygen saturation greater than 94% or at baseline for at least 2 hours before discharge to home [14].

Summary

Considering the increasing complexity of patients undergoing surgery and interventional and diagnostic procedures, anesthesiologists must maintain vigilance in the postanesthetic environment as well as to pre- and intraoperatively. Anesthesia providers should be familiar with the various assessment tools used in PACU management as well as the common complications seen in the PACU in order to decrease morbidity and mortality associated with the perioperative period, increase efficiency and safety in patient recovery and discharge, and increase patient satisfaction.

References

1. Aravapalli A, Norton HJ, Rozario N, et al. Increased anesthesia usage in a large-volume endoscopy unit: patient acuity is not the main predictor. *South Med J.* 2015;108(9):547–52. doi: 10.14423/SMJ.0000000000000338. PMID:26332480

2. Yamamoto H, Shido A, Sakura S, Saito Y. Monitored anesthesia care based on ultrasound-guided subcostal transversus abdominis plane block for continuous ambulatory peritoneal dialysis catheter surgery: case series. *J Anesth.* 2016;30 (1):156–60. doi: 10.1007/s00540-015-2074-0. Epub 2015 Sep 4. PMID:26337833

3. Apfelbaum JL, Silverstein JH, Chung FF, et al, Practice guidelines for postanesthetic care: an updated report by the American Society of Anesthesiologists Task Force on Postanesthetic Care. *Anesthesiology.* 2013;118(2):291–307. doi: 10.1097/ALN.0b013e31827773e9. PMID: 23364567

4. American Society of Anesthesiologists. Statement on distinguishing monitored anesthesia care ("MAC") from moderate sedation/analgesia (conscious sedation). Original approval: October 18, 2023. www.asahq.org/standards-and-practice-parameters/statement-on-distinguishing-monitored-anesthesia-care-from-moderate-sedation-analgesia

5. American Society of Anesthesiologists, 2019, Statement on continuum of depth of sedation: definition of general anesthesia and levels of sedation/analgesia. Last amended: October 23, 2019. www.asahq.org/ standards-and-practice-parameters/statement-on-continuum-of-depth-of-sedation-definition-of-general-anesthesia-and-levels-of-sedation-analgesia

6. Kim, S., Chang, B.A., Rahman, A. et al. Analysis of urgent/emergent conversions from monitored anesthesia care to general anesthesia with airway instrumentation. *BMC Anesthesiol.* 2021;21:183. https://doi.org/10.1186/s12871-021-01403-9

7. Liu, H, Asgarian, C, Zebrower, M, Im, M, Kaye, AD. Recovery and discharge after procedural sedation. In Urman R, Kaye A, eds., *Moderate and Deep Sedation in Clinical Practice.* Cambridge: Cambridge University Press, 2017, 166–74.

8. Marshall SI, Chung F. Discharge criteria and complications after ambulatory surgery. *Anesth Analg.* 1999;88(3): 508–17. PMID: 10071996

9. Sachidananda R, Basavaraj K, Shaikh SI, et al. Comparison of prophylactic intravenous magnesium sulfate with tramadol for postspinal shivering in elective Cesarean section: a placebo controlled randomized double-blind pilot study. *Anesth Essays Res.* 2018;12(1):130–4. doi: 10.4103/aer. AER_196_17. PMID: 29628568; PMCID: PMC5872849

10. Gan TJ, Belani KG, Bergese S, et al. Fourth consensus guidelines for the management of postoperative nausea and vomiting. *Anesth Analg.* 2020;131 (2):411–48. doi: 10.1213/ANE.0000000000004833. Erratum in *Anesth Analg.* 2020;131(5):e241. PMID: 32467512

11. Wu J, Gao S, Zhang S, et al. Perioperative risk factors for recovery room delirium after elective non-cardiovascular surgery under general anaesthesia. *Perioper Med (Lond).* 2021;10(1):3. doi: 10.1186/s13741-020-00174-0. PMID: 33531068; PMCID: PMC7856719

12. Horn R, Kramer J. *Postoperative Pain Control.* Treasure Island, FL: StatPearls Publishing, 2022.

13. McLaren JM, Reynolds JA, Cox MM, et al. Decreasing the length of stay in phase I postanesthesia care unit: an evidence-based approach. *J Perianesth Nurs.* 2015;30(2):116–23. doi: 10.1016/j.jopan.2014.05.010. PMID: 25813297

14. Clifford T. Length of stay: discharge criteria. *J Perianesth Nurs.* 2014;29 (2):159–60. doi: 10.1016/j.jopan.2013.12.005. PMID: 24661488

Outcomes, Controversies, and Future Trends

Julia Metzner and Karen B. Domino

Outcomes of Procedural Sedation

Sedation Complications

The incidence of sedation-related complications for procedures is unknown, as mandatory reporting of outcomes is lacking. However, two sources of information are available that can shed light on the risks of sedation encountered in non-operating-room locations.

The Pediatric Sedation Research Consortium is a multi-institutional group that maintains a database of more than 50,000 cases and collects pediatric sedation-related adverse events. It collects outcomes for various diagnostic and therapeutic procedures at different locations, delivered by anesthesiologists, emergency department specialists, intensive care physicians, pediatricians, and trained nurses [1]. Regardless of the sedation protocols and types of drugs used, the most observed complications were of respiratory origin, including stridor, laryngospasm, airway obstruction, and apnea. One in every 200 sedations required airway and ventilation interventions ranging from bag-mask ventilation to oral airway placement to emergency intubation. No deaths occurred (Table 14.1) [1, 2].

Despite the relative safety of sedation when administered by trained personnel, severe adverse events can occur, including brain damage and death. The American Society of Anesthesiologists (ASA) Closed Claims Project collects and analyzes anesthesia malpractice claims to study in detail rare adverse events and improve patient safety. Recently, the claims associated with sedation and monitored anesthesia care (MAC) [3] and care by anesthesiologists in non-operating-room locations [4, 5] have been reviewed (Table 14.2). Respiratory depression from sedative agents was the leading cause of severe patient injury (death or severe brain damage) during sedation/MAC. Propofol, often administered with an opioid or benzodiazepine, increased the incidence of oversedation and respiratory depression. Complications occurred at a higher rate at extremes of age. The anesthetic care was considered substandard in most of these claims, and errors were judged as preventable by better respiratory monitoring, especially capnography, in two-thirds of claims. As a result of these findings, the ASA changed the standards for

Table 14.1 Complications

	Incidence per 10,000	n	95% CI
Adverse events			
Death	0.0	0	0.0–0.0
Cardiac arrest	0.3	1	0.0–1.9
Aspiration	0.3	1	0.0–1.9
Hypothermia	1.3	4	0.4–3.4
Seizure (unanticipated) during sedation	2.7	8	1.1–5.2
Stridor	4.3	11	1.8–6.6
Laryngospasm	4.3	13	2.3–7.4
Wheeze (new onset during sedation)	4.7	14	2.5–7.8
Allergic reaction (rash)	5.7	17	3.3–9.1
Intravenous-related problems/complication	11.0	33	7.6–15.4
Prolonged sedation	13.6	41	9.8–18.5
Prolonged recovery	22.3	67	17.3–28.3
Apnea (unexpected)	24.3	73	19.1–30.5
Secretions (requiring suction)	41.6	125	34.7–49.6
Vomiting during procedure (non-gastrointestinal)	47.2	142	39.8–55.7
Desaturation below 90%	156.5	470	142.7–171.2
Total adverse events	339.6 (1 per 29)	1020	308.1–371.5
Unplanned treatments			
Reversal agent required (unanticipated)	1.7	5	0.6–3.9
Emergency anesthesia consult for airway	2.0	6	0.7–4.3
Admission to hospital (unanticipated; sedation related)	7.0	21	4.3–10.7
Intubation required (unanticipated)	9.7	29	6.5–13.9
Airway (oral; unexpected requirement)	27.6	83	22.0–34.2
Bag-mask ventilation (unanticipated)	63.9	192	55.2–73.6
Total unplanned treatments	111.9 (1 per 89)	336	85.3–130.2
Conditions present during procedure			
Inadequate sedation, could not complete	88.9 (1 per 338)	267	78.6–100.2

This table includes adverse events and other complications reported to the Pediatric Sedation Research Consortium database. Reproduced with permission from Cravero et al. [2]. © 2006 American Academy of Pediatrics. CI, confidence interval.

Table 14.2 Adverse events and mechanisms of injury associated with claims from anesthesia in remote locations compared with claims from operating room procedures

	Non-operating room; N = 87; n (%)	Operating room; N = 3,287; n (%)
Adverse events		
Death	47 (54)*	949 (29)*
Permanent brain damage	12 (14)	321 (10)
Airway injury	10 (11)	309 (9)
Aspiration pneumonitis	6 (7)	117 (4)
Burn injury	5 (6)	141 (4)
Stroke	3 (3)	118 (4)
Eye injury	2 (2)	183 (6)
Myocardial infarction	1 (1)	123 (4)
Mechanism of injury		
Respiratory event	38 (44)*	671 (20)*
Inadequate oxygenation/ ventilation	18 (21)*	94 (3)*
Cardiovascular event	9 (10)	526 (16)
Equipment failure	12 (14)	438 (13)
Medication-related	5 (6)	256 (8)
Other events[a]	21 (24)	1113 (34)

Other events include surgical technique/patient condition, patient fell, wrong operation/location, positioning, failure to diagnose, other known damaging events, no damaging event, and unknown. Adapted from Metzner et al. [4].
*$p < 0.001$ remote location vs. operating room claims (z test).

monitoring ventilation during moderate or deep sedation to require capnography to measure exhaled carbon dioxide, unless precluded or invalidated by the nature of the patient, procedure, or equipment [6].

Pino reviewed sedation outcomes outside the operating room in a single large institution (over 63,000 cases) [7]. The adverse events were comparable to that in other reports and involved respiratory accidents caused by inadequate monitoring, drug overdose, and lack of vigilance. Although rare, sedation-induced respiratory depression may cause brain damage and/or death.

Influence of Monitoring Modalities on Outcomes

Capnography

As respiratory depression is the most crucial side effect of the commonly used sedatives, early recognition and rapid intervention are paramount to avoid potentially serious complications. Pulse oximetry is the standard monitor for desaturation and hypoxemia during sedation/analgesia; however, it is inadequate to detect ventilatory compromise, such as hypoventilation, airway obstruction, or apnea. Significant respiratory compromise can occur despite normal oxygen saturation, particularly when supplemental oxygen is administered. Clinical monitoring of ventilation (chest excursion, respiratory rate, breath sounds) may provide some information, but only monitoring for the presence of carbon dioxide (CO_2) exhaled by the patient (capnography) can detect subtle hypoventilation before it is evident on clinical examination.

Although capnography is now a standard requirement for monitoring ventilation during moderate or deep sedation by anesthesia providers (ASA standard) [6], it is often not employed by non-anesthesia providers. However, its use in detecting adverse respiratory events associated with procedural sedation has been the focus of studies in both anesthesiology [8] and non-anesthesiology literature [9–12]. One study reported that a quarter of patients developed 20 seconds of apnea missed by clinical signs and pulse oximetry but detected by capnography [8]. An emergency medicine group studied sedation with propofol with and without capnography. Continuous end-tidal CO_2 monitoring decreased the incidence of oxygen desaturation ($SpO_2 < 93\%$) from 42% to 25%; the capnography evidence of respiratory depression always occurred before the onset of hypoxia [11]. Similar findings have been reported in gastroenterology [12]. In summary, using capnography with rapid intervention to treat respiratory depression can efficiently prevent adverse respiratory events during sedation.

Brain Function Monitoring

Brain function monitoring, such as using the bispectral index (BIS), first introduced by Aspect Medical Systems Inc., uses a processed electroencephalogram signal to estimate anesthetic or sedation depth. A BIS value of 100 (unit-less scale) is considered complete wakefulness, 0 is cortical silence, 80–90 is associated with sedation, and the range of 40–60 is considered to be consistent with general anesthesia. BIS has been validated for use during general anesthesia in the operating room and the ambulatory setting, and its popularity for procedural sedation is rising. It is widely believed that brain function monitoring may be beneficial in preventing oversedation and in facilitating fast-track recovery. However, the role of brain function monitoring for sedation targeted to the moderate level has not been established. BIS monitoring has shown low accuracy discriminating between mild to moderate and moderate to deep levels of sedation during endoscopy [13] and various emergency department procedures [14, 15]. In summary, brain function monitoring may benefit procedural sedation in the future but requires more investigation.

Controversies of Procedural Sedation

The major controversies in procedural sedation are the choice of sedative agents and propofol administration by non-anesthesia providers.

Traditionally, moderate sedation in the gastrointestinal suite was provided with a benzodiazepine (midazolam or diazepam) used either alone or in combination with an opioid (fentanyl or meperidine). However, during the last few years, there has been increasing use of propofol, a general anesthetic agent. To date, there is no demonstrated difference in endoscopic safety or efficacy with propofol sedation compared to sedation with a benzodiazepine with or without an opioid. However, the studies failed to critically measure adverse respiratory effects. There is a trend towards higher satisfaction levels and cost-effectiveness for using propofol during colonoscopies. Using propofol during upper gastrointestinal endoscopies may expect higher levels of patient satisfaction and improved efficacy.

For routine endoscopic procedures (e.g., colonoscopies and upper endoscopies), the safety of propofol administered by non-anesthesia providers is controversial. Most endoscopy-oriented specialty societies support propofol procedural sedation by non-anesthesia providers. However, the healthcare practitioners (e.g., anesthesia providers) with the most experience with propofol are primarily against propofol administration by sedation nurses and other non-anesthesia providers. While economic concerns may underlie the debate, the major concern is patient safety, as propofol has variable patient responses, resulting in a quick progression of moderate sedation into deep sedation.

Two major types of administration of propofol by non-anesthesia providers have been studied: nurse-administered propofol sedation (NAPS) and proceduralist direction (Table 14.3) [16–21]. While the safety results in healthy, non-obese patients are encouraging, these studies do not thoroughly investigate respiratory depression or hemodynamic compromise, and instead focus only on infrequent severe adverse outcomes, and therefore lack adequate power to detect differences. In a review of more than 36,000 endoscopies performed under NAPS, the rate of clinically significant adverse events (defined as an episode of apnea or other airway compromise requiring bag-mask ventilation) ranged from approximately one event per 500 endoscopies to one per 1,000 [22]. A recent multinational study of 646,000 endoscopist-directed propofol administrations for gastrointestinal procedures reported a relatively low overall risk of cardiopulmonary complications [20]. Only 0.1% of patients needed bag-mask ventilation, and only 11 patients required endotracheal intubation; no patients sustained a permanent neurologic injury, and four patients with underlying severe disabling diseases died (Table 14.3). However, these sedation studies generally did not examine the magnitude and duration of oxygen desaturations, respiratory obstruction, hypoventilation, apnea, or adverse hemodynamic effects. Some new data support the safe use of propofol sedation during endoscopic retrograde cholangiopancreatography (ERCP), particularly in elderly patients with significant comorbidities: the studies showed faster recovery times and lower desaturation events during the procedure [23].

Choice of Drugs: New and Common

Dexmedetomidine

Dexmedetomidine is a selective alpha-2-adrenoceptor agonist that provides cooperative sedation, anxiolysis, analgesia, a reduction of sympathetic outflow, and an increase in vagal tone. The main advantage of dexmedetomidine over other sedatives is that despite deeper levels of sedation, the respiratory function remains preserved. Because of these qualities, dexmedetomidine has been proven useful in sedating adult and pediatric patients in the operating room, intensive care, and out-of-operating-room locations [24]. Dexmedetomidine is often delivered as an initial bolus of 0.5–1 µg/kg over 10–20 minutes, followed by a continuous infusion of 0.2–0.7 µg/kg per hour. As it may cause significant bradycardia and hypotension, careful hemodynamic monitoring is advisable.

Table 14.3 Selected series of administration of propofol by various providers

Authors, year	Study design	Number of patients	ASA physical status	Procedure	Provider	Drug(s)	Complications
Schilling et al., 2009 [16]	Prospective	151	3–4	ERCP, EUS	Nurse	Propofol vs. midazolam/ meperidine	$SpO_2 < 90\%$ in 11.8% vs. 9.3% Hypotension: 5.2% vs. 2.6%
Mcquaid and Laine, 2008 [17]	Meta-analysis	3,918 (36 studies)	N/A	EGD, colonoscopy	Endoscopist	Regimens 1. BDZ 2. BDZ + opioid 3. Propofol	SpO_2 Hypotension $< 90\%$ 0% 18% 7% 6% 5% 11%
Cote et al., 2010 [18]	Prospective case series	799	6% > 3	ERCP, EUS	Anesthesiologist	Propofol alone; propofol combined	$SpO_2 < 90\%$: 12.8% Hypotension: 0.5%
Fatima et al., 2008 [19]	Retrospective case series	806	N/A	EUS	Nurse	Propofol	$SpO_2 < 90\%$: 0.7% PPV: 4 BMV: 1 Hypotension: 13%
Rex et al., 2009 [20]	Retrospective review	646, 080	N/A	EGD, colonoscopy	Endoscopist	Propofol	BMV: 489 patients (0.1%) ETT: 11 patients Death: 4 patients
Singh et al., 2008 [21]	Cochrane meta-analysis	267 studies	1	Colonoscopy	Endoscopist, nurse PCS	Propofol alone; propofol combined	SpO_2, apnea, and respiratory depression comparable

ASA, American Society of Anesthesiologists; BDZ, benzodiazepine; BMV, bag-mask ventilation; EGD, esophagogastroduodenoscopy; ERCP, endoscopic retrograde cholangiography; ETT, endotracheal tube; EUS, esophageal sonographies; N/A, not available; PCS, patient-controlled sedation; PPV, positive-pressure ventilation; SpO_2, oxygen saturation.
Adapted from Metzner and Domino [5].

Lower administration rates may be required in elderly, sicker, or hypovolemic patients (such as after a bowel prep). The recovery time may also be longer than for propofol.

Nitrous Oxide: A New Look at an Old Drug

Nitrous oxide is a sweet-smelling, non-flammable gas of low potency; it has a minimum alveolar concentration (MAC) of 104% and is relatively insoluble in blood. Compared to other inhalational agents, the uptake and elimination time are relatively quick, primarily because of their low blood–gas partition coefficient. Nitrous oxide has a mild analgesic effect and produces drowsiness, amnesia, and anxiolysis at subanesthetic concentrations (25% MAC). While initially rejected by anesthesiologists as a single agent choice due to its lack of potency, nitrous oxide has gained popularity as a sedative/analgesic for various procedures, particularly in the pediatric area [25, 26].

Ketamine: A Revival of an Old Drug

Ketamine, a phencyclidine derivative, was discovered in 1962 and used as a first-line agent for procedural sedation. It is unique because it exerts sedative and analgesic effects without impairing spontaneous respiratory drive or cardiovascular tone. Since its dissociative effects on the central nervous system are well known, ketamine is frequently used in combination with low-dose midazolam to prevent hallucinations and delirium.

The role of ketamine in procedural sedation has been explored in both the anesthesiology and emergency medicine literature. The putative advantage of ketamine is its ability to preserve respiratory drive and airway defense reflexes better when compared to procedural sedation regimens predominantly incorporating opioids for analgesia. When ketamine is used as a single agent, it is associated with a moderately high incidence of adverse effects with one study reporting agitation in 13% and vomiting in 4% of patients [27]. Most of the more recently published randomized controlled trials on this topic have been designed to evaluate the risks and benefits of adding ketamine to propofol-based procedural sedation or using ketamine to replace fentanyl in sedation regimens. One of these studies suggested that adding ketamine did not increase the incidence of respiratory depression compared to propofol alone, while improving the sedation conditions as judged by nurses and physicians [28]. A study evaluating the use of fixed-dose mixtures of ketamine and propofol (ketofol as it has been called), did not show any advantages for ketamine–propofol mixtures when compared to a single-agent propofol regimen. The findings of this study also indicated that a 1:1 (mg per mg) propofol–ketamine mixture was more likely to be associated with agitation during recovery than a 4:1 (4 mg propofol to 1 mg ketamine) or propofol-only regimen [29]. In a study of sedation for endoscopic retrograde cholangiopancreatography, with the substitution of ketamine for fentanyl in a regimen combining midazolam and propofol, there was no difference in the quality of sedation between the two groups [30]. In summary, ketamine has been safely incorporated into procedural sedation regimens with no firm evidence of unique advantage when added to propofol-based regimens.

Oliceridine and Remimazolam

Oliceridine and remimazolam are experimental drugs that could be valuable: both drugs received US Food and Drug Administration (FDA) approval in 2020/2021.

Oliceridine (OLINVYK™) is a novel mu-opioid receptor agonist. Compared with conventional opioids, oliceridine stimulates G protein signaling with significantly less beta-arrestin activation. This mechanism of action permits the provision of analgesia while potentially mitigating the risks of respiratory depression and gastrointestinal adverse effects. Based on a rigorously conducted three-phase trial involving more than 1,500 patients undergoing orthopedic or abdominal procedures, oliceridine presented an efficient reduction in postoperative pain and no major side effects [31, 32]. Although no research has been conducted to evaluate its benefits for moderate/deep sedation outside the operating room, the expectation is that the rapid onset of action within 2-4 minutes and fewer opioid-related side effects will make it suitable for future use in that domain.

Remimazolam is a rapid onset/offset new benzodiazepine. As its name suggests, it combines the unique features of midazolam and remifentanil by acting on the gamma-aminobutyric acid (GABA) receptors as midazolam but being metabolized by non-specific plasma esterases like remifentanil [33]. Subsequently, it has a shorter half-life than midazolam. It achieves better safety with rapid recovery and early restoration of cognitive function: for example, at equi-effective doses of remimazolam with respect to midazolam, the median recovery time was 30 minutes faster with remimazolam [34]. A well-designed study in the phase III trial of this drug carried out by Rex et al. for colonoscopies confirmed that remimazolam could be used safely and efficiently in high-risk ASA-classified patients with no significant side effects. Remimazolam was superior to midazolam, reaching the desired endpoints in 91.3% vs. 25.2% of patients, respectively [35]. In addition to a systemic clearance three times that of midazolam, remimazolam is fully reversible by flumazenil and in modeling studies exhibits minimal extension of its predicted context-sensitive half-life (6–8 minutes after a 4-hour infusion) despite prolonged infusions [32].

New Drug Delivery Methods
Patient-Controlled Sedation/Analgesia

This innovative technique allows the patient to directly control and adjust the sedation level as needed. The patient-controlled sedation/analgesia (PCSA) system resembles a conventional patient-controlled analgesia machine and consists of an infusion pump and a patient-controlled handset (push-button). Lockout intervals (usually 3–5 minutes), bolus doses, and maximum infusion rates are predetermined to avoid oversedation. Patients may trigger intermittent drug boluses or control a variable-rate infusion. In clinical practice, propofol is the drug most often used alone or combined with an opioid. Mandel and colleagues found that colonoscopy could be performed well with PCSA with different drug regimens (midazolam–fentanyl or propofol–remifentanil) [36]. It appears that PCSA is comparable with physician-conducted traditional sedation; generally patients use lower doses, the recovery is faster, and patient satisfaction is high [37].

Computer-Assisted Personalized Sedation

Computer-assisted personalized sedation (CAPS) is designed to deliver propofol safely and effectively when used by a trained physician/nurse team. The best-known device in this category is SEDASYS®, which combines target-controlled infusion of propofol and a physiologic monitoring unit. The device interfaces continuous monitoring of the patient's vital signs, including ECG, pulse oximetry, capnography, blood pressure, and responsiveness with computer-controlled propofol delivery to facilitate precise control of sedation. With signs of oversedation, it automatically decreases or stops the propofol infusion rate while simultaneously increasing oxygen delivery through the nasal cannula attached to the patient. The device is programmed to reduce or stop an infusion in response to either a clinical (unresponsiveness to audible/tactile stimuli) or physiologic (oxygen desaturation, hypoventilation) indication of oversedation.

However, less than a year into a limited rollout and with little explanation, the manufacturer Ethicon announced in March 2016 that it was pulling out SEDASYS® from the market [38]. As research and technological advancements continue, CAPS still holds the potential to revolutionize anesthesia care.

Closed-Loop Anesthesia Delivery System

The closed-loop anesthesia delivery system (CLADS) is a relatively new method that involves automatic, computer-based adjustments of infusion rates of different anesthetic drugs based on BIS or electroencephalography monitoring (Figure 14.1).

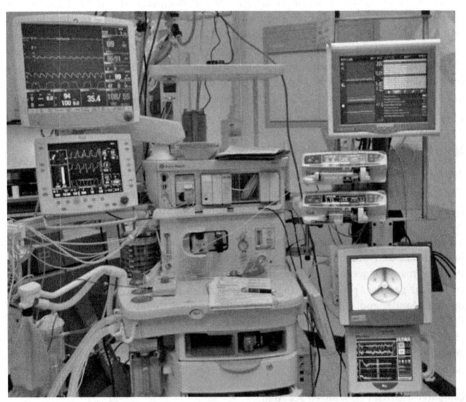

Figure 14.1 Example of a closed-loop anesthesia delivery system. Reproduced from West N, van Heusden K, Görges M, Brodie S, Rollinson A, Petersen CL, Dumont GA, Ansermino JM, Merchant RN. Design and evaluation of a closed-loop anesthesia system with robust control and safety system. *Anesth Analg.* 2018;127(4):883–94. DOI: 10.1213/ANE.0000000000002663

Potential benefits of a CLADS include lower drug dosing, faster postoperative recovery, and stable vital signs. Most studies have focused on proving that a CLADS performs better in maintaining a stable anesthetic depth by infusing propofol/remifentanil than manual control [39].

Although these innovations are remarkable, questions remain regarding patient safety, delivery system reliability, provider training, and regulatory approval.

Summary

Sedation provided by trained personnel is generally safe, with the most frequent adverse event being respiratory depression. When not detected and treated, severe brain damage or death may result. End-tidal capnography improves the early detection of respiratory depression and airway obstruction. Brain function monitoring may also help achieve desired sedation levels, although more studies are required. Controversies include the optimal choice of sedative agents and whether non-anesthesia providers can safely administer them. New sedation agents and computerized techniques are emerging, which may advance the safety, quality, and outcomes of sedation. Still there is a need for standardized metrics to evaluate and improve the practice.

References

1. Havidich JE, Cravero JP. The current status of procedural sedation for pediatric patients in out-of-operating room locations. *Curr Opin Anaesthesiol.* 2012;25:453–60.

2. Cravero JP, Blike GT, Beach M, et al. Incidence and nature of adverse events during pediatric sedation/anesthesia for procedures outside the operating room: report from the Pediatric Sedation Research Consortium. *Pediatrics.* 2006;118:1087–96.

3. Bhananker SM, Posner KL, Cheney FW, et al. Injury and liability associated with monitored anesthesia care: a closed claims analysis. *Anesthesiology.* 2006;104:228–34.

4. Metzner J, Posner KL, Domino KB. The risk and safety of anesthesia in remote locations: the US closed claims analysis. *Curr Opin Anaesthesiol.* 2009;22:502–8.

5. Metzner J, Domino KB. Risks of anesthesia or sedation outside the operating room: the role of the anesthesia care provider. *Curr Opin Anaesthesiol.* 2010;23:523–31.

6. American Society of Anesthesiologists (ASA). Standards for basic anesthetic monitoring. Affirmed December 13, 2020 (last amended October 20, 2010). www.asahq.org/standards-and-practice-parameters/standards-for-basic-anesthetic-monitoring

7. Pino RM. The nature of anesthesia and procedural sedation outside of the operating room. *Curr Opin Anaesthesiol.* 2007;20:347–51.

8. Soto RG, Fu ES, Vila H, Miguel RV. Capnography accurately detects apnea during monitored anesthesia care. *Anesth Analg.* 2004;99:379–82.

9. Krauss B, Hess DR. Capnography for procedural sedation and analgesia in the emergency department. *Ann Emerg Med.* 2007;50:172–81.

10. Anderson JL, Junkins E, Pribble C, Guenther E. Capnography and depth of sedation during propofol sedation in children. *Ann Emerg Med.* 2007;49:9–13.

11. Deitch K, Miner J, Chudnofsky CR, et al. Does end tidal CO_2 monitoring during emergency department procedural sedation and analgesia with propofol decrease the incidence of hypoxic events? A randomized, controlled trial. *Ann Emerg Med.* 2010;55:258–64.

12. Qadeer M, Vargo JJ, Dumot JA, et al. Capnographic monitoring of respiratory activity improves safety of sedation for

endoscopic cholangiopancreatography and ultrasonography. *Gastroenterology.* 2009;136:1568–76.

13. Qadeer MA, Vargo JJ, Patel S, et al. Bispectral index monitoring of conscious sedation with the combination of meperidine and midazolam during endoscopy. *Clin Gastroenterol Hepatol.* 2008;6:102–8.

14. Agrawal D, Feldman HA, Krauss B, Waltzman ML. Bispectral index monitoring quantifies depth of sedation during emergency department procedural sedation and analgesia in children. *Ann Emerg Med.* 2004;43:247–55.

15. Dominguez TE, Helfaer MA. Review of bispectral index monitoring in the emergency department and pediatric intensive care unit. *Pediatr Emerg Care.* 2006;22:815–21.

16. Schilling D, Rosenbaum A, Schweizer S, et al. Sedation with propofol for interventional endoscopy by trained nurses in high-risk octogenarians: a prospective, randomized, controlled study. *Endoscopy.* 2009;41:295–8.

17. McQuaid KR, Laine L. A systematic review and meta-analysis of randomized, controlled trials of moderate sedation for routine endoscopic procedures. *Gastrointest Endosc.* 2008;67:910–23.

18. Cote GA, Hovis RM, Ansstas MA, et al. Incidence of sedation-related complications with propofol use during advanced endoscopic procedures. *Clin Gastroenterol Hepatol.* 2010;8:137–42.

19. Fatima H, DeWitt J, LeBlanc J, et al. Nurse-administered propofol sedation for upper endoscopic ultrasonography. *Am J Gastroenterol.* 2008;103:1649–56.

20. Rex DK, Deenadayalu VP, Eid E, et al. Endoscopist-directed administration of propofol: a worldwide safety experience. *Gastroenterology.* 2009;137:1229–37.

21. Singh H, Poluha W, Cheung M, et al. Propofol for sedation during colonoscopy. *Cochrane Database Syst Rev.* 2008;(4):CD006268.

22. Rex DK, Heuss LT, Walker JA, Qi R. Trained registered nurses/endoscopy teams can administer propofol safely for endoscopy. *Gastroenterology.* 2005;129: 1384–91.

23. Cheriyan DG, Byrne MF. Propofol use in endoscopic retrograde cholangiopancreatography and endoscopic ultrasound. *World J Gastroenterol.* 2014;20:5171–6.

24. Dere K, Sucullu I, Budak ET, et al. A comparison of dexmedetomidine versus midazolam for sedation, pain and hemodynamic control, during colonoscopy under conscious sedation. *Eur J Anaesthesiol.* 2010;27:648–52.

25. The European Society of Anaesthesiology task force on the use of nitrous oxide in clinical anaesthetic practice. The current place of nitrous oxide in clinical practice: An expert opinion-based task force consensus statement of the European Society of Anaesthesiology. *Eur J Anaesthesiol.* 2015;32(8):517–20.

26. Robertson AR, Kennedy NA, Robertson JA, Church NI, Noble CL. Colonoscopy quality with Entonox® vs intravenous conscious sedation: 18608 colonoscopy retrospective study. *World J Gastrointest Endosc.* 2017;9:471.

27. Newton A, Fitton L. Intravenous ketamine for adult procedural sedation in the emergency department: a prospective cohort study. *Emerg Med J.* 2008;25:498–501.

28. David H, Shipp J. A randomized controlled trial of ketamine/propofol versus propofol alone for emergency department procedural sedation. *Ann Emerg Med.* 2011;57:435–41.

29. Miner JR, Moore JC, Austad EJ, et al. Randomized, double-blinded, clinical trial of propofol, 1:1 propofol/ketamine, and 4:1 propofol/ketamine for deep procedural sedation in the emergency department. *Ann Emerg Med.* 2015;65:479–88.

30. Bahrami Gorji F, Amri P, Shokri J, et al. Sedative and analgesic effects of propofol–fentanyl versus propofol–ketamine during endoscopic retrograde cholangiopancreatography: a double-

blind randomized clinical trial. *Anesth Pain Med.* 2016;22:e39835.

31. The Anesthetic and Analgesic Drug Products Advisory Committee. Oliceridine briefing document. www.fda .gov/media/121230/download

32. Goudra B, Mason KP. Emerging approaches in intravenous moderate and deep sedation. *J Clin Med.* 2021;10:1735.

33. Tanious MK, Beutler S, Urman RD. New hypnotic drug development and pharmacologic considerations for clinical anesthesia. Review. *Anesthesiol Clin.* 2017;35:e95–113.

34. Antonik LJ, Goldwater DR, Kilpatrick GJ, et al. A placebo- and midazolam-controlled phase I single ascending-dose study evaluating the safety, pharmacokinetics, and pharmacodynamics of remimazolam (CNS 7056): part I. Safety, efficacy, and basic pharmacokinetics. *Anesth Analg.* 2012;115:274–83.

35. Rex DK, Bhandari R, Desta T, et al. A phase III study evaluating the efficacy and safety of remimazolam (CNS 7056) compared with placebo and midazolam in patients undergoing colonoscopy. *Gastrointest Endosc.* 2018;88:427–37.

36. Mandel JE, Tanner JW, Lichtenstein GR, et al. A randomized, controlled, double-blind trial of patient-controlled sedation with propofol/remifentanil versus midazolam/fentanyl for colonoscopy. *Anesth Analg.* 2008;106:434–9.

37. Rodrigo MR, Irwin MG, Tong CK, Yan SY. A randomised crossover comparison of patient-controlled sedation and patient-maintained sedation using propofol. *Anaesthesia.* 2003;58:333–8.

38. Goudra B, Singh PM, Failure of SEDASYS: destiny or poor design? *Anesth Analg.* 2017;124:686–8.

39. West N, van Heusden K, Gorges M, et al. Design and evaluation of a closed-loop anesthesia system with robust control and safety system. *Anesth Analg.* 2018;127:883–94.

Simulation Training for Sedation

Valeriy Kozmenko, Lyubov Kozmenko, Stacy Lee,
Elyse M. Cornett, and Alan D. Kaye

Introduction

Simulation has been extensively used in military and aviation training. In 2003, the Louisiana State University Health Sciences Center developed and successfully implemented a required simulation curriculum, one of the first of its kind in the United States. Since then, this practice has been widely accepted by many other medical schools, both in the United States and abroad. Simulation has been used for teaching medical students and residents, nursing students and practicing nurses, as well as clinical physicians in many fields of patient care. Simulation is one of the tools that can be effectively used to teach sedation to both anesthesiologists and non-anesthesiologists.

The purpose of simulation is "knowledge application that is an observable behavior based on understanding specific concepts and principles and executed in specific context" [1]. Multiple studies have shown that the best acquisition of new knowledge and skills occurs in environments that are very similar or identical to the conditions in which those skills will be used; this is called situated, or immersive, teaching and learning. Simulation can create highly realistic immersive environments that can greatly enhance learning. In a real clinical setting, all patients undergoing sedation differ in gender, body weight, coexisting medical conditions, distinctive attributes of the anatomy of the upper airways, reaction to medications, etc., which makes providing the same teaching experience to all trainees difficult. In contrast, simulation can deliver standardized experiences to any number of trainees an unlimited number of times by using realistic preprogrammed scenarios. Reducing the level of anxiety associated with learning new skills, which can potentially harm a patient when the skill is learned on a real patient, significantly enhances the clinical value of the simulation experience. Simulation is an ideal tool for learning how to manage both rare clinical events and conditions that a trainee might experience on a routine basis. "Perhaps the best and most valid use of simulation training is to shorten the traditional learning curve and reduce risks" [1].

Simulator Types

There are several classifications of simulators, divided into three major categories, each of which has its advantages and disadvantages:

- computer screen-based simulators
- mannequin-based simulators
- procedural task trainers

Computer Screen-Based Simulators

Screen-based simulators have several obvious positives, such as:

- Cost of technology: For example, one copy of Sedation Simulator, produced by Anesoft Corporation, costs about $99, while an institutional license that allows for unlimited installations of the software costs under $1,000. Therefore, computer screen-based simulators are much less expensive than mannequin-based simulators. Sedation Simulator has a built-in performance assessment tool that can evaluate the quality of virtual patient care (Figure 15.1).
- Low cost of maintenance: No laboratory space is required, and there is no need to purchase an expensive hardware maintenance warranty, which is usually required in the case of mannequin-based simulators. The cost of maintenance for these varies from one simulator brand to another as many developers switch to the subscription models and could be as high as $10,000–$20,000 per simulator.
- No need for a full-time or part-time instructor to operate the simulator: In 2016, an average simulator instructor's salary was $60,000–$80,000 per year in the United States, based on the instructor's experience and qualifications.

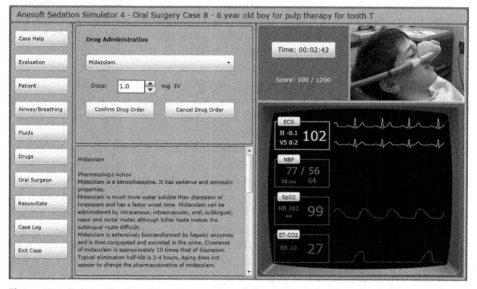

Figure 15.1 Sedation Simulator. Image courtesy Anesoft Corporation with permission to use.

- Convenience and flexibility: The trainees can run the simulator in the convenience of their own homes. This is an especially attractive feature for practicing healthcare personnel, whose schedules are usually too busy to allocate time for attending a simulation center event.
- Flexibility in portraying the patient: Screen-based simulators use a three-dimensional (3D) image to simulate a patient. Changing patient gender, race, body build, as well as simulation of body movements and emotional response, is much easier to accomplish than with the mannequin-based simulation.
- Consistency: Because screen-based simulators do not require an instructor or operator, their responses to the learner's interventions must be preprogrammed, making them very consistent in delivering educational content.
- Ease of updating and upgrading: Screen-based simulators are evolving faster than mannequin-based simulators because they are not constrained by hardware limitations.

Negatives of the screen-based simulators include:

- Lower level of physical realism in comparison to presently available mannequin-based simulators.
- Simulation sessions are not supervised by an instructor, who can debrief the session.
- Efficacy of learning might be affected by the trainee's computer skills.

Mannequin-Based Simulators

Mannequin-based simulators have many positives:

- Higher level of fidelity: mannequin-based simulators have greater physical realism and allow for easier suspension of disbelief and engagement in learning. It is not unusual for participants to get so immersed in the scenario that they forget that they have a simulator rather than a live person as a patient.
- Possibility of use with real clinical equipment: presently, most mannequins are anatomically correct and allow for various types of airway management, invasive procedures such as chest tube placement, placing intravenous access, or Foley catheter insertion. Working in a mixed reality simulation environment, which is a combination of real medical and simulated technology and equipment, creates the most realistic immersive learning setting.
- Can be used for in-situ training in a real clinical environment: the ability to use mannequin-based simulators has been the key factor in advancing simulation beyond academic settings and bringing it to the point of patient care, such as operating and emergency rooms and radiology laboratory.
- Can be used for team training in conjunction with the other simulators and live participants: mannequin-based simulators are often used in conjunction with the other simulators such as surgical or interventional procedural simulators, standardized patients, and virtual reality simulators. Hybrid simulation allows the use of several simulation modalities in such a way that they compensate for each other's deficiencies and enhance the learning potential of the activity.
- Performing procedures on a mannequin-based simulator does not require advanced computer skills: interaction with the mannequins during simulation occurs in a way similar to working with a real patient. This allows for easier translation of skills acquired in the simulated environment to patient care settings.

Negatives of the mannequin-based simulators:

- Cost of the simulator, which can vary between $19,000 and $250,000, depending on the vendor and the type of simulator.
- Designated laboratory space is required. Due to busy hospital schedules and workflows, this could be a challenge for in-situ simulation training. Bringing simulated equipment to the patient care area can compromise patient safety if simulation equipment is mistakenly used during patient care.
- Frequent use of the simulator is associated with extensive wear and tear damage, which may require replacing parts and purchasing expensive maintenance warranties from the manufacturer.
- Interactions between the trainees and the simulator are usually performed via an instructor, which adds to the cost of operating the simulator. In addition to the cost of having designated simulation personnel, mannequin-based simulation is more instructor-dependent than computer-based; thus, not all participants will have the same experience with the scenario.
- As technology advances, upgrades are usually expensive. An average mannequin's life cycle ranges from 5 to 8 years, which requires equipment depreciation to be built into the simulation budget.
- Limitations in changing mannequins' appearances. Even though some props can be used, usually, it is not easy to change the simulator's body mass index, race, or other physical characteristics that provide diagnostic clues in real life.

All mannequin-based simulators can be divided into three groups based on the level of fidelity that they provide:

- low-fidelity simulators and task trainers
- intermediate-fidelity simulators
- high-fidelity simulators

The difference between intermediate- and high-fidelity simulators can be subjective, and sometimes it is difficult to determine to which category a simulator belongs.

Simulators in Sedation Education

Appropriate airway management, which should include endotracheal intubation, is part of teaching the safe administration of sedation. An intubating head, such as Nasco's "Airway Larry" Adult Airway Management Trainer (around $1,000), can be used to teach non-anesthesiologists the basic principles of maintaining patency of the patient's airway and endotracheal intubation. Examples of a combined low-fidelity simulator and a simple vital signs simulator include the UNI-SiM Rigel 333 ECG Patient Simulator, etc. (Rigel Medical), Figure 15.2.

Louisiana State University Health Sciences Center has developed and successfully implemented a 3D avatar-based simulator. A similar simulator could be used as a valuable addition to any simulation system or combination of several simulators. A 3D animated patient is the core of the avatar-based simulator. An avatar can be remotely controlled by an operator, who can trigger different verbal responses from the avatar as well as facial expressions and body movements. An avatar-based simulation can be used for pre-procedural evaluation of the patient as well as for the assessment of the level of sedation/analgesia during or after the procedure.

High-Fidelity Mannequin-Based Simulators

Currently, the following are the main high-fidelity mannequin-based computer-driven simulators utilized for teaching procedural sedation and analgesia (Figures 15.3–15.5):

- Laerdal (www.laerdal.com)
- CAE (www.cae.com)
- Gaumard (www.gaumard.com)

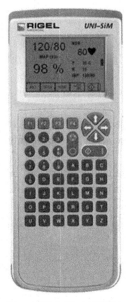

Figure 15.2 Rigel UNI-SiM. Image from the manufacturer's website with permission to use.

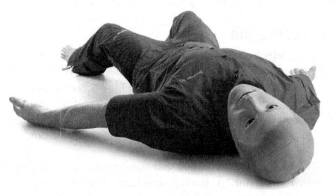

Figure 15.3 Laerdal SimMan 3G. Image provided by the manufacturer with permission to use.

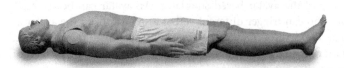

Figure 15.4 CAE Human Patient Simulator. © Image courtesy of CAE Healthcare.

These simulators share some common features, such as the ability to generate the patient's vital signs, including pulse oximetry, cardiac rhythm tracing, and pulses, but they also have unique distinctive properties.

In general, CAE simulators have the most elaborate design, with built-in physiologic and pharmacologic systems that can be used for modeling different clinical conditions, and they have a sophisticated scenario editor/player. The CAE Human Patient Simulator, the most advanced in the CAE family of simulators, has an automated drug recognition system that uses barcode-labeled syringes to detect the type and amount of drug injected. When the simulator detects what drug and how much has been administered to the virtual patient, its pharmacologic model will automatically generate an appropriate pharmacodynamic response. The CAE simulators have tremendous automation capabilities, which make them extremely useful if the same scenarios are used on a daily basis (Figure 15.6).

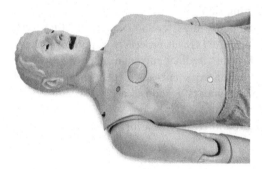

Figure 15.5 High-fidelity Gaumard HAL. Image used with the permission of the manufacturer.

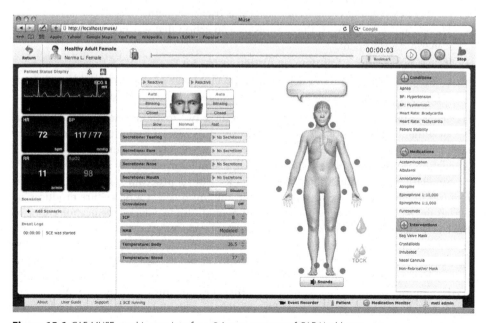

Figure 15.6 CAE MUSE graphic user interface. © Image courtesy of CAE Healthcare.

Laerdal SimMan simulators also have advanced programming features that allow them to run preprogrammed scenarios and scenarios that can be changed on the fly. In its most advanced model, SimMan 3G, Laerdal has implemented the proximity sensors in the syringes and the mannequin, making automatic drug recognition possible. The University of South Dakota Sanford School of Medicine Parry Center for Clinical Skills and Simulation has developed an advanced programming concept called the HUB, which can be used with both classic and LLEAP Laerdal software interfaces. This technique has simplified programming and uses complex clinical scenarios [2, 3].

There are two main ways to run mannequin-based simulators – on the fly and using preprogrammed scenarios. Each method has its own pros and cons, as outlined in the next section [4].

Running Preprogrammed Scenarios

- Developing scenarios is time-consuming.
- It requires some scripting or programming skills.
- It saves time if the same scenario is used frequently (develop it once, use it forever).
- It provides a consistent simulation experience. (This is especially important if the simulation is used for certification or in a longitudinal curriculum.)
- A well-scripted scenario makes the simulation experience less dependent on the level of the instructor's expertise because the simulators' responses are carefully preprogrammed.
- A full-time simulator instructor is required to create scenarios.

Running a Simulator on the Fly

- There is no upfront time investment.
- It can be exhausting if the same scenario is used frequently.
- There is more flexibility if the trainees take an action that was not anticipated during scenario development.
- It does not require a full-time simulation instructor.
- How the scenario plays out depends on the instructor's level of clinical knowledge.
- It is less dependent on the instructor's computer programming skills.

If one takes into account the pros and cons of these two methods, the logical conclusion is that if the same scenarios are going to be used on a regular basis, it will make sense to spend time to preprogram the scenarios because it will save time in the long run. If a simulation is used only occasionally, running a simulator on the fly is the best choice.

Simulating the administration of sedation for clinical procedures is unique because it requires the instructor to correctly assess the amount of stress a procedure produces, as well as the patient's response to a mixture of hypnotic and analgesic medications. One of the challenges of simulating sedation is that often a patient's response to surgical stimuli is via body movements, which mannequins cannot simulate. To compensate for that, the instructor needs to provide the trainees with verbal feedback on how the patient responds to painful stimuli. As the intensity of surgical stress and the amount of medication the patient receives changes, scenario evaluation should be very prompt.

A variety of commercially available simulators with different levels of fidelity and realism raises the question as to which one should be used for a particular course. After many debates at the Society for Simulation in Healthcare, a consensus has been reached that the learning objectives dictate how much realism is sufficient [5]. For example, if the primary goal of the course is to teach procedural sedation and/or analgesia, using expensive surgical lights in the simulation theater will not significantly add to the course's educational value. Equally, if the purpose of the course is to teach surgical residents appropriate chest tube placement, the presence of a real anesthesia machine will not help to reach this specific teaching point.

Recent Clinical Considerations

In recent years, simulation sedation training has become common in many disciplines. Some examples of programs that have been employed include emergency medicine, oral and maxillofacial surgery, radiology, dentistry, interventional radiology, and gastroenterology [5]. Some national organizations have structured this training utilizing board like review courses and examinations. Some examples include the American Society of Anesthesiologists, the American Association of Oral and Maxillofacial Surgeons, the American College of Radiology, the American Dental Association, the American Society of Dentist Anesthesiologists, the Society of Interventional Radiology, and the American Society for Gastrointestinal Endoscopy [5].

Summary

Simulators are very effective in healthcare education, and they can be used for teaching the safe administration of sedation and analgesia. There are a variety of commercially available simulators on the market today, from very affordable part task trainers and vital signs generators to highly sophisticated mannequin-based computer-driven high-fidelity simulators. The selection of an appropriate simulator or combination of simulators can be determined by the teaching and learning objectives of a particular course, as well as by reference to the strategic plans of a given institution. Any simulator is capable of providing learners and instructors with an engaging and worthwhile training experience.

References

1. Kozmenko V, Kaye AD, Hilton C. Theory and practice of developing an effective simulation-based curriculum. In Kyle RR, Murray WB, eds., *Clinical Simulation: Operations, Engineering and Management*. Academic Press, 2007, 135–52.

2. Kozmenko V, Wallenburg B. The HUB concept or How to release the full power of the SimMan3GTM – an automatic mode with manual override. Simulation User Network, San Diego, CA, April, 2014.

3. Kozmenko V, Wallenburg B. Overcoming limitations of the current high-fidelity simulators with the use of an innovative scenario design paradigm. Society for Simulation in Healthcare 5th place technology award, New Orleans, LA, 2015.

4. Kozmenko V, Young M. Programming patient outcomes in simulation: concepts in scenario standardization and automation. *Healthcare Simulation: A Guide for Operations Specialists*. Wiley, 2015.

5. Benzoni T, Cascella M. *Procedural Sedation*. Treasure Island, FL: StatPearls Publishing, www.ncbi.nlm.nih.gov/books/NBK551685 (last update July 3, 2023; accessed April 2024)

Additional Reading

Alhadeff E. Serious games improving training and performance metrics. Serious Games Market. www.seriousgamemarket.com/2010/07/serious-games-improving-training-and.html

Casuer J, Barach P, Williams M. Expertise in medicine: using the expert performance approach to improve simulation training. *Med Educ.* 2014;48:115–23.

Dieckman P, Gaba D, Rall R. Deepening the theoretical foundation of a patient as social practice. Simulation in Healthcare. *Simul Healthc.* 2007;2:183–92.

Guyot P, Drogoul A, Honiden S. Power and negotiation: lessons from agent-based participatory simulations. Proceedings of the Fifth International Joint Conference on Autonomous Agents and Multiagent Systems (AAMAS-06), 2006, 27–33.

Hwang J, Bencken B. Simulated realism: essential, desired, overkill. In Kyle R, Bosseau R, eds., *Clinical Simulation Operations, Engineering and Management.* Elsevier, 2008, 86.

Idaho Bioterrorism Awareness and Preparedness Program. Training methodologies.

Knowles MS, Holton EF, Swanson RA. *The Adult Learner*, 6th ed. Elsevier, 2005.

Kozmenko V, Paige J, Chauvin S. Initial implementation of mixed reality. *Stud Health Technol Inform.* 2008;132:216–21.

Kuhrik N, Kuhrik M, Rimkus C, Tecu N, Woodhouse J. Using human simulation in the oncology clinical practice setting. *J Contin Educ Nurs.* 2008;39(8):345–55.

Radcliff BJ. *Why Soft-Skills Simulation Makes a Hard Case for Sales Training.* CompeteNet, 2005.

Shapiro FE, Pawlowski JB, Rosenberg NM, et al. The use of in-situ simulation to improve safety in the plastic surgery office: a feasibility study. *Eplasty* 2014;14:e2.

Urman RD, Punwani N, Shapiro FE. Office-based surgical and medical procedures: educational gaps. *Ochsner J.* 2012;12(4):383–8.

Sedation in the Interventional Radiology Suite

Ezra Burch and Ryan Reichert

Introduction

A growing number of interventional procedures and diagnostic studies performed in the radiology department require moderate sedation. During the past decades interventional radiology has evolved from a referral-based specialty to a clinical specialty, a change reflected in its recognition as an independent medical specialty by the American Board of Medical Specialties [1]. This paradigm shift has been accompanied by an increase in the scope and volume of practice, and in the commensurate requirement for moderate sedation.

Moderate sedation is used in the interventional radiology suite for a wide variety of image-guided procedures. Interventional radiologists treat a broad range of conditions utilizing diverse techniques, including endovascular and direct percutaneous interventions. Imaging modalities include fluoroscopy, ultrasound, CT, MRI, and positron emission tomography. Patients undergoing strictly diagnostic imaging studies, such as MRI, also sometimes need moderate sedation, as they are required to stay still for prolonged periods of time in an enclosed space.

The American College of Radiology (ACR) and the Society of Interventional Radiology have jointly published practice guidelines for the administration of minimal and/or moderate sedation/analgesia, which can assist providers in safely providing moderate sedation during interventional and diagnostic examinations.

This chapter discusses additional screening that is required for patients undergoing radiologic studies, including pertaining to contrast and renal function. Common interventional procedures are then reviewed. Finally, special considerations around MRI are discussed.

Contrast Media in Radiology

Contrast media are often used in radiology imaging. Iodinated contrast is employed in fluoroscopy and CT, and gadolinium-based contrast agents (GBCAs) are used in MRI. Although contrast is used millions of times per year, like all other pharmaceuticals there is an associated risk. It is important to have knowledge of the indications for contrast use, potential adverse events, and management of adverse reactions. Potential adverse events include allergic-like and physiologic reactions to administered agents, renal injury with iodinated contrast, and nephrogenic systemic fibrosis (NSF) with gadolinium contrast.

Allergic-like reactions to iodinated and gadolinium contrast agents are uncommon and range from mild reactions such as hives to life-threatening anaphylactic reactions. Aggregate rates of allergic-like reactions with iodinated contrast are 0.6% and with GBCAs are 0.01–0.22% [2, 3]. The mechanism for adverse reactions to contrast are incompletely understood. Prior sensitization is not required for a reaction to occur, and most reactions are due to direct release of histamine and other mediators from circulating basophils and eosinophils. Immunoglobulin-E-mediated allergy is uncommon, occurring in less than 4% of patients having anaphylactic symptoms [4].

A pre-procedure assessment of the following conditions is helpful to identify patients at an increased risk for contrast reactions:

- Allergy: Patients with unrelated allergy are at a 2–3 increased risk of having a contrast reaction. Patients with a prior reaction to the same class of contrast agent (e.g., iodinated contrast) have a five-fold risk of an adverse reaction [3].
- Asthma: Patients with asthma are at an increased risk of bronchospasm.
- Anxiety: There is some evidence that anxiety increases the risk of a contrast reaction [5].

Below is a brief overview of clinical signs and possible treatment methods of contrast reactions. For a more thorough understanding of contrast reactions, the authors suggest referring to the ACR contrast manual.

- Mild reactions such as limited urticaria and pruritus often require no treatment, but the patient should be observed to ensure that the symptoms resolve and do not progress to a more severe reaction. Diphenhydramine 25–50 mg PO (per os; by mouth) may be given for patient comfort and relief of symptoms.
- Moderate reactions – which have the potential to become severe if untreated – and severe reactions require urgent attention. These reactions may include diffuse edema or erythema, bronchospasm, and laryngeal edema, and could be associated with hypotension and hypoxia. Vitals signs should be monitored and intravenous (IV) access maintained. Treatment depends on the specific symptoms and may include diphenhydramine for cutaneous symptoms or beta agonists for bronchospasm.
  In cases of hemodynamic instability or airway compromise, epinephrine should be administered. Auto-injector delivery systems, such as an EpiPen, are quite useful to have available, as they are appropriately dosed and ready for immediate use.

Current guidelines do not support screening patients for seafood and shellfish allergies, as this has not been shown to increase the risk for an adverse reaction. Patients who will receive the same contrast to which they had a prior reaction to are at risk for a recurrent reaction and should receive premedication prior to any future administration. Premedication should only be considered in patients with prior mild or moderate reactions, as it may not be effective in preventing recurrent severe reactions.

There are several premedication protocols available, and they should be confirmed with the patient prior to the procedure. For emergency procedures, IV steroids have not been shown to be helpful when given less than 4–5 hours prior to contrast administration.

Table 16.1 Prevention strategies for contrast media reactions

	Elective procedures	Emergency procedures
Option 1	Methylprednisolone 50 mg PO at 13 hours, 7 hours, and 1 hour before contrast injection, and diphenhydramine 50 mg IV, IM, PO 1 hour before contrast.	Methylprednisolone sodium succinate 40 mg IV or hydrocortisone sodium succinate 200 mg IV immediately and then every 4 hours until contrast given, and diphenhydramine 50 mg IV 1 hour prior to contrast injection.
Option 2	Methylprednisolone 32 mg PO at 12 hours and 2 hours before contrast injection, with the addition of diphenhydramine 50 mg IV, IM, PO 1 hour before contrast as an option.	If allergic to methylprednisolone, may use dexamethasone sodium sulfate 7.5 mg immediately and then every 4 hours until contrast injection, and diphenhydramine 50 mg IV 1 hour prior to contrast administration.

Some patients' diseases may be exacerbated by administration of iodinated contrast media. These include cardiac arrhythmia, congestive heart failure, myasthenia gravis, and severe hyperthyroidism.

Iodinated contrast is sometimes associated with kidney injury, although it is rarely the causative agent. When iodinated contrast causes renal injury, it is called contrast-induced acute kidney injury (CI-AKI). The largest risk factor for contrast-induced AKI is preexisting severe renal insufficiency. Patients with a glomerular filtration rate (GFR) below 30 mL/min/1.73 m^2 are at potential risk [6].

The ACR suggests that patients who have the following risk factors may warrant laboratory screening for renal insufficiency: history of renal disease including chronic kidney disease (CKD), remote history of AKI, dialysis, kidney surgery, kidney ablation, albuminuria, history of diabetes mellitus, and those taking metformin or metformin-containing drug combinations. Although there is no absolute renal function threshold below which iodinated contrast is absolutely contraindicated, the risk–benefit ratio must be considered in patients with poor renal function. In some cases, alternative contrast agents such as carbon dioxide may be used.

GBCAs are conversely associated with NSF, which is a disease that affects the skin and soft tissues but may affect other organs such as the lungs, esophagus, heart, and skeletal muscles. NSF presents initially as skin thickening and/or pruritis, but may progress rapidly, leading to joint immobility and contractures, and in some cases it may be fatal. It is hypothesized that the etiologic agent of NSF is gadolinium, which is released from chelates that constitute GBCAs. Symptoms may develop within days of exposure but usually take years [7].

GBCAs are divided into groups I-III based on their molecular structure, and group II GBCAs are considered unlikely to cause NSF. Patients at risk of NSF include those on dialysis, those with severe end-stage CKD (CKD 4 or 5), and AKI. Patients may be screened prior to administration of GBCAs. Histories of renal disease, including dialysis, kidney transplant, single kidney, kidney surgery, kidney cancer, CKD or prior AKI, and also diabetes mellitus are considered risk factors. In at-risk patients, renal function should be assessed. In those at risk, high-risk GBCAs (group I and group III) should be avoided, and the risk–benefit ratio of GBCA administration should be explored [8].

Procedures in Interventional Radiology Requiring Moderate Sedation

Arteriography/Venography

A percutaneous catheter is inserted, often through a sheath placed in a peripheral artery or vein. The contrast medium is injected and images are captured using direct X-ray or fluoroscopy. Indications for angiography include diagnosis of vessel stenoses, thromboses, aneurysms, bleeding, and vascular malformations, within the viscera or in the extremities. When an abnormality is found, additional interventional procedures to treat the vessel are often performed immediately following angiography.

The most common sites for arterial puncture are the right or left femoral arteries, but other sites such as the radial artery are increasingly being used. The most common sites for venous puncture are the right or left femoral veins or internal jugular veins. Once the skin puncture is made, a vascular sheath is often inserted using the Seldinger technique. The vascular sheath contains a hemostatic valve that allows the passage of guidewires and various catheters to the intended location while minimizing loss of blood. Contrast is then injected by hand or power injector, and radiographic images are acquired.

Procedural and Recovery Considerations

- Pain assessment and management of anxiety are essential throughout the procedure and must be provided while at the same time allowing for the patient to cooperate with breath holds and/or to answer basic neurologic assessment questions.
- Moderate sedation should be administered prior to local anesthetic injection and skin puncture and maintained throughout the procedure.
- Patients may experience nausea, warmth, and heat sensation during contrast injection.
- While contrast injection into the large vessels does not cause pain, special attention should be given during contrast injections to peripheral vasculature of the extremities and head, as these can be quite painful, and analgesia should be administered prior to injection.
- The patient must remain still during image acquisition because movement will negatively affect image quality.
- Contrast media volume varies depending on the number of vessels imaged or interventions deployed.
- A urinary catheter may be needed if the planned procedure and recovery period are long and require activity restrictions. Most arteriography examinations last several hours, but additional time can be expected if interventional procedures follow the diagnostic examination.
- With arteriography, post-procedure activity restrictions include bed rest with immobilization of the femoral arterial-puncture-site limb for 6 hours unless a closure device is deployed at the end of the procedure. When these devices are placed, bed rest is usually limited to 2 hours or per specific manufacturer guidelines. Radial access requires shorter bed rest.

Complications of arteriography include bleeding from the puncture site, thrombosis at the insertion site or other accessed vessel, contrast reaction, embolus, and dissection.

Arterial Interventions

When an artery becomes occluded or is abnormal, the treatment options are determined by the occlusion or abnormality type, location, and desired technical and clinical end point. There are several types of interventions, including:

- percutaneous transluminal angioplasty with or without stent placement
- thrombolysis
- embolization

Percutaneous Transluminal Angioplasty

Percutaneous transluminal angioplasty is used to treat narrowed or occluded arteries and veins in the periphery or viscera. A catheter with a balloon attached is inserted through a sheath into a peripheral artery or vein and directed to the stenotic or occluded site under fluoroscopic guidance. The balloon is inflated and blood flow is restored. If appropriate, a stent is placed to maintain vessel patency.

Procedural and recovery considerations include the following:

- Arteriography or venography will precede interventional therapy. Monitor for contrast reaction.
- Patients need to maintain position and remain still, especially during imaging, balloon inflation, and stent deployment.
- Patients will most likely experience increased pain during angioplasty of peripheral vessels and may require additional analgesia prior to balloon inflation and stent deployment.
- Spasm may occur during artery manipulation, requiring administration of nitroglycerine to the affected vessel.
- Post procedure, the puncture site should be assessed for bleeding, hematoma, and pain.

Mild pain responsive to non-opioid analgesics at the vessel access site is normal but severe pain at the access site intervention site should be evaluated immediately for complications such as bleeding, dissection, or thrombus.

Thrombolysis

A patient with acute or chronic peripheral arterial or bypass graft vessel occlusion with thrombus may present with acute pain and decreased or absent pulses in the affected limb. A thrombolytic drug such as tissue plasminogen activator (TPA) is infused at a specific rate over several hours through a catheter positioned at the site of the occlusion. Repeat angiography is performed to assess vessel patency. The catheter may be left in place for an additional 24–48 hours to deliver a low dose of a thrombolytic agent. A thrombectomy catheter may be placed to mechanically remove the thrombus as well.

Thrombolysis and thrombectomy may also be performed for venous occlusion. Increasingly, mechanical thrombectomy systems are being employed that reduce the need for TPA. Systems using rheolytic thrombectomy can cause myoglobinuria and AKI. In these cases, renal function should be monitored post procedure.

Percutaneous Transcatheter Embolization

Embolization of an artery or vein is performed to occlude a vessel by administering an embolic agent made of coils, sclerosants, absolute ethanol, particles, or glue to the site of the vessel abnormality. Choice of embolic agent is based on the clinical application, target lesion, and specific technical and clinical considerations. Examples of indications for embolization therapy include treatment of bleeding, arteriovenous malformations, aneurysms, uterine fibroids, and varicoceles. In addition, embolization is used for preoperative devascularization of hypervascular organs and lesions to reduce intraoperative blood loss. All embolization procedures begin with selective angiography with contrast to evaluate the target.

Procedural and recovery considerations for common arterial embolization procedures are shown in Table 16.2.

Interventional Oncology Procedures

In addition to arterial embolization procedures such as chemoembolization and radioembolization, percutaneous ablation techniques such as microwave ablation (MWA) and cryoablation are used to treat cancerous lesions of the liver, kidney, lung, and bone. CT, ultrasound, or MRI imaging is used to guide specialized probes to the tumor site, where ablative therapy is then delivered.

Microwave Ablation

With MWA, an antenna connected to a microwave generator is placed through the skin and directly into the tumor. The antenna, which resembles a needle, is connected by a wire to a microwave generator. Electromagnetic energy is delivered via the antenna, resulting in high tumoral temperatures and cell death. Ablation takes approximately 10–15 minutes depending on the target.

Although some MWA procedures can be performed with moderate sedation, deep sedation or general anesthesia are often needed to manage pain, discomfort due to positioning, and patient movement. The sedation plan is often determined by operator preference and patient choice. Patients can experience moderate pain immediately after MWA and are managed with opioid analgesics. Patients are often discharged home the same day if pain can be controlled with oral medication. Procedure time can range from 1–3 hours.

Immediate post-procedure complications include:

- Lung MWA: Pneumothorax is reported in 32% of patients, and serial chest X-rays are needed during the recovery phase for those who are small or asymptomatic [9]. About half of pneumothoraxes are self-limiting and do not require a chest tube. Other complications include intercostal nerve injury and bleeding.
- Liver MWA: Bleeding, especially in patients with abnormal coagulation, and non-target tissue injury of the bowel or gallbladder. Metabolic derangements including myoglobinuria can occur. Brief or long-lasting shoulder pain is also reported.
- Renal MWA: Significant bleeding requiring transfusion occurs in 1–2% of cases [10]. Intercostal nerve injury can occur during the procedure and is noted when the patient complains of pain, but if the patient is deeply sedated this will often go undetected.

Cryoablation

Most commonly employed for the treatment of renal cell carcinoma, lung cancer, and liver cancer, this procedure involves the placement of several cryoprobes under CT,

Table 16.2 Procedural and recovery care considerations for some common arterial embolization procedures

Procedure	Procedural considerations	Recovery considerations
Uterine fibroid embolization	Moderate sedation is typically adequate for procedural management of pain and anxiety. Contrast media is utilized during arteriography for catheter placement. Abdominal pain and cramping generally occurs minutes after the uterine artery is embolized and fibroid tumor necrosis begins.	Pain and cramping may be severe peaking 8–12 hours following the procedure. IV non-steroidal anti-inflammatory drugs and tylenol in addition to patient-controlled analgesia are usually good options for patients. Assess respiratory status closely while patient-controlled pain medications are being titrated to avoid oversedation.
Trans-arterial chemoembolization	Used for liver lesions taking advantage of the dual blood supply to the liver. Selective angiography is performed to locate the lesion. A chemotherapeutic agent(s) is delivered directly to the tumor site often loaded on an embolic particle. This induces direct ischemia to the tumor and direct delivery of the chemotherapeutic agent, resulting in high local drug concentration. Because the chemotherapeutic agents are not delivered systemically, side effects are reduced. Patients are given antiemetic agents, steroids, and prophylactic antibiotics prior to the procedure. The procedure length is 2–3 hours.	Patients can develop post-embolization syndrome characterized by abdominal pain, nausea, vomiting, fever, and fatigue. Antiemetics, pain medications, and IV fluids should be continued during recovery. Patients will be admitted to the hospital for about 24 hours for symptom management and observation.
Radioembolization for non-surgical treatment of liver tumors	A selective hepatic angiogram is performed and a catheter is guided to a branch of the hepatic artery and placed near the liver tumor. Tiny microsphere beads containing yttrium-90, a radioisotope that emits beta-radiation, are infused into the blood supply of the tumor. The procedure can take 60–90 minutes. A pre-planning hepatic angiogram is performed prior to radioembolization to identify blood supply to the lesion. Coils may be inserted into vessels supplying the intestine or stomach to prevent migration of radioactive microspheres.	Abdominal pain, nausea, and fatigue are common after treatment. Patients are discharged home after they have recovered from sedation and the groin puncture site is stable.

ultrasound, or MRI guidance into the tumor. Argon gas is delivered to the tip, where it expands and cools to temperatures below –100 °C, creating an "ice ball" and destroying cancerous cells and surrounding tissue. Two to three freeze–thaw cycles are recommended depending on the tissue type to increase the efficacy of tumor ablation. Cryoablation may be performed under moderate sedation but is often performed under deep sedation or general anesthesia because of positioning requirements and to limit any patient movement during cryoprobe placement.

Vascular Access

Placement of central venous catheters in the interventional radiology department is typically accomplished with the use of both ultrasound and fluoroscopic guidance. The most common sites for tunneled central catheter insertion are the internal jugular and external jugular veins, in addition to the brachial and basilic veins for peripherally inserted central catheters. Catheters are placed for a variety of indications such as hemodialysis, chemotherapy, long-term IV antibiotic therapy, parenteral nutrition, or poor vascular access in an acutely ill patient. Several types of central venous catheters are available from various manufacturers (Table 16.3).

Procedural Considerations

- Procedure length is usually minimal, and light to moderate sedation is all that is required in most cases.
- Non-tunneled catheters may be placed with local anesthetic only; however, patients must maintain a turned neck position during catheter insertion and may require analgesia.
- Peripherally inserted central catheters are usually placed with local anesthetic only.
- Regardless of the use of sedation or local anesthetic, patients should be placed on ECG monitoring during the procedure to assess for arrhythmias, which can occur during placement due to mechanical irritation from the catheter or guidewires near the right atrium.

Table 16.3 Central venous catheters: types and indications

Catheter type	Indications	Duration
Non-tunneled catheters: peripherally inserted central catheters, standard triple-lumen central catheters, temporary dialysis catheters	IV antibiotic therapy and IV medications requiring central venous access Poor peripheral venous access Parenteral nutrition Hemodialysis access in acutely ill patient	Short to intermediate use
Tunneled catheters	Chemotherapy Hemodialysis Apheresis	Long-term use
Implanted ports	Chemotherapy Intermittent IV therapy	Long-term intermittent use

Percutaneous Needle Biopsy/Core Needle Biopsy

Although fluoroscopy may be used, most needle biopsies are performed using ultrasound or CT guidance. The type of image modality used depends upon the location, size, and accessibility of the lesion. While most superficial and many liver lesions are amenable to ultrasound guidance, biopsies of the lung and bone are usually performed using CT guidance. A trans-jugular approach to liver biopsy may be required for patients with coagulopathy, whereby a core tissue sample is obtained by a catheter inserted in the jugular vein and guided to the hepatic venous system. Various biopsies, imaging techniques usually employed, and potential complications are listed in Table 16.4.

Hemodialysis and Fistula/Graft Maintenance Procedures

Patients receiving dialysis will often develop occlusions and stenosis of the fistula or graft. Several treatment options are available, including angioplasty, stenting, thrombolysis, and thrombectomy. If a fistula is thrombosed, the particular treatment is based on individual patient considerations but the most important issues for prolonged access patency are removal of clot, successful treatment of stenoses, and restoration of adequate graft blood flow [11, 12]. Once treated, fistulas and grafts can often re-stenose, requiring re-treatment.

Procedural Considerations

- Prior to any hemodialysis access intervention, the patient's potassium level and fluid volume status must be assessed if hemodialysis has not been performed recently due to fistula/graft dysfunction.

Table 16.4 Biopsies: imaging techniques and sedation-related procedural considerations

Organ/site	Imaging modality	Procedural considerations
Superficial (including thyroid)	Ultrasound	Local anesthetic. Moderate sedation not needed in cooperative patients.
Liver	Ultrasound, CT, MRI, fluoroscopy	Analgesia is usually minimal, but patient may require sedation to limit movement and promote comfort. Major complications include hemorrhage, and it may be life-threatening. Bed rest required post procedure for 2–4 hours.
Abdominal (kidney, pancreas, spleen)	Ultrasound, CT, MRI	Based on location of lesion, sedation may be required to maintain patient position and provide analgesia.
Chest (lung)	CT	Local analgesia may be preferable to maintain normal respirations. Assess respiratory status closely, as patient is at risk for pneumothorax and bleeding. May note a small amount hemoptysis after tissue sample obtained. Post-procedure chest -rays needed to evaluate for pneumothorax.
Bone	CT, fluoroscopy	May be positioned supine or prone and require increased analgesia during procedure.

- The procedure begins with a venogram of the native venous system from the hemodialysis circuit to the heart.
- Once all areas of stenosis and occlusion are identified, moderate sedation should be administered and maintained prior to any balloon inflation or catheter manipulation, to minimize unwanted movement and provide analgesia.
- The procedure can take 1–2 hours if the hemodialysis circuit is occluded or multiple sites of stenosis are addressed.
- Once the procedure has been successfully completed, patients may receive dialysis immediately. If the procedure is not successful, or if continuous thrombolytic therapy is required, a temporary central catheter may be placed to perform hemodialysis until the fistula is fully functional.

Drainage Catheter Placement

There are many types of drainage catheters placed under radiologic guidance to remove fluid accumulations from the body, such as chest tubes, nephrostomy tubes, and biliary tubes. In addition, a drainage catheter may be placed to remove fluid from an abscess located in the abdominal or pelvic cavity. Moderate sedation is used in most cases, because of the location and depth of the fluid collection, and discomfort related to catheter insertion. Specific procedural considerations are noted in Table 16.5.

Moderate Sedation in MRI

Providing moderate sedation in the MRI suite presents both patient and environmental challenges. The most common need for moderate sedation in MRI arises from severe anxiety from claustrophobia while in the scanner. Reports in the literature indicate that 4–30% of patients undergoing an MRI examination experience anxiety that results in a non-diagnostic examination due to frequent movement [13]. Even when they are given oral anxiolytic agents, it is still difficult for patients to complete the study [14]. Other indications for moderate sedation include:

- interventional procedures performed under MRI guidance
- severe pain that limits the ability to maintain body position during the examination
- Neurologic or behavior disorders that prevent the patient from tolerating the examination

It is important to limit patient movement in order to acquire clear diagnostic images, and in some instances patients require deep sedation or general anesthesia administered by an anesthesiologist.

Compliance with MRI safety rules is paramount in order to protect both patients and staff. An important point to remember is that the magnet is always "on" whether or not there is an examination in progress. The MRI area is divided into four zones:

- Zone I: General public areas outside the MRI environment.
- Zone II: Interface area between public area and zone III. Typical activities include registration, safety screening, patient history, and insurance questions. Area is supervised by MRI personnel.
- Zone III: Area is physically restricted to MRI personnel by key locks or other locking systems. This zone has free access to zone IV.
- Zone IV: Scanner magnet room.

Table 16.5 Drainage catheters: procedural and sedation considerations

Catheter type	Description	Procedural considerations	Sedation considerations
Biliary	A catheter is placed through the skin and liver into the bile ducts to drain bile, either externally into a drainage bag or internally into the small bowel.	Prophylactic antibiotics are given. Contrast is administered to aid with and to confirm placement. Patients with underlying liver disease may have coagulopathy and are at risk for bleeding. If appropriate, a stent may be placed for areas of stricture.	Acute bacteremia may develop during the procedure or in the recovery phase, leading to acute hemodynamic instability. Placement may be painful requiring anesthesia care. Patients who are critically ill require anesthesia care. Patients may have altered mental status due to acute liver dysfunction.
Nephrostomy	A catheter is placed through the skin and kidney to the renal pelvis or calyx.	Prone position is used. Prophylactic antibiotics are given. Contrast is injected into the catheter to guide and confirm placement. Patients must be cooperative and follow directions.	Respiratory status must be monitored closely because of positioning. Obese and elderly patients are at risk for hypoventilation. Transient bacteremia may occur, causing altered hemodynamics during the procedure or immediately post- procedure. May require anesthesiology consultation in patients who are septic or who are unable to follow direction and maintain position.
Gastrostomy/ jejunostomy	Catheter is placed through the abdominal wall directly to the stomach with fluoroscopic guidance.	There are two techniques for catheter placement, one directly through the skin and the other through the patient's mouth and pulled out the stomach through the abdominal wall using a snare catheter.	May be performed with local anesthetic, but often given moderate sedation as may be uncomfortable.
Abscess	Catheter is placed through the skin directly to the area of fluid collection.	Positioning dependent on fluid location, most likely supine.	Monitor respiratory status closely. Transient bacteremia may develop during catheter placement.

Ferromagnetic objects and equipment at the interface of zones III and IV and within zone IV produce a "missile effect" injury as they are pulled into the bore of the scanner at a rapid speed. Commonly reported objects include infusion pumps and poles, wheelchairs, and scissors, and there is a report of an oxygen tank that led to a pediatric patient death [15]. Other injuries include skin burns from objects that produce heat while in the scanner, such as coiled monitor leads and certain medical implants, wires and staples, and objects such as bullets and shrapnel. Implanted objects such as certain aneurysm clips and surgical staples are also at risk of becoming dislodged. Acoustic injury can occur from the loud knocking sound made by the scanner, and patients should wear appropriately fitting earplugs and headphones. For MRI-guided percutaneous procedures such as biopsies of the breast, all equipment, catheters, needles, and supplies must be non-ferromagnetic and compatible for use in the scanner. The US Food and Drug Administration (FDA) labeling system for portable objects taken into the scanning room, as developed by the American Society for Testing and Materials International, is as follows:

- MRI safe (green square label): non-metallic objects
- MRI conditional (yellow triangular label): no or negligible attractive forces
- MRI unsafe (red round label): not safe

While some equipment and medical devices may be deemed safe or conditional at lower magnet strength, such as 1.5 tesla, they may be found to be unsafe at higher strength, such as in the newer 3.0-tesla scanners. A listing of medical devices and implants tested for safety is available from the Institute for Magnetic Resonance Safety, Education, and Research [16, 17]. Any item not listed as MRI safe or conditional must not be allowed in zone IV until testing is completed.

The ACR has published safety guidelines and alerts, and all personnel working in the MRI environment must review these guidelines and receive facility-specific safety training and screening prior to caring for patients in the MRI environment [18]. It is important to review the most current listing of approved medical devices, as this is updated frequently. For example, a recent review of the literature on patients with cardiac pacemakers and defibrillators and guidelines from professional groups clearly outline procedures that must be followed in order to safely perform imaging on these patients, and the benefits and risks must be clearly understood and discussed with the patient [19, 20, 21, 22].

Prior to sedation, the patient must complete an MRI safety questionnaire and medical history. If the patient is not competent, a family member, guardian, or primary physician with knowledge of the patient's medical history must complete and sign the form. Direct visualization of the patient's respiratory status is not possible while the patient is in the scanner, and therefore the following MRI-safe monitoring equipment must be available: ECG, pulse oximetry, blood pressure, and capnography. The magnetic field will produce intermittent ECG tracing distortions despite filter settings, but heart rate and oxygenation are available by pulse oximetry. For patients with heart rhythm concerns, assessments may be made between imaging sequences. The capnograph provides a respiratory waveform and can be used as a respiratory-rate monitor.

Specific MRI examination protocols that require the patient to maintain a supine or prone position for several hours typically are performed under monitored anesthesia care. Breast biopsies, on the other hand, are typically performed with local anesthesia and minimal anxiolysis.

Emergency equipment should be stored in zones II or III; however, in the event of an emergency, the patient should be removed from zone IV immediately before resuscitative effort begins. Most emergency equipment, such as defibrillators, are ferromagnetic and could lead to a dangerous and possibly lethal situation for patient and staff. Emergency responders should not be allowed in zone IV unless they have been previously screened and trained in MRI safety.

Acknowledgments

We acknowledge Brenda Schmitz, author of the previous version of this chapter.

References

1. di Marco L, Anderson MB. The new Interventional Radiology/Diagnostic Radiology dual certificate: "higher standards, better education." Insights Imaging. 2016;7(1):163–5. doi:10.1007/S13244-015-0450-9

2. Wang CL, Cohan RH, Ellis JH, et al. Frequency, outcome, and appropriateness of treatment of nonionic iodinated contrast media reactions. AJR Am J Roentgenol. 2008;191(2):409–15. doi:10.2214/AJR.07.3421

3. Katayama H, Yamaguchi K, Kozuka T, et al. Adverse reactions to ionic and nonionic contrast media. A report from the Japanese Committee on the Safety of Contrast Media. Radiology. 1990;175 (3):621–8. doi:10.1148/RADIOLOGY.175.3.2343107

4. Trcka J, Schmidt C, Seitz CS, et al. Anaphylaxis to iodinated contrast material: nonallergic hypersensitivity or IgE-mediated allergy? AJR Am J Roentgenol. 2008;190(3):666–70. doi:10.2214/AJR.07.2872

5. Lalli AF. Urographic contrast media reactions and anxiety. Radiology. 1974;112(2):267–71. doi:10.1148/112.2.267

6. Davenport MS, Khalatbari S, Cohan RH, Dillman JR, Myles JD, Ellis JH. Contrast material-induced nephrotoxicity and intravenous low-osmolality iodinated contrast material: risk stratification by using estimated glomerular filtration rate. Radiology. 2013;268(3):719–28. doi:10.1148/RADIOL.13122276

7. Shabana WM, Cohan RH, Ellis JH, et al. Nephrogenic systemic fibrosis: a report of 29 cases. AJR Am J Roentgenol. 2008;190 (3):736–41. doi:10.2214/AJR.07.3115

8. American College of Radiology. ACR Manual on Contrast Media, 2023. www.acr.org/-/media/ACR/Files/Clinical-Resources/Contrast_Media.pdf

9. Belfiore G, Ronza F, Belfiore MP, et al. Patients' survival in lung malignancies treated by microwave ablation: our experience on 56 patients. Eur J Radiol. 2013;82(1):177–81. doi:10.1016/J.EJRAD.2012.08.024

10. Kim KR, Thomas S. Complications of image-guided thermal ablation of liver and kidney neoplasms. Semin Intervent Radiol. 2014;31(2):138–48. doi:10.1055/S-0034-1373789

11. Bent CL, Sahni VA, Matson MB. The radiological management of the thrombosed arteriovenous dialysis fistula. Clin Radiol. 2011;66(1):1–12. doi:10.1016/J.CRAD.2010.05.010

12. Lok CE, Huber TS, Lee T, et al. KDOQI clinical practice guideline for vascular access: 2019 update. Am J Kidney Dis. 2020;75(4):S1–164. doi:10.1053/j.ajkd.2019.12.001.

13. Meléndez JC, Mccrank E. Anxiety-related reactions associated with magnetic resonance imaging examinations. JAMA. 1993;270(6):745–7. doi:10.1001/JAMA.1993.03510060091039

14. Middelkamp JE, Forster BB, Keogh C, Lennox P, Mayson K. Evaluation of adult outpatient magnetic resonance imaging sedation practices: are patients being

sedated optimally? *Can Assoc. Radiol J.* 2009;60(4):190–5. doi:10.1016/ J.CARJ.2009.06.002

15. Kanal E, Barkovich AJ, Bell C, et al. ACR guidance document on MR safe practices: 2013. *J Magn Reson Imaging.* 2013;37 (3):501–30. doi:10.1002/JMRI.24011

16. Institute for Magnetic Resonance Safety, Education, and Research. www.imrser.org

17. Shellock F. MRI safety. www.mrisafety.com

18. American College of Radiology. ACR Manual on MR Safety. www.acr.org/-/ media/ACR/Files/Radiology-Safety/MR-Safety/Manual-on-MR-Safety.pdf

19. Nazarian S, Hansford R, Rahsepar AA, et al. Safety of magnetic resonance imaging in patients with cardiac devices. *N Engl J Med.* 2017;377(26):2555–64. doi:10.1056/NEJMOA1604267

20. Russo RJ, Costa HS, Silva PD, et al. Assessing the Risks Associated with MRI in Patients with a Pacemaker or Defibrillator. *N Engl J Med.* 2017;376 (8):755–64. doi:10.1056/ NEJMOA1603265

21. Vigen KK, Reeder SB, Hood MN, et al. Recommendations for imaging patients with cardiac implantable electronic devices (CIEDs). *J Magn Reson Imaging.* 2021;53(5):1311–17. doi:10.1002/ JMRI.27320

22. Indik JH, Gimbel JR, Abe H, et al. 2017 HRS expert consensus statement on magnetic resonance imaging and radiation exposure in patients with cardiovascular implantable electronic devices. *Heart Rhythm.* 2017;14(7): e97–153. doi:10.1016/ J.HRTHM.2017.04.025

Sedation in Endoscopy

Maryam Mubashir and James D. Morris

Introduction

With the technological advancement in medicine, a paradigm shift has been noted in what can be achieved with the minimally invasive endoscopic procedures with equal, and in some cases superior, outcomes as the conventional modalities due to lower procedure and recovery time and markedly reduced adverse outcomes. Approximately 50 million gastrointestinal endoscopic procedures were performed in 2017. Of these, over 19 million were lower gastrointestinal endoscopies (sigmoidoscopies and colonoscopies) [1, 2], and most of these procedures were performed under varying levels of sedation. The advancement in the endoscopic sedation has been equally tremendous, from the unsedated procedures early on, to over 98% of endoscopies being performed under sedation in the United States, with similar trends elsewhere in the world [3]. The most notable change over the last couple of decades has been the shift from hospital to office-based practices and the slow but growing use of sedatives like propofol by non-anesthesiologists despite the ongoing debate on who the appropriate provider for this administration should be [4]. Even though some procedures can be performed unsedated, it is recommended that sedation should be offered to every patient before endoscopy [5], especially since patient satisfaction, in addition to other factors affected by adequate sedation, is considered a quality indicator of endoscopy [3, 6]. As a result, sedation and analgesia are now an integral part of the practice of gastrointestinal endoscopy.

Pre-sedation Patient Assessment

All patients undergoing endoscopic procedures require pre-procedural evaluation to assess their risk for sedation and to manage potential problems related to preexisting medical conditions [5, 6, 7]. This is also the opportunity to discuss the details of the procedures, including possible adverse events associated with the procedure and sedation. This evaluation increases the likelihood of satisfactory sedation and decreases the likelihood of adverse outcomes. The American Society of Anesthesiologists (ASA) recommends a classification of patients according to their individual risk factors, as it has been shown to correlate well with the risk of adverse events (see Table 17.1) [8].

Clinicians administering sedation/analgesia should be familiar with sedation-oriented aspects of the patient's medical history and how these might alter the patient's response to sedation/analgesia. These include abnormalities of the major organ systems and previous adverse experience with sedation/analgesia and anesthesia. The presence of underlying cardiopulmonary disease must be assessed, as these patients may not tolerate shifts in heart rate, blood pressure, and oxygen saturation that can occur with sedation. A history of obstructive sleep apnea and snoring should be assessed for presence of active or undiagnosed obstructive disease [9]. It is also important to review drug allergies, current medications for potential drug interactions, and history of tobacco, alcohol, or recreational drugs, as well as determining the time and nature of the last oral intake. Even though there is no clear standard, the ASA practice guidelines for sedation and analgesia by non-anesthesiologists recommend patients should have enough time to allow a sufficient period for gastric emptying, which is usually a minimum of 2 hours for clear liquids and 6 hours for a light meal. In urgent, emergent, or when gastric emptying is impaired, the potential for pulmonary aspiration of gastric contents must be considered in determining (1) the target level of sedation, (2) whether the procedure should be delayed, or (3) whether the trachea should be protected by endotracheal intubation [10].

A focused physical examination, including vital signs, auscultation of the heart and lungs, and evaluation of the neck and airway should always be done along with the focused history to help predict the likelihood of airway obstruction during spontaneous ventilation. Furthermore, a difficult airway in case of positive-pressure ventilation, with or without tracheal intubation, is required in the event of respiratory compromise during sedation/analgesia (see Box 17.1 and Figure 17.1) [11]. Attention must especially be paid to individuals with oropharyngeal and laryngeal malignancies as stimulation of this already tight space during esophageal intubation may lead to significant edema, resulting in complete obstruction of airway. With meticulous clinical evaluation, endoscopists can anticipate most potential complications, which leads to swift and appropriate responses to such events.

Pre-procedure laboratory testing should be guided by the patient's underlying medical condition and the likelihood that the results will affect the management of sedation/analgesia. These evaluations should be confirmed immediately before sedation is initiated.

Personnel and Equipment for Patient Monitoring

According to the American Society for Gastrointestinal Endoscopy (ASGE) *Guidelines for Conscious Sedation and Monitoring during Gastrointestinal Endoscopy*, patients undergoing endoscopic procedures with moderate or deep sedation must have continuous monitoring before, during, and after the administration

Table 17.1 American Society of Anesthesiologists physical status classification system

ASA physical status level	Patient description	Patient conditions
ASA I	A normal healthy patient	Healthy, non-smoking, no or minimal alcohol use
ASA II	A patient with mild systemic disease	Mild diseases only without substantive functional limitations. Examples include (but not limited to): current smoker, social alcohol drinker, pregnancy, obesity ($30 <$ BMI < 40), well-controlled diabetes mellitus or hypertension, mild lung disease
ASA III	A patient with severe systemic disease	Substantive functional limitations; one or more moderate to severe diseases. Examples include (but not limited to): poorly controlled diabetes mellitus or hypertension, chronic obstructive pulmonary disease, morbid obesity (BMI ≥ 40), active hepatitis, alcohol dependence or abuse, implanted pacemaker, moderate reduction of ejection fraction, end-stage renal disease undergoing regularly scheduled dialysis, premature infant post-conceptual age < 60 weeks, history (> 3 months) of myocardial infarction (MI), cerebrovascular accident (CVA), transient ischemic attack (TIA) or coronary artery disease (CAD)/stents
ASA IV	A patient with severe systemic disease that is a constant threat to life	Examples include (but not limited to): recent (< 3 months) MI, CVA, TIA or CAD/stents; ongoing cardiac ischemia or severe valve dysfunction; severe reduction of ejection fraction; sepsis; disseminated intravascular coagulation; acute respiratory distress syndrome; or end-stage renal disease not undergoing regularly scheduled dialysis
ASA V	A moribund patient who is not expected to survive without the operation	Examples include (but not limited to): ruptured abdominal/thoracic aneurysm, massive trauma, intracranial bleed with mass effect, ischemic bowel in the face of significant cardiac pathology or multiple organ/system dysfunction

Table 17.1 (cont.)

ASA physical status level	Patient description	Patient conditions
ASA VI	A declared brain-dead patient whose organs are being removed for donor purposes	

Box 17.1 Factors that may be associated with difficulty in airway management

History
  Previous problems with anesthesia or sedation
  Stridor, snoring, or sleep apnea
  Advanced rheumatoid arthritis (limited neck extension)
  Chromosomal abnormality, e.g., trisomy 21 (atlantoaxial instability)

Physical examination

Habitus
Significant obesity (especially involving the neck and facial structures)

Head and neck
  Short neck, limited neck extension
  Decreased hyoid–mental distance; less than 3 cm (about 1.18 in) in an adult
  Neck mass
  Cervical spine disease or trauma
  Tracheal deviation
  Dysmorphic facial features (e.g., Pierre Robin syndrome)

Mouth
  Small opening; less than 3 cm (about 1.18 in) in an adult
  Edentulous
  Protruding incisors
  Loose or capped teeth
  Dental appliances
  High arched palate
  Macroglossia
  Tonsillar hypertrophy
  Nonvisible uvula

Jaw
  Micrognathia/retrognathia
  Trismus
  Significant malocclusion

---

of sedatives and is paramount in minimizing the potential risks [12]. The rooms need to be large enough to accommodate all of the endoscopic equipment and the following monitoring equipment, while still allowing for staff to move around the patient.

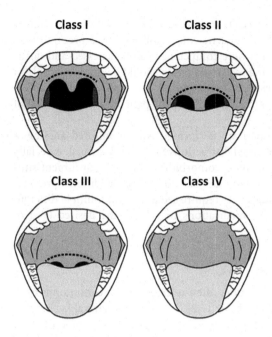

Figure 17.1 The Mallampati classification. Class I: soft palate, fauces, uvula, pillars; class II: soft palate, fauces, portion of uvula; class III: soft palate, base of uvula; class IV: hard palate only. The original figure was first published in the article "Multisociety sedation curriculum for gastrointestinal endoscopy" *Gastrointest Endosc.* 2012;76:el–25 and is reused with permission.

Standard non-invasive monitoring involves the following:
- blood pressure*
- ECG*
- oxygen and gas analyzer
- pulse oximetry (SaO_2)*
- continuous quantitative capnography*
- body temperature

Note that for the items with an asterisk above, these are the minimal monitoring requirements for gastrointestinal endoscopy [13]. In addition, the required emergency and resuscitation equipment should be located within the unit.

Furthermore, the following emergency equipment is required to be immediately available to the patient:
- bag-valve mask and source of 100% oxygen
- suction equipment and portable suction machine
- airway and intubation equipment
- reversal medications

Finally, the unit is required to have emergency equipment
- defibrillator and crash cart
- additional resuscitation medications required for advanced cardiac life support

Patients should be under constant surveillance by trained medical or nursing personnel from the start of sedation until the patient's consciousness returns to the pre-sedation baseline. In addition to the endoscopist, a trained registered nurse exclusively assigned to the administration and monitoring of the sedation should be present. A technician can be assigned to assist the endoscopist with equipment needs during the procedure.

Most states require the nurse to demonstrate competency in this skill through annual training. This education usually includes a didactic course followed by a preceptorship with an experienced healthcare provider, where competency can be assessed and documented [14]. Both the endoscopist and the registered nurse should be knowledgeable in advanced cardiac life support techniques. Freestanding units are required to have access to an advanced cardiac life support team that can transfer the patient to a higher level of care should the need arise.

A considerable number of endoscopies are performed with monitored anesthesia care. An advantage of this process is decreased distractions for the endoscopist, especially in patients with complex and multiple medical comorbidities or emergent/urgent situations. Additionally, complex procedural techniques benefit from the additional provider managing sedation issues. Such individuals may require sedation with multiple different sedatives in addition to other adjunctive medications to achieve the desired level of sedation.

Choosing the Level of Sedation

The ASA has classified four "levels" of sedation, often referred to as a continuum, from minimal sedation to general anesthesia (see Table 17.2) [8]. There are several factors that dictate the appropriate level of sedation for an endoscopic procedure. Some of these factors include patient anxiety and fear, complexity, duration, and type of procedure. Most upper endoscopies and colonoscopies can be performed satisfactorily under moderate sedation, whereas most advanced procedures (endoscopic ultrasound, endoscopic retrograde cholangiopancreatography [ERCP]) require deep sedation or in some cases general anesthesia. ASA class IV and higher ASA scores should be done by an anesthesia professional [7]. In addition, individuals with increased risk for airway obstruction because of anatomic variants or neck masses such as enlarged thyroid or otorhinolaryngological malignancies should undergo endoscopic procedures under monitored

Table 17.2 The sedation continuum

	Minimal sedation (anxiolysis)	Moderate sedation (conscious sedation)	Deep sedation	General anesthesia
Responsiveness	Normal response to verbal stimulation	Purposeful response to verbal or tactile stimulation	Purposeful response after repeated or painful stimulation	Unarousable even with painful stimulus
Airway	Unaffected	No intervention required	Intervention may be required	Intervention often required
Spontaneous ventilation	Unaffected	Adequate	May be inadequate	Frequently inadequate
Cardiovascular function	Unaffected	Usually maintained	Usually maintained	May be impaired

anesthesia care. Another factor that plays a key role is experience and preference of the individual practitioner; the requirements or constraints imposed by the patient, procedure, or institution; and the type of advanced airway management available in the event that a deeper level of sedation than anticipated occurs. Individuals differ in their responses to sedation and may require different levels of sedation at different steps during the same procedure. Therefore, practitioners should possess the skills necessary to resuscitate or rescue a patient whose level of sedation is deeper than initially intended.

It is estimated that over half of colonoscopies currently performed are completed with monitored anesthesia care [15]. Potential advantages to the use of anesthesia-provider-administered sedation for routine colonoscopy and upper endoscopy may include improved patient satisfaction and decreased distractions for the endoscopist. In addition, patients with medical comorbidities may require monitored anesthesia care that typically involves administration of propofol with or without adjunctive sedatives to achieve moderate sedation, deep sedation, or general anesthesia. Anesthesia-provider-administered sedation may be considered for complex endoscopic procedures or patients with multiple medical comorbidities or are at risk for airway compromise.

Unsedated/Minimal Sedation

Unsedated gastrointestinal endoscopic procedures are more common outside of North America and Europe [16]. Select patients may be able to undergo endoscopic procedures without sedation and providing education may increase patient willingness to consider this option. Older patients, men, patients who are not anxious, and patients without a history of abdominal pain may be more willing to undergo upper endoscopy or colonoscopy with little or no sedation [17, 18].

Standard pre-procedural preparations for sedation and monitoring, including intravenous insertion, should be followed. If the patient does not tolerate the procedure or develops a cardiopulmonary unplanned event, sedation is required.

To facilitate the procedure, small-diameter endoscopes (<6 mm) and topical anesthesia may be used for upper endoscopy and for colonoscopy. Water-assisted or carbon dioxide insufflation may reduce pain during and after the procedure [19, 20].

Moderate Sedation

Moderate sedation provides high patient satisfaction for gastrointestinal endoscopy. Moderate sedation with opioids and benzodiazepines can be administered by a registered nurse who is directed by a physician [7, 8].

Multiple societies in the United States and around the world, such as the American Gastroenterological Association (AGA), American Society for Gastrointestinal Endoscopy (ASGE), Spanish Society of Gastrointestinal Endoscopy, Canadian Association of Gastroenterology, International Society of the Diseases of the Esophagus, among others, consider propofol administration by non-anesthesiologists to not only be safe but, according to the ASGE, its administration by non-anesthesiologists improves practice efficiency for healthy, low-risk patients undergoing routine gastrointestinal endoscopy. Propofol should, however, not be administered by nurses.

Because it is not always possible to predict how a specific patient will respond to sedative and analgesic medications, practitioners intending to produce a given level of sedation should be able to rescue patients whose level of sedation becomes deeper than initially intended [10, 11, 21]. For moderate sedation, this implies the ability to manage a compromised airway or hypoventilation in a patient who responds purposefully after repeated or painful stimulation [11].

Deep Sedation and General Anesthesia

A patient undergoing deep sedation cannot be aroused easily but may respond purposefully to repeated stimulation or painful stimulation. Airway support maneuvers, such as performance of chin lifts or jaw thrusts, as well as insertion of oral or nasal airways, may be required during deep sedation [7, 8]. Deep sedation, like general anesthesia, should be administered by an anesthesia professional, which could be either an anesthesiologist, certified registered nurse anesthetist, or anesthesiologist assistant. In addition, multiple societies like the AGA, ASGE [7], and the Society for Gastrointestinal Nurses and Associates have been consistent in their recommendation that, during deep sedation, the individual monitoring the sedated patient should not have any other responsibilities [21]. This necessitates an additional individual to assist the endoscopist with technical aspects of the procedure. The ASGE [7] recognizes that the institutional policy in some places require an anesthesia professional for administration of deep sedation and recommended that the same individual can also monitor the patient during the procedure.

If the level of sedation becomes deeper than initially intended, as in a movement to deep sedation, it is implied that the sedation provider should have the ability to manage respiratory or cardiovascular instability in a patient who does not respond purposefully to painful or repeated stimulation [11, 13].

Medication of Choice

The choice of the appropriate sedation modality is always a balance between optimizing the benefits of sedation and minimizing the potential risks. Multiple surveys and studies revealed that the most used regimen is an opioid combined with a benzodiazepine for sedation [14]. Propofol is, however, used more often for deep sedation and complex/advanced endoscopic procedures. Patients undergoing sedation for gastrointestinal endoscopy may be premedicated with benzodiazepine, preferably midazolam. Analgesia is usually accomplished with fentanyl, a short-acting potent opioid. Propofol is preferred over other anesthetics because of its rapid onset and short duration of action. However, multiple frequently repeated dosing of any of the drugs can lead to drug accumulation and oversedation.

Benzodiazepines

Benzodiazepines act within the central nervous system (CNS) at specific benzodiazepine receptor sites. Occupation of these receptors results in augmentation of gamma-aminobutyric acid, which is an inhibitory neurotransmitter resulting in depression of cortical function. Thus, benzodiazepines result in a dose-dependent continuum of effect from mild sedation through drowsiness and sleep to deep sedation. In addition to sedation, benzodiazepines have anxiolytic and amnesic effects [3].

The most used benzodiazepine is midazolam because of its fast onset, short duration, and high amnesic properties. Doses are titrated to patient tolerance depending upon age, other illnesses, use of additional medications, and the sedation requirements of the procedure. See Table 17.3 for a list of some benzodiazepines commonly used for sedation.

Table 17.3 Benzodiazepines used for sedation

Drug (brand name); action	Mode of administration	Pharmacokinetics	Comments
Midazolam hydrochloride (Versed); short-acting benzodiazepine that produces sedation, anxiolysis, and amnesia	0.5–2.5 mg initial bolus IV. Additional midazolam may be given in 0.25–1 mg IV doses to maintain the desired level of sedation. For an otherwise healthy patient, the initial dose is 0.03 mg/kg, not to exceed 2.5 mg IV. Administer slowly with adequate time interval (2–3 min) between doses to assess for the effect of the previously administered dose. Decrease subsequent doses.	*Onset*: 1–2.5 min *Peak*: 3–5 min *Duration*: 1–5 h *Elimination*: 1.8–6.4 h	Duration doubles in elderly and obese patients. *Respiratory*: Central respiratory depressant and may produce apnea with rapid administration. Effects are pronounced with concomitant opioid administration. *Cardiovascular*: Hypotension in hypovolemic patients, incidence increased with concomitant opioid administration. *Caution:* Do not use midazolam when the patient is taking a protease inhibitor.
Lorazepam (Ativan); longer-acting benzodiazepine with amnesic and anticonvulsant properties	0.5–1 mg initial bolus IV. Additional lorazepam may be given in 0.25–0.5 mg doses IV to maintain desired level of sedation. **Not an FDA-approved indication.**	*Onset*: 15–20 min *Peak*: 60–90 min *Amnesic effects*: 6–8 h after a single dose *Elimination*:12 h	Must be diluted prior to administration in a peripheral vein. Give slowly to reduce side effects. *Caution:* Reduce dosage in the elderly or debilitated patient. The safety of lorazepam in pediatric patients has not been established.
Diazepam (Valium)	Up to 10 mg initial bolus IV (usually given in 1–2 mg doses). Up to 20 mg max IV dose.	*Onset*: 1–2 min *Peak*: 8 min *Elimination*: 0.83–2.25 d (18–54 h)	*Respiratory*: Minimal respiratory depression. *Cardiovascular*: Minimal depressant effects *Caution*: May cause pain on injection, local irritation, and phlebitis.

Opioids

The analgesic effect of opioids (Table 17.4) is exerted mostly from binding to the mu-opioid receptor, which results in an analgesic effect as well as euphoria. Opioids also cause respiratory depression in a dose-dependent manner that may be reversed by opioid antagonists. Respiratory depression can occur with doses smaller than the dose needed to achieve altered consciousness. Opioids depress both the hypoxic and hypercarbic respiratory drive [22].

Table 17.4 Opioids used for sedation

Drug (brand name); action	Mode of administration	Pharmacokinetics	Comments
Fentanyl citrate (Sublimaze); short-acting narcotic analgesic	The initial dose is 25–100 µg IV administered over a 2-min period. Titrate 25–50 µg IV to patient response. Titration to desired level of sedation should be performed with adequate time interval (3–4 min) between doses.	*Onset*: 3–5 min *Duration*: 3 h	*Respiratory*: Potent respiratory depressant alone and when combined with benzodiazepines. *Cardiovascular*: Vagotonic producing bradycardia and hypotension in the hypovolemic patient. *Caution*: Rapid administration may cause chest wall rigidity, leading to difficult ventilation.
Meperidine (Demerol)	Dilute and titrate 5–10 mg IV in increments.	*Onset*: 3–5 min *Duration*: 1–3 h	In equal analgesic doses will produce same sedation, respiratory depression, and incidence of nausea and vomiting as morphine. Use caution with patients with renal insufficiency, liver failure, or CNS dysfunction. May exacerbate seizure disorder.
Morphine sulfate	1 mg IV increments; peak clinical effects not apparent for up to 20 min. Because of the late onset and long duration, morphine is not an ideal agent for sedation and therefore not commonly used.	*Onset*: 5–10 min, peak CNS effect delayed up to 20 min *Duration*: 2–4 h	*Respiratory*: Potent respiratory depressant in presence of other sedatives. *Cardiovascular*: Hypotension may follow administration to the hypovolemic patient. *Gastrointestinal*: nausea and vomiting. *Genitourinary*: Urinary retention. Use with caution on patients with sphincter of Oddi dysfunction as it may increase pancreatic spasms.

Most endoscopic procedures do not require strong analgesics, as there are usually only limited periods of modest stimulation. Fentanyl may be given in small boluses as an adjunct to the anesthetic regimen. The ventilatory-depressant effects of opioids should be noted, especially when they are used in combination with other sedatives [23]. Patients undergoing sedation for endoscopy have an unprotected airway, and thus may become apneic and have the potential for aspiration. However, it is noted that individuals who have a combination of fentanyl with benzodiazepines like midazolam usually require smaller doses of benzodiazepines, have a shorter duration of procedure, and do not have any additional adverse events [24].

Propofol

Propofol (2,6-diisopropofol) is a phenolic derivative which is highly lipophilic, and thus can rapidly cross the blood–brain barrier, resulting in an early onset of action. Its rapid metabolism makes it a short-acting agent with a short recovery profile, regardless of the depth or length of the sedation period. It has sedative and amnesic properties

According to published values, endoscopist-directed propofol has a lower mortality rate than endoscopist-delivered benzodiazepines and opioids, and a comparable rate to general anesthesia by anesthesiologists [25]. The major adverse effects are respiratory depression, hypotension, and pain on injection. Hypotension results from the cardiovascular effects of propofol, which include decreased cardiac output and systemic vascular resistance. With overdosing, respiratory depression generally precedes clinically significant hypotension [26]. There is no pharmacological antagonist to reverse its effect, although hypotension and respiratory depression typically respond rapidly to a dose reduction or interruption of drug infusion.

The safety and efficacy of non-anesthesiologist-administered propofol sedation has been well established through multiple studies and is now used in multiple centers [27]. However, the practice is still not widespread/nationwide given differences in state level regulations [28]. Typically, loading doses of an opioid and benzodiazepine are given, followed by intermittent bolus dosing of propofol to target moderate sedation. This is called balanced propofol sedation. When propofol is used alone for endoscopy, its lack of analgesic properties may require larger doses and, therefore, result in deep sedation, for which there is no specific reversal agent [25, 26]. In contrast, the use of benzodiazepines or opioids should be considered in certain situations as this allows for a reduced dose and adverse effects, particularly hypotension in cardiac patients or in hypovolemia, but recovery is delayed [7]. Regardless, analgesia and amnesia can be achieved with less than hypnotic doses, mitigating the potential for deep sedation. Furthermore, more precise dose titration is possible with smaller bolus doses of propofol (5–15 mg), and the potential for partial pharmacologic reversibility is retained by using naloxone or flumazenil [26, 29].

Usually an initial bolus of propofol (0.5–1 mg/kg) is administered intravenously, followed by a repeated bolus (10–20 mg) according to the patient's condition. A continuous propofol infusion is not usually recommended. However, it is used at some centers (2–6 mg/kg per hour, with an additional bolus administered as needed).

For this sedation, the team must have appropriate education and training in advanced life support skills (i.e., airway management, defibrillation, and the use of resuscitative medications). Trained personnel must be dedicated to the uninterrupted monitoring of the patient's clinical and physiologic parameters throughout the procedure. In addition to the routine monitoring, continuous quantitative capnography should be considered because it may decrease the risks during deep sedation. The team should be aware that monitoring oxygenation by pulse oximetry is not a substitute for monitoring ventilatory function.

Adjunct Medications

Adjunct medications enhance the effects of opioids and sedatives, especially in opioid-tolerant patients, and in patients with a history of alcohol and substance abuse. Some adjunct medications also have antiemetic qualities. Examples of adjunct medications include promethazine and diphenhydramine (Benadryl). Due to their superior antiemetic properties in comparison to older agents, serotonin-receptor antagonists (e.g., ondansetron), these are increasingly being used. Use of adjunct medications for long procedures will decrease the need for larger amounts of opioid analgesics, thereby reducing risks associated with these doses. Therefore, the identification of high-risk patients and the potential for longer therapeutic procedures is useful for optimal sedation practices. For one of the adjunctive agents, droperidol, the Food and Drug Administration (FDA) issued a black box warning due to the potential for cardiac arrhythmias during drug administration.

Ketamine can preserve spontaneous ventilation and minimize the risk of airway compromise. It can be used by anesthesia personnel as an additive to propofol to reduce the propofol dosing requirements, thereby decreasing the risk of hypoxemia and hypotension in patients with poor cardiovascular reserve. Some of the adverse effects of ketamine are increased salivation and emergence phenomenon (e.g., hallucinations) [30].

Dexmedetomidine can be considered in patients with potential for airway obstruction as it preserves spontaneous ventilation. However, due to its slow onset and offset of effect, its use is not widespread. Hypotension and bradycardia are noted with its use.

Pharyngeal Anesthesia

Commonly used topical anesthetics include benzocaine, tetracaine, and lidocaine, which are administered by aerosol spray or gargling. Topical benzocaine is effective to prevent gag reflexes during insertion of the endoscope. The application should be limited to a single spray of 1-second duration to avoid methemoglobinemia, a systemic side effect that may result if multiple doses are administered topically.

Adverse Events Related to Sedation

Sedation for gastrointestinal endoscopy is considered safe, with only minimal risk for the patient. However, cardiopulmonary complications account for most of all reported complications. These complications mostly result from aspiration from suppressed laryngeal reflex, oversedation, hypoventilation, vasovagal episodes, and airway obstruction [10, 31]. Adverse events have been significantly correlated with patient age and body mass index (BMI), with an increased likelihood of adverse events in ASA class III and IV patients [5]. Hypoxemic events require interventions such as chin lift, jaw thrust, and increasing supplemental oxygen. These are more commonly noted in obese individuals and the rate of complications and adverse events from sedation in this subset is slightly higher than general population [32]. A retrospective review of 21,011 procedures found the rate of cardiovascular complications was 5.4 per 1,000 procedures [33]. The reported complications varied from mild transient hypoxemia to severe cardiorespiratory compromise and death [31, 33].

Colonic perforation occurs with higher frequency in patients undergoing colonoscopy with propofol deep sedation [34].

Recovery

Patients may continue to be at significant risk for developing complications even following completion of the procedure. The critical period is usually the initial 15 minutes after removal of the endoscope. Patients should be continuously observed in an appropriately staffed and equipped area until they are near their baseline level of consciousness and no longer at risk for hypoxemia and cardiorespiratory depression. Discharge criteria should follow the institutional guidelines.

Sedation in Special Populations

Certain types of patients are at increased risk for developing complications related to sedation/analgesia unless special precautions are taken. In patients with significant underlying medical conditions (e.g., extremes of age; severe cardiac, pulmonary, hepatic, or renal disease; pregnancy; drug or alcohol abuse) a pre-procedure consultation with an appropriate medical specialist (e.g., cardiologist, pulmonologist) may decrease the risks associated with moderate and deep sedation. In patients with significant sedation-related risk factors (e.g., uncooperative patients, morbid obesity, potentially difficult airway, sleep apnea), consultation with an anesthesiologist should be considered to help minimize adverse outcomes. When administering moderate or deep sedation to these challenging patients, the provider may request that an anesthesiologist be immediately available should problems arise. Most of the patients on this list fall on the high ASA physical status scale and should be considered for procedures under monitored anesthesia care even if undergoing elective, short, or straightforward procedures.

Chronic Obstructive Pulmonary Disease

Special attention must be given to patients with severe chronic respiratory insufficiency as any complication like aspiration pneumonia or carbon dioxide narcosis can lead to fatal consequences due to poor respiratory reserve.

For patients with type 2 respiratory failure (hypoxemia with hypercapnia), the oxygen saturation (SpO_2) should be maintained at 88–92% to avoid carbon dioxide narcosis.

Procedures for patients with advanced disease especially should be done under monitored anesthesia care as deep sedation can induce hypoxemia or hypotension, and suitable management from an anesthesiologist is required.

Obstructive Sleep Apnea

Patients with obstructive sleep apnea are at increased risk of having sedation-related adverse events and are especially susceptible to the respiratory-depressant and airway effects of sedatives and opioids. The susceptibility is due to propensity for airway collapse and sleep deprivation. This risk is not only high during the procedure but also post-procedurally. Therefore, the potential for post-procedural respiratory compromise should be considered in selecting medications [9].

Heart Disease

Prior assessments of cardiac function and consultation with cardiologist are recommended for invasive or long duration procedures on patients with ischemic heart disease, as they can cause anginal attacks or heart failure.

Chronic Renal Failure

Avoid use of medications with high renal clearance to avoid prolonged and higher than intended depth of sedation, which can cause hypoxemia or respiratory insufficiency. Use of short-acting and liver-metabolizing drugs (e.g., propofol) are recommended in this population.

Liver Cirrhosis

As the benzodiazepines undergo glucuronidation in the liver to become deactivated, patients who have decreased liver function may have an unpredictable response due to prolonged half-life and are more prone to have sedation-related adverse events [5]. Therefore, extra caution must be exercised while administering benzodiazepines and short-acting drugs (e.g., midazolam) are recommended. Furthermore, due to the risk of hepatic encephalopathy, moderate rather than deep sedation must be considered [32].

Psychotropic Drug Administration

Patients who are on benzodiazepine drugs, opioid analgesics, or psychotropic drugs require higher doses of benzodiazepine and opioid medications due to tolerance and often have an unsatisfactory experience.

Myasthenia Gravis

Myasthenia gravis is an autoimmune disease that disrupts synapse transmission at the neuromuscular junction. Assessments of the voluntary and respiratory muscles are carried out in order to safely conduct sedated endoscopic examinations. For respiratory muscle examination, sedated endoscopy is not recommended under conditions where negative expiratory pressure and forced vital capacity are used in lung function examinations and spare respiratory functions are virtually non-existent. Benzodiazepine drugs like midazolam and diazepam have muscle relaxation effects and are contraindicated due to their tendency to exacerbate symptoms. Reports have indicated the efficacy of propofol due to its short-acting effects, which do not influence the neuromuscular junction.

Seniors

Due to age-related functional decline in various body systems, senior patients are more prone to sedation-related adverse events. Due to higher sensitivity, lower doses of shorter-acting medications along with closer monitoring are recommended to avoid procedural and post-procedural problems. Lower initial doses of sedatives than standard adult dosing should be considered in the elderly and that titration should be more gradual to allow assessment of the full dose effect at each dose level [35].

Pregnant Patients

Endoscopic procedures should usually be avoided in pregnancy unless there's a strong indication; however, they are safe during the second trimester. Diagnostic esophagogastroduodenoscopy or colonoscopy carried out for gastrointestinal bleeds and ERCP for required for decompression of biliary tree, have not shown to induce any premature labor. Propofol is a Category B drug whereas narcotics and benzodiazepines are Category C and D, respectively. These procedures should be performed under monitored anesthesia care with careful monitoring due to altered physiological parameters in pregnancy, and particular attention must also be paid to the effect of hypoxemia, hypercarbia, and hypotension on the uteroplacental circulation. In addition, the teratogenic effect of some of the agents should also be considered. Effort should be made to shorten the procedure and hence the sedation time, as much as possible [36].

Generally, breastfeeding can be safely done 4–5 hours after sedation as this is the time it takes for midazolam to be completely metabolized. After propofol, usually once the mother has completely recovered from the effects of sedation, lactation can be resumed whereas fentanyl is considered compatible with lactation [36, 37].

HIV Patients on Antiretroviral Therapy

Protease inhibitors and non-nucleoside reverse transcriptase inhibitors have an excellent inhibitory activity against HIV-1. These are metabolized by cytochrome 450 (CYP) isoenzymes, which have several clinically significant interactions that have been described [38]. Midazolam, which is the most used sedative, is extensively metabolized by CYP3A4. Therefore, coadministration of these medications and midazolam leads to significantly prolonged and accumulative effects of midazolam, leading to severe prolonged respiratory depression [39]. Use of efavirenz, fosamprenavir, and nelfinavir is contraindicated with midazolam. Increases in the concentration of midazolam are expected to be significantly higher with oral than parenteral administration but caution should also be exercised with intravenous use. It is preferred that alternatives, like propofol, should be used when performing endoscopic procedures for such patients.

Future Directions

The need to have anesthesia providers adds a significant financial burden, especially for smaller private practices. Efforts have been made by both drug and device manufacturers to find alternative drugs that can be safely administered by non-anesthesiologists. Fospropofol is one such effort that did not live up to the expectations due to respiratory depressant properties similar to propofol. This was followed by a new tool to administer propofol in the form of Sedasys® but the device failed due to inadequate sedation. The latest effort is remimazolam, a new benzodiazepine that has a quicker recovery profile [40]. In the interim, many drug combinations such as propofol–dexmedetomidine and propofol–ketamine are improving safety without compromising the quality of sedation.

Patient controlled anesthesia with propofol has been shown to have higher patient satisfaction, but the use is still not widespread [7].

Summary

Sedation and anesthesia have evolved along with endoscopic advances of the digestive tract. The pharmacological agents not only make the procedures tolerable and safe but a myriad of options available with a range of different mechanisms of actions allow sedation to be tailored to each individual clinical situation.

References

1. Rex, DK. US GI endoscopy volumes: biggest change is increases in upper endoscopic ultrasound. Douglas K. Rex, MD, MASGE, reviewing Peery AF, et al. Gastroenterology 2021 Oct 19. www .endoscopy-campus.com/en/ec-news/u-s-gi-endoscopy-volumes-biggest-change-is-increases-in-upper-endoscopic-ultrasound

2. IData Research. An Astounding 16.6 million Colonoscopies are Performed Annually in The United States. https:// idataresearch.com/an-astounding-19-million-colonoscopies-are-performed-annually-in-the-united-states

3. Gotoda T, Akamatsu T, Abe, S, et al. *Guidelines for Sedation in Gastroenterological Endoscopy*, 2nd ed. Wiley, 2020.

4. Birk J, Kaur Bath R. Is the anesthesiologist necessary in the endoscopy suite? A review of patients, payers and safety. *Expert Rev Gastroenterol Hepatol.* 2015;9(7):883–5.

5. Riphaus A, Wehrmann T, Hausmann J, et al. Update S3-guideline: "sedation for gastrointestinal endoscopy" 2014 (AWMF-register-no. 021/014). *Z Gastroenterol.* 2016;54(01):58–95.

6. Rizk MK, Sawhney MS, Cohen J, et al. Quality indicators common to all GI endoscopic procedures. *Gastrointest Endosc.* 2015;81(1):3–16. doi: 10.1016/ j.gie.2014.07.055

7. ASGE Standards of Practice Committee; Early DS, Lightdale JR, et al. Guidelines for sedation and anesthesia in GI endoscopy. *Gastrointest Endosc.* 2018;87(2):327–37. doi: 10.1016/j. gie.2017.07.018

8. American Society of Anesthesiologists. Statement on ASA Physical Status Classification System. www.asahq.org/ standards-and-practice-parameters/ statement-on-asa-physical-status-classification-system

9. American Society of Anesthesiologists Task Force on Perioperative Management of patients with obstructive sleep apnea. Practice guidelines for the perioperative management of patients with obstructive sleep apnea: an updated Report by the American Society of Anesthesiologists Task Force on Perioperative Management of Patients with Obstructive Sleep Apnea. *Anesthesiology.* 2014;120(2):268–86. doi: 10.1097/ ALN.0000000000000053

10. American Society of Anesthesiologists. Practice guidelines for preoperative fasting and the use of pharmacologic agents to reduce the risk of pulmonary aspiration: application to healthy patients undergoing elective procedures: an updated report by the American Society of Anesthesiologists Task Force on Preoperative Fasting and the use of pharmacologic agents to reduce the risk of pulmonary aspiration. *Anesthesiology.* 2017;126:376–93.

11. Practice guidelines for moderate procedural sedation and analgesia 2018: a report by the American Society of Anesthesiologists Task Force on Moderate Procedural Sedation and Analgesia, the American Association of Oral and Maxillofacial Surgeons, American College of Radiology, American Dental Association, American Society of Dentist Anesthesiologists, and Society of Interventional Radiology. *Anesthesiology.* 2018;128:437–79.

12. American Society for Gastrointestinal Endoscopy. Guidelines for sedation and anesthesia in GI endoscopy. www.asge .org/docs/default-source/education/

practice_guidelines/
piis0016510717321119.pdf?sfvrsn=4

13. American Society of Anesthesiologists. Statement on respiratory monitoring during endoscopic procedures. Last amended: October 23, 2019. www.asahq .org/standards-and-practice-parameters/ statement-on-respiratory-monitoring-during-endoscopic-procedures

14. American Society of Anesthesiologists. Statement of granting privileges for administration of moderate sedation to practitioners who are not anesthesia professionals. Last amended: October 13, 2021. www.asahq.org/standards-and-practice-parameters/statement-on-granting-privileges-for-administration-of-moderate-sedation-to-practitioners-who-are-not-anesthesia-professionals

15. Adams MA, Saleh H, Rubenstein JH. A systematic review of factors associated with utilization of monitored anesthesia care for gastrointestinal endoscopy. *Gastroenterol Hepatol (N Y)*. 2016;12 (6):361–70.

16. Wang TH, Lin JT. Worldwide use of sedation and analgesia for upper intestinal endoscopy. Sedation for upper GI endoscopy in Taiwan. *Gastrointest Endosc*. 1999;50(6):888–9; discussion 889–91. doi: 10.1016/s0016-5107(99) 70188-4

17. Mahajan RJ, Johnson JC, Marshall JB. Predictors of patient cooperation during gastrointestinal endoscopy. *J Clin Gastroenterol*. 1997;24:220.

18. Paggi S, Radaelli F, Amato A, et al. Unsedated colonoscopy: an option for some but not for all. *Gastrointest Endosc*. 2012;75:392.

19. Leung FW, Aharonian HS, Leung JW, et al. Impact of a novel water method on scheduled unsedated colonoscopy in U.S. veterans. *Gastrointest Endosc*. 2009; 69:546.

20. Radaelli F, Paggi S, Amato A, Terruzzi V. Warm water infusion versus air insufflation for unsedated colonoscopy: a randomized, controlled trial. *Gastrointest Endosc*. 2010;72:701.

21. Dossa F, Megetto O, Yakubu M, Zhang DDQ, Baxter NN. Sedation practices for routine gastrointestinal endoscopy: a systematic review of recommendations. *BMC Gastroenterol*. 2021;21(1):22. doi: 10.1186/s12876-020-01561-z

22. Moon SH. Sedation regimens for gastrointestinal endoscopy. *Clin Endosc*. 2014;47(2):135–40. doi: 10.5946/ ce.2014.47.2.135

23. Lin OS. Sedation for routine gastrointestinal endoscopic procedures: a review on efficacy, safety, efficiency, cost and satisfaction. *Intest Res*. 2017;15(4):456–66. doi: 10.5217/ ir.2017.15.4.456

24. Khan KJ, Fergani H, Ganguli SC, et al. The benefit of fentanyl in effective sedation and quality of upper endoscopy: a double-blinded randomized trial of fentanyl added to midazolam versus midazolam alone for sedation. *J Can Assoc Gastroenterol*. 2019;2(2):86–90.

25. Nishizawa T, Suzuki H. Propofol for gastrointestinal endoscopy. *United European Gastroenterol J*. 2018;6 (6):801–5.

26. Fassoulaki A, Theodoraki K, Melemeni A. Pharmacology of sedation agents and reversal agents. *Digestion*. 2010;82(2):80–3. doi: 10.1159/000285351

27. Cohen LB, Wecsler JS, Gaetano JN, et al. Endoscopic sedation in the United States: results from a nationwide survey. *Am J Gastroenterol*. 2006;101:967–74.

28. American Society of Anesthesiologists. Statement on granting privileges to non-anesthesiologist physicians for personally administering or supervising deep sedation. www.asahq .org/standards-and-practice-parameters/ statement-on-granting-privileges-for-deep-sedation-to-non-anesthesiologist-physicians

29. American Society of Anesthesiologists. Statement on safe use of propofol. Last amended: October 23, 2019. www.asahq .org/standards-and-practice-parameters/ statement-on-safe-use-of-propofol

30. Goudra B. Big sleep: beyond propofol sedation during GI endoscopy. *Dig Dis Sci.* 2019;64(1):1–3. doi: 10.1007/s10620-018-5287-x

31. U.S. Food and Drug Administration collaborative study on complication rates and drug use during gastrointestinal endoscopy. *Gastrointest Endosc.* 1991;37:421–7.

32. Triantafillidis JK. Merikas E, Nikolakis D, Papalois AE. Sedation in gastrointestinal endoscopy: current issues. *World J Gastroenterol.* 2013;19(4):463–81. doi: 10.3748/wjg.v19.i4.463

33. Cooper GS, Kou TD, Rex, DK. Complications following colonoscopy with anesthesia assistance: a population-based analysis. *JAMA Intern Med.* 2013;173(7):551–6. doi: 10.1001/jamainternmed.2013.2908

34. Adeyemo A, Bannazadeh M, Riggs T, et al. Does sedation type affect colonoscopy perforation rates? *Dis Colon Rectum.* 2014;57(1):110–4.

35. Early DS, Acosta RD, Chandrasekhara V, et al. Modifications in endoscopic practice for the elderly. *Gastrointest Endosc.* 2013;78(1):1–7.

36. Kronenfeld N, Berlin M, Shaniv D, Berkovitch M. Use of psychotropic medications in breastfeeding women. *Birth Defects Res.* 2017;109(12):957–97. doi: 10.1002/bdr2.1077

37. ASGE Standard of Practice Committee, Shergill AK, Ben-Menachem T, et al. Guidelines for endoscopy in pregnant and lactating women. *Gastrointest Endosc.* 2012;76(1):18–24. doi: 10.1016/j.gie.2012.02.029

38. Keubler A, Weiss J, Haefeli WE, Mikus G, Burhenne J, Drug interaction of efavirenz and midazolam: efavirenz activates the CYP3A-mediated midazolam 1'-hydroxylation in vitro. *Drug Metab Dispos.* 2012;40(6):1178–82. doi: 10.1124/dmd.111.043844

39. Backman ES, Triant VA Ehrenfeld, JM, et al. Safety of midazolam for sedation of HIV-positive patients undergoing colonoscopy. *HIV Med.* 2013;14(6):379–84. doi: 10.1111/hiv.12014

40. Goudra B, Gouda G, Mohinder P. Recent developments in drugs for GI endoscopy sedation *Dig Dis Sci.* 2020;65(10):2781–8. doi: 10.1007/s10620-020-06044-5

Sedation in the Interventional Cardiology Suite

Katherine S. Cox, Dev Vyas, and Bryan Lynn

Introduction

As new medical techniques and technologies develop, the number of non-surgical interventions continue to evolve. The anesthesiologists' role in non-operating room anesthesia (NORA) locations continues to expand. In a study of the National Anesthesia Clinical Outcomes Registry, Nagrebetsky et al. found that the proportion of NORA cases increased from 28% in 2010 to 36% in 2014 alone [1]. Interventional cardiology and electrophysiology procedures are no exception to this, as they have continued to develop into fields that offer advanced and comprehensive therapies to treat a wide variety of cardiac pathologies. With the ever-growing success rate of percutaneous approaches to pathologies that once needed surgical intervention, the target patient population has broadened. As such, the increased need for anesthesia services in the interventional cardiology suite reflects a major expansion of our practice perimeter.

Procedures performed in the cardiology suite range from stenting of narrowed or occluded vessels to the implantation of prosthetic heart valves. Percutaneous coronary interventions with both bare metal stents and drug-eluting stents can be performed with nurse-administered sedation under the direction of the cardiologist. Most pacemaker and implantable cardioverter-defibrillators (ICD) placements are done with local anesthetic infiltration, combined with mild to moderate sedation, but can be done under a pectoralis plane block with or without monitored anesthesia care (MAC) when not well tolerated [2, 3]. Implantation of biventricular ICDs may be complex and lengthy because of difficulty positioning the left ventricular lead into the coronary sinus, and tunneling of the relatively large lead can be quite painful for the patients. This often requires deep sedation or general anesthesia for the intraoperative testing of defibrillating thresholds. Many patients who qualify for these cardiac resynchronization devices have extensive cardiac histories with cardiomyopathy, coronary artery disease, low ejection fraction, and ventricular arrhythmias; this means these patients are generally at high risk for intraoperative and postoperative cardiac complications. Therefore, the anesthesiologist's presence is crucial in facilitating these procedures while maintaining the patient's airway and hemodynamic stability [4].

The growth within the field of electrophysiology has allowed for the management of cardiac arrhythmias that may have otherwise been refractory to medical treatment. An example of this is the employment of radiofrequency ablation in the treatment-resistant arrhythmias. Patients range from young and healthy to those with extensive comorbidities. The complexity and length of these procedures have evolved dramatically and frequently mandate the administration of general anesthesia to ensure patient comfort and optimal mapping [5, 6].

Since the first percutaneous heart valve for human use was implanted in Europe in 2002, transcatheter valve placement has revolutionized the treatment of structural cardiac valve diseases [7, 8]. Over the last decade, there has been tremendous improvement in the research and technologies regarding transcather aortic valve replacement (TAVR) for high-risk surgical patients, drastically changing the management of severe aortic stenosis. Recent clinical trials, namely the Evolut Low Risk trial sponsored by Edwards's life sciences, and the Placement of Aortic Transcatheter Valves (PARTNER) 3, evaluating Medtronic's TAVR device, suggest that the use of TAVR should be expanded into low-risk aortic stenosis patients [9]. With the increasing number of patients eligible for TAVR, it is important that anesthesiologists be familiar with the devices and with the management of this specific patient population.

These procedures are typically performed in hybrid operating rooms (ORs) with cardiopulmonary bypass or percutaneous ventricular assist device support on standby. As studies show the non-inferiority of transcatheter valve replacement to surgical aortic valve replacement at 1 year in terms of survival, TAVR has been viewed as a suitable alternative in patients in whom the risk of cardiac surgery is deemed too high [10, 11]. As such, anesthesiologists must be prepared to treat this challenging patient population and import our OR safety standards to these new venues [12].

The Cardiology Suite

As the scope of anesthesiology practice expands beyond the familiar domain of the OR, we should seek to establish the same standards of safety and reliability in the NORA locations. Typically, non-OR procedure suites, including cardiology suites, are designed with the proceduralist in mind. The layout of the typical catheterization and electrophysiology laboratory differs significantly from that of the OR. They are built with separate control stations and procedure rooms. The control room contains a fully functional workstation that allows the technician to control the fluoroscopy machine, record digital data, and monitor the patient's vital signs and ECG readings. The control room is shielded from radiation and the person inside the control room has visual access to the procedure room, which enables him to communicate frequently with the cardiologist. The procedure room is where the intervention is carried out. Equipment in the procedure room includes the fluoroscopy machine, a procedure table, screens for viewing the procedure, a sterile table for the catheters and supplies, a blood analysis machine, and infusion pumps [13]. These take up a lot of space and the anesthesia equipment (machine, cart, pumps, monitors), often an afterthought, are frequently pushed to the back of the room, in functionally less ergonomic positions than in the

OR. Electrical and gas outlets, suction, monitors for vital signs, and emergency equipment, including cardioverter-defibrillator, may not be optimally placed. This will require anesthesiologists to spatially reorient themselves and re-configure the necessary equipment and setup. Accessibility to the patient's head is limited by the often rotating fluoroscopy C-arm. Longer tubing and extensions are needed for ventilator circuits and intravenous lines, and they must be secured away from the moving fluoroscopy equipment. It is necessary to have an anesthesia cart stocked with the necessary airway equipment, extra intravenous lines, medications, and other essential supplies, given the usual remote location of the cart. Additionally, imaging screens can limit visual access to the procedure. This makes it difficult for the anesthesiologist to anticipate events, emphasizing the need for familiarity with the procedure and maintaining good communication with the cardiologist. Anesthesiologists must be aware of the occupational hazards of ionizing radiation and should take the necessary precautions against radiation exposure [14].

The anesthetic and monitoring equipment used for NORA locations must meet the same standards as equipment provided in the OR, and the anesthesia machines and monitors in these locations need to undergo routine maintenance. Some institutions utilize portable machines and monitors. This underscores the importance of a standardized pre-procedural checklist and ensuring proper functioning of all equipment prior to administering the anesthetic [15]. Data from the American Society of Anesthesiologists (ASA) closed claims database suggest that respiratory depression secondary to oversedation accounted for over one-third of remote location claims [16]. The facilities most involved in remote location claims were the gastrointestinal suite (32%) and cardiology catheterization and electrophysiology laboratories (25%). In addition to the standard ASA monitors (pulse oximetry, non-invasive blood pressure, heart rate, and rhythm), utilizing capnography significantly increases the detection of adverse respiratory events [17]. Effective as of July 2011, the ASA guidelines mandate the use of exhaled end-tidal carbon dioxide monitoring during both moderate and deep sedation [18]. Patient acuity and certain procedures like TAVR may require additional monitoring, including placement of arterial lines and trans-esophageal echocardiography.

Anesthesiologists should function collaboratively with the cardiologists in establishing institution specific protocols and guidelines to ensure patient safety and improve procedural efficiency and outcomes. The Society of Non-Operating Room Interventionalists and Anesthesiologists was created with the aim of increasing efforts and dialogue affecting patient safety and clinical outcomes. While NORA locations are frequently cited to be less safe than the OR, studies are increasingly finding improved safety and outcomes with NORA procedures [19].

Patient Evaluation

Patients undergoing interventional cardiac procedures require a detailed preoperative evaluation for medical risk factors. Patients must be screened preoperatively and medically optimized when necessary. Compliance with preoperative assessment standards must be met before providing procedural sedation by both anesthesiologists and non-anesthesia providers. Patients undergoing interventional cardiac procedures range from being essentially healthy (e.g., structurally normal heart undergoing radio frequency ablation for atrioventricular nodal reentry tachycardia) to hemodynamically unstable patients (e.g., ventricular tachycardia ablations for frequent ICD discharges in patients with end-stage heart failure [20]). It is essential for the anesthesiologist to have a thorough understanding of the goals of the procedure performed. Some cardiac laboratory procedures may require unusual patient positioning or the duration of the procedure may be long, warranting general anesthesia. The anesthesiologist caring for these patients should be aware of positioning requirements as this may change the anesthetic plan [21].

Patients with obstructive sleep apnea, morbid obesity, chronic obstructive pulmonary disease (COPD), congestive heart failure, and potentially difficult airways are considered as high risk for sedation and general anesthesia. Patients who meet criteria for difficult bag-mask ventilation or difficult intubation must be assessed by an anesthesiologist and the dangers of oversedation should be stressed upon. Airway access may be difficult as the fluoroscopy machine surrounds the patient's head and chest. This limits visualization of respiratory movements. The amount of space available is limited to maneuver equipment for respiratory assistance, as previously mentioned [22]. Additionally, most cardiac patients have multiple comorbidities [20]. Some examples are listed in Box 18.1.

A pre-procedure evaluation enables anesthesiologists to intervene early and to prepare the patient for sedation, and possibly avoiding general anesthesia, for instance by the use of diuretics and improving respiratory function days before the procedure. Consideration should be given to patients receiving a radiocontrast dye. Nephrotoxicity is a potential complication in patients with preexisting renal disease or diabetes mellitus [21]. Patients with gastroesophageal reflux disease are prone to silent aspiration with an unprotected airway and sedation is difficult in patients with poor respiratory status such as COPD, obstructive sleep apnea, and chronic oxygen use. All patient medications must be reviewed prior to the procedure.

The anesthetic drug plan is patient specific as patients could be on chronic pain and anxiolytic medications that may make providing effective sedation difficult [23]. A previous anesthetic and sedation record is frequently available and should be reviewed preoperatively. Often patients have a history of previous cardiac diagnostic catheterizations, stent placements, arrhythmia ablations, and intra-cardiac device placement surgeries [23]. General anesthesia is preferable if a previous cardiac intervention failed due to oversedation, difficulty in adequately sedating the patient, hemodynamic instability, or problems with airway management.

Box 18.1 Common comorbidities in cardiology patients

Poor functional status
Hypertension
Cardiomyopathy
Congestive heart failure
Valvular heart disease
Coronary artery disease
Cerebrovascular disease
Arrhythmias
Hyperlipidemia
Diabetes mellitus
Obstructive sleep apnea

Interventional Procedures in the Cardiology Suite

Advancements in cardiology procedures and imaging have allowed procedures that were once only able to be completed surgically, now to be completed via minimally invasive techniques. Electrophysiology procedures that can be performed include permanent pacemaker (PPM) insertion, ICD placement, cardiac resynchronization therapy (CRT), cardioversion, electrophysiology studies for diagnosis, and catheter ablation procedures for multiple types of dysrhythmias [24].

PPM or ICD implantation is one of the most common procedures performed in the electrophysiology laboratory [20]. Some examples of indications for PPM insertion include high-degree atrioventricular blocks, symptomatic bradycardia, sick sinus syndrome, recurrent syncope from carotid stimulation, heart failure, hypertrophic obstructive cardiomyopathy, idiopathic dilated cardiomyopathy, and heart transplantation with resulting bradycardia [25]. The placement of an ICD can be for primary prevention of sudden cardiac death in patients with an impaired left ventricular function ejection fraction (EF) ($< 30\%$), hypertrophic cardiomyopathy, idiopathic cardiomyopathy, long QT syndrome, or Brugada syndrome with syncope or history [25]. The placement of an ICD can also be for secondary prevention in patients with a history of cardiac arrest or sustained ventricular tachycardia. CRT is indicated when the patient meets all the following criteria: EF $\leqslant 35\%$, QRS > 120 ms, sinus rhythm, and New York Heart Association (NYHA) class III or IV symptoms on optimal medical therapy.

The placement of a PPM or ICD can usually be done with minimal sedation and local anesthesia. A subcutaneous pocket is made for the device in the upper chest below the clavicle [20]. The procedure can typically be completed via vascular access for lead placement via a cephalic vein cutdown or subclavian vein cannulation using the Seldinger technique [20]. One or two leads are then placed in the right ventricle and atrium, respectively. CRT requires biventricular leads with one lead in the right ventricle and the other in the coronary sinus, to allow synchronized pacing of both ventricles. The placement of an ICD involves similar techniques, except the device is tested under deep sedation after induction of ventricular fibrillation. Complication rates are rare with mortality less than 0.1% but can be greater than 1% in very moribund patients. Pneumothorax, intrathoracic bleeding, and cardiac perforation with tamponade are the most common complications of PPM and ICD placement [25]. Other complications include infection of the device pocket and complications related to vascular access (3–4%), such as bleeding, infection, and vascular injury [25].

Another common procedure completed in the electrophysiology suite is cardioversion. Indications for cardioversion include supraventricular tachycardia, reentrant tachyarrhythmias such as atrial fibrillation, atrial flutter, atrioventricular nodal reentry tachycardia (AVNRT), and ventricular tachycardia [25]. External cardioversion usually requires deep sedation, but only briefly for the cardioversion. Adverse events include the R on T phenomenon, which may precipitate ventricular arrhythmias. Also, transient myocardial depression, recurrent arrhythmias, thermal injury, and thromboembolisms may occur. Protection of providers is also important as the current may pass if safety measures are not taken.

In the United States, the rate of ablations for arrhythmias has significantly increased over the past four decades. For example, from 1990 to 2005, the rate of ablations for atrial fibrillation in the United States has increased from 0.06% in 1990 to 0.79% in 2005.

Since then, more patients are undergoing ablation for atrial fibrillation, as more modern techniques (use of antiarrhythmic drug and multiple ablations) have shown to be as successful as 69% in long-term conversion to sinus rhythm [26, 27]. Outcome data derived from recent randomized controlled trials support catheter ablation as a first-line therapy in certain patients with paroxysmal atrial fibrillation [28, 29]. Indications for other types of catheter ablations include AVNRT, ectopic and reentrant atrial tachycardia, Wolff–Parkinson–White syndrome, and other dysrhythmias. Due to the procedure's length, tedious nature, and requirement for a motionless patient, general anesthesia is usually warranted, but may not be in some instances. Electrophysiology studies are contraindicated for patients with acute myocardial infarction, contraindications to anticoagulation, inability to lie flat due to underlying cardiorespiratory disease, and contraindications to general anesthesia [25]. Large amounts of radiation are used during electrophysiology procedures, therefore personnel involved in them should take great care to shield themselves and stay as far away as possible from the radiation source.

Performing the electrophysiology study and determining the three-dimensional electroanatomical mapping is the basis on which the catheter ablation takes place [24]. Positioning of catheters in various locations allows arrhythmias to be induced and the electrophysiologist to determine the etiology behind them. Catheters are typically placed in the right atrium, right ventricle, and the bundle of His via the femoral vein. The ablation is performed by applying radiofrequency energy to the cardiac tissue to create a transmural lesion [26]. A test is done at the conclusion of the procedure to confirm the results of the ablation. Complications of electrophysiology studies are similar to those of PPM or ICD placement, with some additional risks. Difficulties with vascular access contribute to about 3–4% of these complications, and those related to oversedation, loss of airway, placement of an advanced airway, or conversion to general anesthesia have been reported to occur in 40 percent of non-general anesthesia electrophysiology procedures. Additional risks specific to ablative procedures include hemodynamic instability due to unstable arrhythmias requiring immediate intervention or vasopressor support. Thermal injuries to the esophagus and formation of atrioesophageal fistulas occur in 0.01–0.02% of patients. Cardiac perforation and tamponade can also occur in electrophysiology procedures, with an incidence of 1–2%. If suspected, an echocardiogram can be useful for diagnosis. Thromboembolism with resulting stroke is a rare occurrence as the patient will be heparinized with an activated clotting time of greater than 300 seconds [25].

Advancements in electrophysiology diagnostics and interventions have led to less invasive options for management of certain arrhythmias. These procedures have their own risks and considerations for anesthesiologists and knowledge of the physiology and techniques of the various procedures will be beneficial in optimal patient management.

Sedation and Pharmacology

Sedation is often offered to patients undergoing procedures to allow for a more pleasurable perioperative experience. However small or daunting a procedure is, a patient's anxiety is typically elevated during a surgical procedure, which makes sedation a key component of a successful operation. Sedation in the cardiology catheterization and electrophysiology suite can involve procedures lasting a few minutes to those that continue for several hours and the sedation requirements range from minimal sedation to the induction of general anesthesia. The choice of sedation by the anesthesiologist is multifactorial and is dependent on the patient's comorbidities, type of procedure, length of the procedure, location of the procedure, and recovery period from the procedure [15].

When providing sedation to a patient, it is of utmost importance to understand the varying stages of sedation and the transition from one stage of conscious sedation to a deeper level of sedation. The levels of sedation are in a continuum; practitioners providing sedation should always be prepared to rescue the patient from the next level of sedation. If a provider is not comfortable in doing so, they should not be providing the sedation. Per the ASA guidelines, a procedure necessitating deep sedation should involve a practitioner trained in securing the airway so that, if a state of general anesthesia occurs, the provider should be able to ventilate and secure the patient's airway [26].

A non-anesthesia provider can provide sedation/analgesia; however, an anesthesiologist must be consulted if the patient will require MAC. The differentiating factors between the two are that an anesthesia provider will conduct a preoperative evaluation, maintain continuous intraoperative monitoring, and will be able to conduct a deep anesthetic, continuing to a general anesthetic if required [15]. Once again, the interventionist performing the procedure will need to make the decision of the necessity to involve the anesthesia team in their patient's care. For example, a patient having an outpatient diagnostic catheterization may do well with local anesthetic and minimal sedation, but a patient coming in for an intervention for structural heart disease may require MAC with the possibility of converting to a general anesthetic.

There is no one correct way to provide conscious sedation; a minute dose in one patient compared to a sizable dose in another patient could easily shift conscious sedation to general anesthesia in a matter of seconds. The first measure of safety is to have adequate monitors in place; this includes at least continuously assessing perfusion, oxygenation with oxygen saturation, capnography, as well as monitoring a patient's hemodynamics with blood pressure and heart rate [22]. Early recognition of changes in these values allows for prompt recognition and, most importantly, immediate intervention. Vigilance by the provider is of paramount importance during sedation or MAC; the notation of vital signs and the patient consciousness as frequent as every two and a half minutes helps to establish that the provider is aware and in tune with the current level of sedation [30].

Patient comfort is best achieved by targeting the three pillars of an ideal anesthetic: analgesia, anxiolysis, and hypnosis [15]. There is no one ideal drug to use in sedation; therefore, a combination of pharmaceutical agents is usually used for optimal results. The benefit of using multiple agents is that there is synergy between the various classes of drugs and the overall dose of each drug is decreased, but the primary drawback is that the rate of drug interactions and resulting cardiorespiratory complications is increased. Additionally, the breadth of cases performed in the cardiology suites is extensive; an anesthesia or non-anesthesia provider should have a sound understanding of the type and length of the case to be performed, to provide the patient with adequate sedation or anesthesia. In most circumstances, it will be ideal for shorter-acting drugs to be selected, which can be easily titrated as the demand of the procedure and patient dictate.

Propofol is easily titratable and has become an ideal choice in sedation for anesthesia and non-anesthesia providers. Propofol is primarily used for hypnosis and provides optimal patient comfort during a procedure. It can be titrated in small doses or given as an infusion. Propofol's short context-sensitive half-life allows for a rapid awakening of the patient. Other benefits of propofol include decreased postoperative nausea and vomiting, and a faster return to baseline mentation than with other sedative medications. The drawbacks of using propofol include no lasting analgesic properties, pain on injection, cardiovascular depression, and the risk of an overdose that could result in conversion to an apneic patient without a secured airway [31].

Benzodiazepines are frequently used during MAC cases, because of their ability to provide amnesia, anxiolysis, and hypnosis [32]. The most frequently used benzodiazepine in anesthesia is midazolam due to its fast onset of action and short elimination half-life compared to other drugs in its category. To have a more balanced sedation, midazolam will often be combined with an opioid to provide analgesia. The addition of an opioid puts the patient at an increased risk of respiratory depression. Selection depends on the patient and type of procedure. Fentanyl is the most used opioid for sedation due to its rapidness in onset of action and its shorter duration of action. It is also crucial to understand that both benzodiazepines and opioids can be reversed in the event of an overdose. Flumazenil is used to reverse a benzodiazepine overdose and naloxone to reverse an opioid.

Dexmedetomidine, a highly selective alpha-2 agonist, has become a popular agent for conscious sedation in the cardiac suite as it is able to provide analgesia, sedation, and hypnosis with minimal effects on respiration [33]. It has been shown to decrease the incidence of postoperative delirium and may play a protective role in ischemia/reperfusion injury in animal models. Adverse effects of dexmedetomidine are due to its sympatholytic effects and include bradycardia, hypotension, and paradoxical hypertension when given in bolus dose. This drug should be avoided in patients with advanced heart block and severe ventricular dysfunction due to its effects at the pre- and post-synaptic alpha-2 receptors [33].

Overall, there are many sedation/anesthesia options to consider when providing care for a patient having an intervention in the cardiac suite. Therefore, it is imperative for the anesthesiologist to form a plan in conjunction with the cardiologist to optimize care for the patient.

Summary

Cardiology is a dynamic field that has advanced tremendously over the past 30 years. While cardiology and electrophysiology were once considered to be diagnostic specialties, advances in technology have allowed for the major expansion of this field into progressive and comprehensive therapies for heart conditions. The patient population in this field has also expanded due to these advances in technology, and for these reasons there is an increased need for anesthesiologists in the field of cardiology. Anesthesiologists in the cardiology suite must be prepared to encounter a variety of heart-related conditions in addition to being familiar with the guidelines, regulations, and procedures associated with the proper treatment of a cardiovascular patient case. There are a variety of anesthetics that are appropriate for use in the OR for cardiology cases. The anesthesiologist must take into consideration the patient's heart condition and health history when choosing the appropriate sedative and/or pain medication.

References

1. Nagrebetsky A, Gabriel RA, Dutton RP, Urman RD. Growth of nonoperating room anesthesia care in the United States: a contemporary trends analysis. *Anesth Analg.* 2017;124:1261–7.

2. Mavarez AC., Ripat CI, Suarez MR. Pectoralis plane block for pacemaker insertion: a successful primary anesthetic. *Front Surg.* 2019; 6. https://doi.org/10.3389/fsurg.2019.00064

3. Faillace RT et al. The role of the out-of-operating room anesthesiologist in the care of the cardiac patient. *Anesthesiol Clin.* 2009;27(1):29–46.

4. Michael A. Gropper MD, Lars I. Eriksson MD, et al. *Miller's Anesthesia.* Philadelphia, PA: Elsevier Health Sciences, 2019.

5. Chua J, Patel K, Neelankavil J, Mahajan A. Anesthetic management of electrophysiology procedures. *Curr Opin Anaesthesiol.* 2012;25(4):470–81.

6. Shook DC, Savage RM. Anesthesia in the cardiac catheterization laboratory and electrophysiology laboratory. *Anesthesiol Clin.* 2009;27(1):47–56.

7. Cribier A. Percutaneous transcatheter implantation of an aortic valve prosthesis for calcific aortic stenosis: first human case description. *Circulation* 2002;106(24):3006–8.

8. Pavcnik D, Wright KC, Wallace S. Development and initial experimental evaluation of a prosthetic aortic valve for transcatheter placement. Work in progress. *Radiology* 1992;183(1): 151–4.

9. Spears J, Al-Saiegh Y, Goldberg D, et al., TAVR: a review of current practices and considerations in low-risk patients. *J Interv Cardiol.* 2020;2582938. doi:10.1155/2020/2582938

10. US Food and Drug Administration. Recently-approved devices – Edwards SAPIEN transcatheter heart valve (THV) – P100041. www.accessdata.fda.gov/scripts/cdrh/cfdocs/cfpma/pma.cfm?id=p100041

11. Smith CR, et al. Transcatheter versus surgical aortic-valve replacement in high-risk patients. *N Engl J Med* 2011;364(23):2187–98.

12. Reardon MJ, Mieghem NM, Popma JJ, et al. Surgical or transcatheter aortic-valve replacement in intermediate-risk patients. *N Engl J Med.* 2017;376(14):1321–31.

13. Haines DE, et al. Heart Rhythm Society expert consensus statement on electrophysiology laboratory standards: process, protocols, equipment, personnel, and safety. *Heart Rhythm.* 2014;11F(8): e9–51.

14. Chaffins JA. Radiation protection and procedures in the OR. *Radiol Technol.* 2008;79(5):415–28;quiz 429–31.

15. Morgan GE, Mikhail MS, Murray MJ. *Clinical Anesthesiology.* New York: McGraw Hill, 2005.

16. Metzner J, Posner KL, Domino KB. The risk and safety of anesthesia at remote locations: the US closed claims analysis. *Curr Opin Anaesthesiol.* 2009;22(4):502–8.

17. Waugh JB, Epps CA, Khodneva YA. Capnography enhances surveillance of respiratory events during procedural sedation: a meta-analysis. *J Clin Anesth.* 2011;23(3):189–96.

18. Merchant R, Chartrand D, Dain S, et al. Guidelines to the practice of anesthesia: revised edition 2015. *Can J Anaesth.* 2015;62(1):54–67.

19. Chang B, Kaye AD, Diaz JH, et al. Interventional procedures outside of the operating room: results from the National Anesthesia Clinical Outcomes Registry. *J Patient Saf.* 2018;14:9–16

20. Drabek T, Němec J. Anesthetic management of electrophysiological procedures for heart failure. *Int Anesthesiol Clin.* 2012;50(3):22–42.

21. Bader AM, Pothier MM. Out-of-operating room procedures: preprocedure assessment. *Anesthesiol Clin.* 2009;27(1):121–6.

22. Faillace R, Kaddaha R, Bikkina M. The role of the out-of-operating room

anesthesiologist in the care of the cardiac patient. *Anesthesiol Clin.* 2009;27:29–46.

23. Caplan JP, Querques J. Consultation, communication, and conflict management by out-of-operating room anesthesiologists: strangers in a strange land. *Anesthesiol Clin.* 2009;27(1):111–20.

24. Price A, Santucci P. Electrophysiology procedures: weighing the factors affecting choice of anesthesia. *Semin Cardiothorac Vasc Anesth.* 2013;17(3):203–11.

25. Anderson R, Harukuni I, Sera V. Anesthetic considerations for electrophysiologic procedures. *Anesthesiol Clin.* 2013;31(2):479–89.

26. Nicoara A, Holmquist F, Raggains C, Mathew JP. Anesthesia for catheter ablation procedures. *J Cardiothorac Vasc Anesth.* 2014;28(6):1589–603.

27. Clarnette JA, Brooks AG, Mahajan R, et al. Outcomes of persistent and long-standing persistent atrial fibrillation ablation: a systematic review and meta-analysis. *Europace.* 2018;20(FI_3): f366–76. doi:10.1093/europace/eux297

28. Andrade JG, Wells GA, Deyell MW, et al. Cryoablation or drug therapy for initial treatment of atrial fibrillation. *N Engl J Med.* 2021;384(4):305–15.

29. Kirchhof P, Camm AJ, Goette A, et al. Early rhythm-control therapy in patients with atrial fibrillation. *N Engl J Med.* 2020;383(14):1305–16.

30. Practice guidelines for sedation and analgesia by non-anesthesiologists. *Anesthesiology.* 2002;96(4):1004–17.

31. McKeage K, Perry CM. Propofol: a review of its use in intensive care sedation of adults. *CNS Drugs.* 2003;17(4):235–72.

32. O'Boyle CA. Benzodiazepine-induced amnesia and anesthetic practice: a review. *Psychopharmacol Ser.* 1988;6:146–65.

33. Peng K, Ji FH, Liu HY, et al. Effects of perioperative dexmedetomidine on postoperative mortality and morbidity: a systematic review and meta-analysis. *Clin Ther.* 2019;41(1):138–54.e4. doi:10.1016/j.clinthera.2018.10.022

Chapter 19

Sedation and Anesthesia for Interventional Pulmonary Procedures

Micaela Zywicki, Nicholas M. Bacher, Andrea Poon, and Eric Hsu

Introduction

Interventional pulmonology is a subspeciality of pulmonology focusing on minimally invasive endoscopic and percutaneous procedures that can be effective, less invasive alternatives to thoracic surgery. The sedation and analgesia considerations are important to understand given how this field is rapidly expanding and these procedures are becoming increasingly more common. In addition, a strong understanding of the sedation requirements is critical in performing safe anesthesia. Perioperative considerations for patients with acute or chronic pulmonary disease undergoing interventional procedures include:

- smoking cessation
- knowledge of the time of last food/drink consumption
- venue of procedure: intensive care unit (ICU) versus floor versus outpatient
- pulmonary rehabilitation
- treat any underlying pulmonary infection(s)
- optimization of patient's comorbidities
- adequate hydration
- management of secretions
- premedication with bronchodilators, if indicated

General Anesthetic Plan for Interventional Pulmonary Procedures

The following sections discuss the specific anesthetic considerations for the most common pulmonary procedures, which include flexible bronchoscopy, rigid bronchoscopy, robotic or navigational bronchoscopy, endobronchial ultrasound, pleuroscopy (or medical thoracoscopy), and tunneled indwelling pleural catheter placement. However, the general anesthetic plan is similar for all of these procedures and so an overview is provided in this section. Specific considerations for each procedure are included in the relevant sections below [1].

For all monitored anesthesia care (MAC) and general anesthesia (GA) cases, the American Society of Anesthesiologists (ASA) recommends standard monitors including pulse oximetry, inspired oxygen content, end-tidal carbon dioxide, temperature, blood pressure and telemetry. For interventional pulmonary procedures and, specifically, flexible bronchoscopy, MAC or GA may be utilized depending on the patient and procedural characteristics. Several factors that are important to consider when deciding between the two forms of anesthesia are the specific type of procedure, the severity of the patient's underlying lung disease, patient comorbidities, and the preferences of the anesthesiologist, patient and pulmonologist [2].

There is a continuum in terms of the depth of anesthesia/sedation (see Table 1.1 in Chapter 1). A sedation nurse is able to perform minimal sedation, anxiolysis, and conscious sedation but a trained anesthesia provider must perform deep sedation/analgesia and GA. This chapter focuses on deep sedation (MAC) in addition to GA [3].

If MAC is chosen for flexible bronchoscopy, topicalization of the airway is performed using lidocaine and, sometimes, superior laryngeal and recurrent laryngeal nerve blocks. Midazolam and fentanyl are given for anxiolysis and analgesia and propofol is given to induce anesthesia and maintain unawareness. Another medication often used is dexmedetomidine as it can maintain a patient's respiratory drive, unlike propofol. Similarly, ketamine maintains respiratory drive but is generally avoided as it can lead to increased secretions and hallucinations. During MAC with flexible bronchoscopy, oxygen delivery is achieved through a nasal cannula or a high-flow nasal cannula.

In addition, there are instances when a provider starts with MAC and needs to switch to GA during the procedure, such as if the patient does not tolerate sedation. Refer to Box 19.1 for a summary of situations when GA is preferred for interventional pulmonary procedures.

Box 19.1 Situations when GA is recommended for interventional pulmonary procedures

General anesthesia is preferred:

- If patient is unable to tolerate bronchoscopy with light or moderate levels of sedation due to anxiety, severe lung disease or morbid obesity
- If there is a requirement of paralysis to prevent movement
- For longer procedures that are not a quick inspection of the airway

  ○ endobronchial ultrasound
  ○ electromagnetic navigation bronchoscopy

- For bronchial thermoplasty procedures
- For rigid bronchoscopy

Table 19.1 Choice of route for maintenance of anesthesia

Benefits and drawbacks	Inhalational anesthesia (typically sevoflurane)	TIVA
Benefits	Bronchodilation Anti-inflammatory Rapid elimination during emergence	Ability to administer anesthetic independent of ventilation without wasting agents or polluting the operating room
Drawbacks	More difficult to control depth of anesthesia given frequent interruptions in the delivery of anesthetic Pollution of the operating room due to frequent removal of bronchoscope Higher amounts of anesthetic required due to higher fresh gas flows and frequent suctioning	Inability to monitor blood concentration Higher risk of awareness Higher cost

When using GA for a flexible bronchoscopy, there are two routes of induction – inhalation and intravenous (IV). Thereafter, total intravenous anesthesia (TIVA) with a propofol infusion is generally used for maintenance of anesthesia as opposed to maintenance with a volatile anesthetic. Table 19.1 summarizes factors that are considered when deciding between maintenance of anesthesia with inhalational agents or TIVA.

Regardless of the choice of induction or maintenance of anesthesia, airway control is an important consideration. Generally, anesthesiologists will use a laryngeal mask airway (LMA) or an endotracheal tube (ETT). Several factors that favor the selection of an LMA include if there is a desire to avoid muscle relaxation; if there will be biopsies of the glottis, upper airway, or adjacent structures; if the procedure is short; and if there are low anticipated ventilator pressures. On the other hand, factors that will lead to the decision to use an ETT include high risk of aspiration, long anticipated duration of the procedure, and high anticipated ventilator pressures. Regardless of the selection between an LMA or ETT, the provider needs to ensure the internal diameter of the tube will accommodate passage of the bronchoscope.

In terms of emergence from anesthesia, providers must prepare for ample suctioning of the oropharynx due to the risk of aspiration, particularly if topical lidocaine was used as it leads to vocal cord paralysis lasting 2–4 hours.

For post-procedural care of patients undergoing flexible bronchoscopy, patients must be monitored until the effects of sedation have worn off. Some of the metrics utilized to measure if the patient is ready for either discharge or returning to their inpatient floor include alertness, blood pressure, cardiac rhythm, heart rate, respiratory rate, oxygen saturation, baseline ambulation, and eating/drinking once gag reflex returns. If the patient is going to the ICU after the procedure, the anesthesiologist will accompany during transport there and provide a handoff to the ICU team, including the nurse and physician. Further, patients undergoing flexible bronchoscopy often have chest X-rays afterwards particularly if they underwent transbronchial biopsy, balloon bronchoplasty, stent placement, rigid bronchoscopy, and if any barotrauma is suspected.

Flexible Bronchoscopy

Overview and Indications

Bronchoscopy refers to an endoscopic procedure allowing for visualization of the tracheobronchial tree by placement of an optical instrument inside the airway. The most common type of bronchoscopy is flexible bronchoscopy, which uses a flexible endoscope permitting access to the lower airways.

There are several indications for flexible bronchoscopy and these can be grouped into diagnostic and therapeutic categories.

Diagnostic indications:

- symptoms such as cough, hemoptysis, wheezing
- unresolved pneumonia
- diffuse lung disease
- rule out metastases
- preoperative evaluation
- assess local disease recurrence
- acute inhalation injury
- during mechanical ventilation (such as during one lung ventilation in thoracic surgery)

Therapeutic indications:

- foreign body
- accumulation of secretions
- atelectasis, aspiration
- lung abscess
- reposition of ETT
- placement of endobronchial tubes
- laser surgery of the airway

Anesthetic Recommendation

The anesthetic recommendations for flexible bronchoscopy are described in the introduction of this chapter.

Intra-procedural Considerations

Specifically for flexible bronchoscopy, there are common complications, less common complications, and rare, serious adverse effects as listed in Table 19.2.

Complications/Post-procedural Care

The postoperative care recommendations for flexible bronchoscopy are similar to those described for all interventional pulmonary procedures in the general anesthetic plan above.

Special Cases

There are several special cases for flexible bronchoscopy and these can be grouped into either diagnostic or therapeutic interventions (see below). Several of the more common interventions listed below are described in further detail in the next sections.

Table 19.2 Flexible bronchoscopy intra-procedural complications

Common	Less common	Rare
Mild, transient hypotension and hypoxia related to sedation Bleeding Pneumothorax Nasal discomfort Sore throat Mild hemoptysis 1–2 days afterwards	Bronchospasm or laryngospasm Aspiration given increased respiratory secretions/decreased airway protective reflexes Epistaxis due to nasal trauma Nausea and vomiting Cardiac arrhythmias Infection or bacteremia Vasovagal syncope Seizure Methemoglobinemia (from lidocaine) Laryngeal edema/injury	Cardiopulmonary arrest Tension pneumothorax Respiratory failure requiring intubation and mechanical ventilation Airway perforation Airway fire

- Diagnostic:
  - ○ endobronchial brushing
  - ○ bronchoalveolar lavage
  - ○ bronchial washings
  - ○ endobronchial biopsy
  - ○ transbronchial biopsy
  - ○ needle aspiration or biopsy

- Therapeutic:
  - ○ endobronchial ultrasound
  - ○ laser resection
  - ○ argon plasma coagulation photodynamic therapy
  - ○ electrocautery
  - ○ cryosurgery
  - ○ balloon dilatation
  - ○ brachytherapy
  - ○ valve placement
  - ○ thermoplasty
  - ○ airway stenting

Rigid Bronchoscopy

Brief Overview, Indications

Rigid bronchoscopy uses a larger, more rigid endoscope than a flexible endoscope, which, as a result, can only access the proximal airways. This form of bronchoscopy is used for evaluating hemoptysis and for performing intrabronchial procedures like mechanical dilation of tracheal or bronchial strictures, laser or mechanical tumor debridement, and removal of foreign bodies that cannot be removed with a flexible bronchoscope.

Anesthetic Recommendation

GA is recommended for this procedure as the scope is rigid. IV induction is preferred, unless the pulmonologist's ability to secure the airway with a rigid scope is uncertain. This is due to the ability of sevoflurane (the inhalational induction agent) to maintain spontaneous ventilation. After the airway is secured, the route of maintenance of anesthesia is with TIVA. In addition, neuromuscular blocking agents are utilized if the pulmonologist needs periods of apnea.

There are two main options for ventilation techniques during rigid bronchoscopy and these include standard positive pressure ventilation (PPV) and jet ventilation. Standard PPV occurs when you connect the patient to the circuit via a side connector on the rigid scope. However, this is not ideal since there will be a significant leak around the scope. Jet ventilation requires TIVA since inhaled anesthetics cannot be administered in this manner.

Emergence from GA after rigid bronchoscopy can occur multiple ways. Some providers will prefer to remove the rigid scope while the patient is deep and replace it with either an ETT or LMA. Otherwise, providers can remove the scope and place a face mask until spontaneous ventilation resumes.

Intra-procedural Considerations

Rigid bronchoscopy involves all of the same intra-procedural considerations of flexible bronchoscopy (refer to the previous section and Table 19.2) along with these considerations specific to rigid bronchoscopy:

- hypoxia
- laryngospasm
- laryngeal edema
- atelectasis
- pneumothorax
- damage to structures of the mouth and oropharynx
- spinal cord injury (if cervical spine disease and severe osteoporosis)
- airway perforation and injury to the vocal cords and arytenoids

Complications/Post-procedural Care

Postoperative care is similar to flexible bronchoscopy (refer to the previous section).

Special Cases

Similarly, the special cases are similar to flexible bronchoscopy and have been previously discussed.

Robotic and Navigational Bronchoscopy

Brief Overview, Indications

Robotic-assisted bronchoscopy is a technique utilizing a small, location-sensing catheter, which is inserted in the airways. In contrast with endobronchial ultrasound or electromagnetic navigation, this technique allows for both direct visualization and virtual guidance. Because of this navigational ability, this type of bronchoscopy is primarily used to obtain tissue diagnosis, especially of more peripheral lesions.

Anesthetic Recommendation

For this procedure, ASA standard monitoring is recommended, and a similar approach to sedation, anesthesia, and analgesia for flexible bronchoscopy (see above) is the method of choice. The longer procedure duration of robotic-assisted or navigational bronchoscopy may make GA with a secured airway preferable, particularly in patients with an elevated risk of aspiration, obstructive sleep apnea, or other pulmonary complications.

MAC for robotic-assisted or navigational bronchoscopy is fundamentally similar to that of flexible bronchoscopy (refer to the flexible bronchoscopy section).

In the case of GA, TIVA is again preferred for more reliable delivery of anesthetic when compared with inhalational anesthesia. Robotic-assisted and navigational bronchoscopy are not typically painful, and thus minimal analgesia is required if adequate depth of anesthesia is achieved

Intra-procedural Considerations

In addition to the intraprocedural considerations of flexible bronchoscopy (Table 19.2), the potentially longer procedure increases the risk of aspiration or airway obstruction if performed under MAC. Use of general anesthesia with an ETT offers a secured airway and helps minimize these risks.

Endobronchial Ultrasound

Brief Overview, Indications

Endobronchial ultrasound is an imaging technique that uses a bronchoscope equipped with a specialized probe that can provide ultrasound images of structures in and adjacent to the airway in addition to the visual data from the bronchoscope itself. This technique is useful in visualization of the lung, airway, and mediastinal structures.

Endobronchial ultrasound is often performed alongside other procedures for diagnostic purposes including bronchoalveolar lavage and endobronchial biopsy. Use of different probe types allows the pulmonologist to biopsy in real time or visualize more peripheral or distal lesions as part of the study [4].

Anesthetic Recommendation

For endobronchial ultrasound, the anesthetic considerations and complications are fundamentally the same as for flexible bronchoscopy. The anticipated length of procedure and planned interventions, along with patient-specific comorbidities, should be considered when establishing an anesthetic plan.

Complications/Post-procedural Care

Complications of endobronchial ultrasound itself are rare and similar to those of flexible bronchoscopy. However, the performance of endobronchial biopsies confers additional risks, including:

- airway bleeding
- pneumothorax
- pneumomediastinum

Though rare, these are potentially serious complications and prompt evaluation with a chest X-ray or repeat bronchoscopy is warranted if shortness of breath or hemoptysis are noted in the recovery area.

Pleuroscopy

Brief Overview, Indications

Pleuroscopy (or thoracoscopy) is a procedure in which a rigid endoscope is passed through an incision in the chest wall to directly visualize the lung and pleura. Pleuroscopy offers a variety of diagnostic and therapeutic options, sparing patients from more invasive thoracic surgeries.

Diagnostic procedures include biopsy (pleura, lung, lymph node) and pleural fluid sampling, which can be useful in the diagnosis of infection or malignancy. Pleurodesis, the intentional fixation of the visceral and parietal pleura, is often performed with pleuroscopy in order to eliminate recurrent pleural effusions. In cases of refractory effusions or in certain other clinical situations, pleuroscopy can also be used as an aid in placement of an indwelling pleural catheter. For more invasive procedures, video-assisted thoracoscopic surgery is used in an operating room setting.

Preprocedural and Intraprocedural Considerations

Pleuroscopy can be a painful procedure, and in cases involving additional interventions there can be significant discomfort for the patient. The common associated comorbidities can often lead to dyspnea while lying flat, and the ability to tolerate this positioning is an important consideration in patient selection. Often pleuroscopy and its related interventions are intended to reduce these symptoms or offer a definitive treatment, but a discussion with the patient and proceduralist to assess the ability to lie flat safely is critical to performing successful and safe pleuroscopy.

Anesthetic Recommendation

The preferred method of analgesia and sedation involves IV sedative infusion with emphasis on good local anesthetic infiltration by the proceduralist at the incision site and during the intrathoracic portion. Importantly, the painful nature of pleuroscopy and its associated interventions may necessitate adjunct therapies for adequate analgesia. Maintenance of spontaneous ventilation is important, as is the avoidance of excessive coughing or movement by the patient. As such, a multimodal approach to monitored anesthesia care should be considered.

Propofol as a primary agent can provide adequate hypnosis but offers little to no analgesia and may cause significant respiratory or cardiovascular depression at the high doses required to tolerate pleuroscopy. The addition of ketamine can offer analgesia without compromising respiratory drive and can be a good choice in patients with reasonable cardiac function. This can be coupled with a peripheral anticholinergic such as glycopyrrolate to reduce secretions. Premedication with midazolam may also be appropriate both to deepen sedation and minimize emergence phenomena associated with ketamine. The incorporation of small doses of opioids provides additional analgesia and can also suppress cough, which in turn improves procedural conditions and patient comfort.

Complications/Post-procedural Care

Postoperatively, it is important to monitor oxygenation and respiratory status as the lungs and pleura are manipulated during pleuroscopy and may be injured. Particular attention should be paid to worsening respiratory distress and a chest X-ray should be obtained to evaluate for effusion or an expanding pneumothorax. While uncommon, these complications can be serious and require further intervention. Chest tube output, if present, should also be closely monitored for both volume and content.

Pain following pleuroscopy and its related interventions is often due to pleural inflammation, and infiltration of local anesthetic by the proceduralist can be helpful in preventing postoperative pain. Oral or IV opioids can be used in the recovery area if severe pain persists, with care to avoid respiratory depression or increased sedation. In the case of severe or refractory pain, regional or neuraxial anesthetic techniques can be used for rescue therapy. This requires an anesthesiologist proficient in regional anesthesia and involves further risks to the patient, and as such is rarely used in routine cases.

Tunneled Indwelling Pleural Catheter Placement

Brief Overview, Indications

The tunneled (indwelling) pleural catheter is an intrapleural catheter that is placed for long-term drainage of recurrent effusion, most often in the case of infection or malignancy. As an alternative to pleurodesis, the indwelling pleural catheter is favored in patients with shorter expected survival or in cases of failed pleurodesis. It carries with it a risk of infection, but can offer a respite from repeated thoracentesis in the case of symptomatic pleural effusions, especially those seen in late-stage malignancy.

Anesthetic Recommendation

Though often performed in conjunction with pleuroscopy (see section above), the placement of an indwelling pleural catheter can be performed on its own in cases where pleuroscopy is not necessary. In these cases, liberal use of local anesthetic at the insertion site is often sufficient for placement. Adjunct agents such as midazolam, fentanyl, or propofol can be used on a case-by-case basis if a patient is unable to lie still or tolerate the procedure.

Intra-procedural Considerations

Typically a short procedure, the placement of an indwelling pleural catheter involves supine or lateral positioning depending on the location of catheter placement. Care should be taken to maintain oxygenation and spontaneous ventilation, as patients often have significant lung disease with discomfort lying flat. The use of intraprocedural opioids or short-acting sedatives can be considered if the patient is unable to tolerate this positioning, but care should be taken to preserve respiratory status.

Complications/Post-procedural Care

Postoperatively, intrapleural catheter placement is a low-risk procedure when done in isolation, and infection at the insertion site or along the tract is the greatest risk associated with the procedure. Post-procedural pain is typically minimal and managed with non-opioid pain medications. If performed with pleuroscopy, the same risks and complications exist as with any pleuroscopy-associated procedure.

Clinical Updates in Literature and Patient Care

Bronchoscopy is a rapidly evolving field with newer technologies being used than a decade prior to now. In addition, bronchoscopy is a very high-risk procedure in terms of spreading infectious diseases to medical personnel due to the aerosolization of secretions during intubation and bronchoscopy itself. This was an important consideration during the COVID-19 pandemic [5]. The first step was determining if the procedure had to happen or could be delayed until the patient was no longer contagious. If bronchoscopy had to be performed in a COVID-19 patient (i.e., for removal of airway mucus plugs or to obtain diagnostic microbial samples), important considerations included [6, 7]:

- performing the procedure in a negative pressure room
- having a multidisciplinary discussion regarding infectious disease risk and infection control measures
- securing the appropriate personal protective equipment (PPE)
- using disposable equipment as much as possible
- avoiding atomized spraying, which can lead to more aerosolization
- considering GA with adequate neuromuscular blockade to avoid coughing
- minimizing the duration the airway is open to the environment
- using high efficiency particulate air (HEPA) filters when possible
- avoiding jet ventilation and disconnection of the circuit
- using measures to avoid postoperative coughing and vomiting

As the COVID-19 pandemic evolved, newer technologies to limit aerosolization and exposure to viral particles were discovered. An example of this is a transparent "airway box" to limit exposure of operating room personnel to the aerosols that are dispersed during intubation/airway manipulation [5]. In addition, there are now masks with antiviral and antimicrobial filters that can be secured to the face, effectively creating a closed circuit.

An online survey was conducted among interventional pulmonology centers with the aim to assess practices in response to COVID-19. They found there was compliance with most international recommendations and postponement of elective procedures. There were a decreased number of flexible and rigid bronchoscopies, and an upscale of PPE during the COVID-19 pandemic [8].

A randomized double-blind controlled study on fixed dexmedetomidine infusion versus fixed dose midazolam bolus in endobronchial ultrasound– guided transbronchial needle aspiration (EBUS–TBNA) found a reduced need for rescue sedation, slightly faster recovery, significantly greater satisfaction for bronchoscopist in the dexmedetomidine group. This study also noted significantly more hypotension and bradycardia in the dexmedetomidine group, though there was no need for specific intervention [9]. However, another randomized, double-blind study compared dexmedetomidine with midazolam sedation during EBUS–TBNA and found that dexmedetomidine was not superior to midazolam in the incidence of oxygen desaturation [10]. There were similar levels of sedation and procedure satisfaction scores for both agents. One observational study to compare dexmedetomidine versus midazolam during medical thoracoscopy found that use of dexmedetomidine led to higher pulmonologist satisfaction, reduced pain, cough, and fentanyl requirements [11].

In a retrospective review on consecutive EBUS–TBNA under moderate sedation versus deep sedation/MAC, there was similar diagnostic yield and procedure duration with both techniques. MAC was associated with more desaturations and episodes of hypotension; however, this did not lead to an increased escalation of care. The study also found that the increased cost associated with deep sedation was modest [12].

A review article covering controversies and updates in anesthesia for bronchoscopy procedures discussed anesthetic options for electromagnetic navigation bronchoscopy and bronchoscopy cryotherapy. A dose of IV fentanyl 100 µg at induction of GA was given to shorten and lessen the severity of post-procedural coughing. Remifentanil infusion may be less favorable due to limited effective duration after termination and less beneficial in prevention of coughing. There were potential adverse reactions of bradycardia, hypotension and hyperalgesia after remifentanil infusion [13].

Summary

In summary, effective communication between interventional pulmonology and anesthesiology teams is mandatory for patient safety in non-operating room anesthesia provided for interventional pulmonology.

References

1. Yang Y, Murphy NE, Long MT. Pandemic bronchoscopy: a technique to improve safety. *Anesthesiology*. 2020;133(3):689–90.

2. de Lima A, Kheir F, Majid A, Pawlowski J. Anesthesia for interventional pulmonology procedures: a review of advanced diagnostic and therapeutic bronchoscopy. *Can J Anaesth J Can Anesth*. 2018;65(7):822–36.

3. Dabu-Bondoc SM. Standard procedures in nonoperating room anesthesia. *Curr Opin Anaesthesiol*. 2020;33(4):539–47.

4. Chen AC, Pastis NJ, Mahajan AK, et al. Robotic bronchoscopy for peripheral pulmonary lesions: a multicenter pilot and feasibility study (BENEFIT). *Chest*. 2021;159(2):845–52.

5. Toda C, Abdelmalak BB. COVID-19 and anesthetic considerations for head and neck surgeries and bronchoscopic and dental procedures. *J Head Neck Anesth*. 2020;e28–e28.

6. Patrucco F, Failla G, Ferrari G, et al. Bronchoscopy during COVID-19 pandemic, ventilatory strategies and procedure measures. *Panminerva Med*. 2021;63(4):529–38.

7. Guedes F, Ferreira AJ, Dionísio J, Rodrigues LV, Bugalho A. Pre- and post-COVID practice of interventional pulmonology in adults in Portugal. *Pulmonology*. 2022;S2531–0437(22) 00070-8.

8. Selzer AR, Murrell M, Shostak E. New trends in interventional pulmonology. *Curr Opin Anaesthesiol*. 2017;30(1):17–22.

9. Kumari R, Jain K, Agarwal R, et al. Fixed dexmedetomidine infusion versus fixed-dose midazolam bolus as primary sedative for maintaining intra-procedural sedation during endobronchial ultrasound-guided transbronchial needle aspiration: a double blind randomized controlled trial. *Expert Rev Respir Med*. 2021;15(12):1597–604.

10. Kim J, Choi SM, Park YS, Lee CH, Lee SM, Yoo CG, et al. Dexmedetomidine versus midazolam for sedation during endobronchial ultrasound-guided transbronchial needle aspiration: a

randomised controlled trial. *Eur J Anaesthesiol.* 2021;38(5):534–40.

11. Sirohiya P, Kumar V, Mittal S, et al. Dexmedetomidine versus midazolam for sedation during medical thoracoscopy: a pilot randomized-controlled trial (RCT). *J Bronchol Interv Pulmonol.* 2022;29(4):248–54.

12. Boujaoude Z, Arya R, Shrivastava A, Pratter M, Abouzgheib W. Impact of moderate sedation versus monitored anesthesia care on outcomes and cost of endobronchial ultrasound transbronchial needle aspiration. *Pulm Med.* 2019;2019:4347852.

13. Abdelmalak BB, Doyle DJ. Updates and controversies in anesthesia for advanced interventional pulmonology procedures. *Curr Opin Anaesthesiol.* 2021;34(4):455–63.

Chapter 20

Sedation for Ophthalmological Procedures

Liang Huang, Alan D. Kaye, Charles J. Fox, and Henry Liu

Introduction

Perioperative anesthesia care for the patients undergoing ophthalmologic procedures is unique and sometimes challenging. Many of the ophthalmologic procedures can often be done with sedation/monitored anesthesia care (MAC) [1]. Intravenous sedatives combined with topical/local/regional anesthesia during eye surgery can alleviate patients' pain, fear, anxiety, thus improving outcomes [2]. In this chapter we review the current practices and trends in anesthesia service with respect to MAC for ophthalmologic procedures with topical/local/regional anesthesia [1, 2, 3]. The nerve blocks performed for eye surgery determine, to some extent, the techniques and requirement of the sedation level by the anesthesia service. And the traditions of surgery teams and hospitals also affect the choice of sedation technique. The evolvement of surgical techniques seems to facilitate the trend that sedation is more and more used in the eye surgical procedures. Anesthesia care options are also based on surgeons' skill and anesthesia providers' comfort level, and the patients' expectations and demands. Regardless, patients' safety and perioperative care quality are the key determinants [1, 3, 4].

Topical/Regional Block Techniques in Ophthalmological Procedures

1. *Topical anesthetic for eye surgery*: The most commonly used topical anesthetic agents include proparacaine, tetracaine, cocaine, lidocaine, bupivacaine, and oxybuprocaine. These agents can be in liquid or gel in various concentrations [3, 5].
2. *Retrobulbar block*: Retrobulbar block is achieved by injecting local anesthetic agents into the muscle cone. It blocks the ciliary ganglion, the ciliary nerves, and cranial nerves III, IV, and VI. The ciliary ganglion is a parasympathetic ganglion.

Retrobulbar block may induce allergic reactions, retrobulbar hemorrhage, central retinal artery occlusion, penetration or perforation, subconjunctival edema (chemosis), oculocardiac reflex, central spread of local anesthetic, and postoperative strabismus [6].

3. *Peribulbar block*: Peribulbar block involves injecting anesthetics to above and below the orbit, in the orbicularis oculi muscle. This approach blocks the ciliary nerves and cranial nerves III and VI. Compared to retrobulbar block, peribulbar block is easier to perform and less likely to cause intraocular or intradural injection because the local anesthetic agent(s) are supposedly deposited outside the muscle cone. However, it is more difficult to achieve a complete and dense surgical anesthesia with the peribulbar technique [6].

4. *Facial nerve block*: Facial nerve block is usually used as the sole technique or in combination with general anesthesia. This block for ocular surgery blocks the periocular branches of the facial nerve aiming to prevent excessive eye movement during surgery via orbicular muscle akinesia [7].

5. *Supraorbital block*: The supraorbital nerve is from the ophthalmic branch of the cranial nerve V trigeminal nerve (V1). The nerve runs through a supraorbital notch (majority) or foramen, then courses into a superficial medial branch and a deep lateral branch. The supraorbital block provides anesthesia to the upper eyelid, brow, forehead, and anterior scalp [8].

6. *Nasociliary block*: This block aims at the anterior and posterior ethmoidal foramina, additionally delivering some anesthetics to the infratrochlear nerve. The nasociliary nerve normally branches off the ophthalmic nerve within the orbit and supplies the mucosal surface of the sphenoid, ethmoid, frontal sinuses, and the anterior septum, lateral nasal cavity, ala, and apex of the nose. Epinephrine is not used in this block to reduce the risk of retinal artery spasm [9].

7. *Supratrochlear block*: The supratrochlear nerve exits the supraorbital margin medially to the supraorbital nerve. This block is often used in conjunction with the supraorbital block to maximize anesthesia of the forehead [10].

Ophthalmological Procedures Usually Done with Sedation

1. *Cataract surgery*: This type of surgery is probably the most commonly performed intraocular procedure [3]. As the prevalence of cataracts continuously increases, the volume of cataract extraction surgery by phacoemulsification technique has also steadily increased [3]. The anesthesia choice is usually topical anesthesia. Topical anesthesia is applied as drops or gels and may be supplemented by intracameral injection by the surgeon for better intraoperative pain control [4, 5].

2. *Vitreoretinal surgery*: Vitrectomy and retinal detachment repair procedures, including scleral buckling, usually require both anesthesia of the posterior segment and akinesia of the eye. Thus, topical and subconjunctival techniques are often times inadequate. Therefore, a sub-Tenon's, retrobulbar, or peribulbar nerve block, or even general anesthesia, will be needed [11]. A sub-Tenon's block usually involves a local anesthetic agent injection below the surface of the globe by using a blunt cannula. Some of the local anesthetic agents will diffuse to the retrobulbar space [5]. Conventional injection blocks involve injecting local anesthetics into the periorbital space, thus called a peribulbar block, or into the eye muscle cone, when it is called a

retrobulbar block. Sometimes a separate facial nerve block may be performed to limit eyelid movement and sensation and optimize the surgical condition [5].

3. *Corneal surgery including corneal transplantation*: The most common procedures on the cornea usually involve trauma, conjunctival flap, removal of foreign bodies, corneal transplantation, pterygium surgery, and keratoprosthesis. Only the anterior segment is needed to be anesthetized typically for these procedures. Most surgeons will require akinesia for penetrating corneal surgery, such as trauma, transplant, prosthetic surgery, and re-do procedures. Some surgeons will use subconjunctival anesthesia to separate the conjunctiva from the sclera in pterygium surgery [11]. Other procedures like corneal ablation, incisional refractive surgery, and intracorneal ring insertion, are also performed usually under topical anesthesia [11].

4. *Laser-assisted in situ keratomileusis (LASIK) procedures*: Topical anesthesia is usually used for LASIK procedures. The anesthetic agents will be similar to those used for cataract surgery [5].

5. *Glaucoma surgery*: Some glaucoma surgeons use local/topical anesthesia and MAC while others may require general anesthesia. There are multiple possibilities of choices from facility to facility. Both glaucoma filtration surgery and trabeculectomy usually involve creating a fistula between the anterior chamber and the subconjunctival space. Only anesthetizing the anterior segment is needed. Some surgeons perform peribulbar anesthesia for these procedures. However, both topical anesthesia, with or without intracameral lidocaine, and subconjunctival anesthesia can potentially avoid the volume injections behind or around the orbit on pulsatile ocular blood flow in patients with advanced glaucoma [5, 11]. On the contrary, non-penetrative glaucoma surgery, such as deep sclerotomy, will usually be longer and maybe more difficult technically, general anesthesia may be a preferable technique, which will guarantee a longer nerve block with akinesia [11]. Cyclophotocoagulation is a relatively painful procedure, which can be done under local anesthesia as sub-Tenon's blocks with MAC; akinesia is not essential, and some surgeons find general anesthesia is preferable [5, 11].

6. *Oculoplastic surgery*: Procedures to the soft tissues of the eye include the following: correction of eyelid malpositions, such as entropion and ectropion, ptosis surgery, eyelash malpositions, eyelid reconstruction, eyelid tumor surgery, tear duct surgery, blepharoplasty, orbital decompression, and enucleation and evisceration. Although local infiltration anesthesia with MAC is indicated for many of these procedures, the choice of anesthetic technique for specific surgery is determined after discussion with specific surgeons [5, 11].

7. *Extraocular muscle surgery*: Strabismus surgery can sometimes be performed with regional/local anesthesia and MAC, although most commonly the procedure is done under general anesthesia in both children and adults. While akinesia is helpful for strabismus surgery, the key requirement is enough anesthesia of the muscle cone, because pulling on extraocular muscles is usually pretty painful, and it may induce an oculocardic reflex. If carrying out only simple suture adjustments, this can be done under topical anesthesia [5, 11].

8. *Surgery for open-globe injuries*: These procedures are usually done under general anesthesia in order to avoid the risks of infection, retrobulbar hemorrhage, and increased intraocular pressure. Higher intraocular pressure may cause more damage.

However, some surgeons advocate to repair open-globe injury under regional/local anesthesia and MAC [5, 11].

9. *Ophthalmic oncology*: Though most procedures to remove eye tumors are performed under general anesthesia, sometimes the surgeons may perform the procedures under just regional/local anesthesia and MAC [5, 11].

Unique Considerations for Ophthalmologic Surgical Anesthesia

1. *Overall sensations*: With topical anesthetic agents applied to the eye(s), patients may perceive light, colors, the surgeon's hand movements, and surgical instruments [12].

2. *Optimizing surgical condition*: If akinesia is critical for the surgical success, regional anesthesia or general anesthesia should be provided.

3. *Visual ability after surgery*: Visual improvement is usually significant after phacoemulsification procedures for cataract patients. This can vary with different local/topical anesthetic techniques, with about 3–16% patients complaining that the experience is frightening [3].

4. *Extraocular movements during surgery*: It would be disastrous if patient moved during an ophthalmologic operation. So, if there is any doubt, general anesthesia should be provided to ensure a stand-still patient intraoperatively.

5. *Eyelid function*: To preserve the eyelid function is very important.

6. *Airway access*: One very challenging issue is the airway access during an eye operation.

Associated/Intrinsic Complications in Ophthalmologic Procedures

1. *Cystoid macular edema*: This is a relatively common pathologic condition of the retina. It occurs in several pathological conditions as central or branch retinal vein occlusion, intraocular inflammation, diabetic retinopathy, and post-cataract extraction.

2. *Lens dislocation*: Intraocular lens dislocation is a rare problem that usually affects patients who underwent cataract surgery. Lens dislocation is the displacement of the implanted lens moving towards the vitreous cavity. The lens sometimes becomes decentered from the visual axis, but usually does not fall into the vitreous cavity. Lens dislocation will cause some changes to patient's vision. If somehow the lens does fall into the vitreous cavity, the lens may produce some traction leading to retinal detachment and/or vitreous hemorrhage [13].

3. *Posterior capsule rupture/vitreous loss*: This is one of the major complications after cataract surgery and is a serious complication. It may also induce retinal detachment, uveitis, glaucoma, cystoid macular edema, uveitis, glaucoma, and intraocular lens dislocation [14].

4. *Vitreous/suprachoroidal hemorrhage*: This has a higher incidence following a second intraocular surgery in a vitrectomized eye, which is often associated with a lack of vitreous support leading to more fluctuations of intraocular pressure. Suprachoroidal hemorrhage may be more localized and has a relatively good prognosis. Usually, the risk factors include high myopia and aphakic/pseudophakic eyes. Active treatment can effectively improve visual prognosis [15].

5. *Endophthalmitis*: This is an inflammation of the inner coating of the eye. It is caused by an intraocular colonization of infectious agents leading to exudation within

intraocular fluids. Endophthalmitis can be postoperative, potentially a blind-causing condition. If untreated or inadequately treated, endophthalmitis will usually progress to panophthalmitis, which will require evisceration or enucleation of the eyeball [16].

Summary

Many ophthalmological procedures can be done with MAC/sedation service. However, sedation of patients undergoing ophthalmological surgery can be challenging because of the anatomical location of the eyes and the delicacy of the surgical procedure. A combination of intravenous sedatives with topical/local/regional blocks can often alleviate patients' anxiety and painful sensations, creating excellent conditions for surgery. However, maintaining a patient's spontaneous ventilation while providing adequate depth of sedation can be difficult, especially because the eye location sometimes does not allow all available means of oxygen supplementation, such as a non-rebreather face mask. Avoiding intraoperative apnea and desaturation is critical in providing MAC in ophthalmological procedures.

References

1. Vann MA, Ogunnaike BO, Joshi GP, Warltier DC. Sedation and anesthesia care for ophthalmologic surgery during local/regional anesthesia. *Anesthesiology*. 2007;107:502–8 doi:10.1097/01.anes.0000278996.01831.8d

2. Pager CK. Randomized controlled trial of preoperative information to improve satisfaction with cataract surgery. *Br J Ophthalmol*. 2005;89:10–13.

3. Waheeb S. Topical anesthesia in phacoemulsification. *Oman J Ophthalmol*. 2010;3(3):136–9. doi:10.4103/0974-620X.71892

4. Rengaraj V, Radhakrishnan M, AuEong KG, et al. Visual experience during phacoemulsification under topical versus retrobulbar anesthesia: results of a prospective, randomized, controlled trial. *Am J Ophthalmol*. 2004;138:782–7.

5. Lodhi O, Tripathy K. Anesthesia for eye surgery. In *StatPearls*, Treasure Island, FL: StatPearls Publishing, 2022. www.ncbi.nlm.nih.gov/books/NBK572131

6. OpenAnesthesia. Retrobulbar vs. peribulbar block. www.openanesthesia.org/retrobulbar_vs-_peribulbar_block (accessed June 25, 2022)

7. Schimek F, Fahle M. Techniques of facial nerve block. *Br J Ophthalmol*. 1995;79(2):166–73. doi:10.1136/bjo.79.2.166

8. Napier A, De Jesus O, Taylor A. Supraorbital nerve block. In *StatPearls* Treasure Island, FL: StatPearls Publishing, 2022.

9. Molliex S, Navez M, Baylot D, et al. Regional anaesthesia for outpatient nasal surgery. *Br J Anaesth*. 1996;76(1):151–3. doi:10.1093/bja/76.1.151

10. Yaghoubian JM, Aminpour S, Anilus V. Supertrochlear nerve block. In *StatPearls*, Treasure Island, FL: StatPearls Publishing, 2022.

11. NYSORA. Local and regional anesthesia for ophthalmic surgery. www.nysora.com/local-regional-anesthesia-ophthalmic-surgery (accessed July 17, 2022)

12. Yaylali V, Yildirim C, Tatlipinar S, et al. Subjective visual experience and pain level during phacoemulsification and intraocular lens implantation under topical anesthesia. *Ophthalmologica*. 2003;217:413–6.

13. Instituto de microcirugia ocular. Intraocular lens dislocation treatment. www.imo.es/en/disorders/intraocular-lens-dislocation-retina-and-vitreous (accessed July 17, 2022)

14. Chen M, Lamattina KC, Patrianakos T, Dwarakanathan S. Complication rate of posterior capsule rupture with vitreous loss during phacoemulsification at a

Hawaiian cataract surgical center: a clinical audit. *Clin Ophthalmol.* 2014;8:375–8. doi:10.2147/OPTH.S57736

15. Mo B, Li SF, Liu Y, et al. Suprachoroidal hemorrhage associated with pars plana vitrectomy. *BMC Ophthalmol.* 2021;21:295.

16. Simakurthy S, Tripathy K. Endophthalmitis. In *StatPearls*, Treasure Island, FL: StatPearls Publishing, 2022.

Procedural Sedation in the Emergency Department

Heikki E. Nikkanen

Introduction

The demands made on a modern emergency department (ED) are such that having an internal capacity to provide a range of procedural sedation is essential to its functioning. Patients arrive at every hour of the day, with pathology that may require sedation for diagnosis or treatment. The requirement for urgent action is greater than in an outpatient office or clinic, where cases are typically planned. Patients in the ED may be critically ill, or have a threat to an organ or limb that must be dealt with rapidly. Imposing on colleagues from the department of anesthesia to provide sedation for these patients is unnecessary and logistically difficult, given the after-hours and unplanned nature of these cases. Emergency physicians with training and board certification in emergency medicine have the skills to recognize these situations, and to assess the risks and benefits of procedural sedation in caring for these patients. In addition, the emergency physician has advanced airway management and resuscitation training to manage complications arising from sedation [1, 2].

Cases requiring sedation in the ED include, but are certainly not limited to, reduction of a dislocation or fracture, especially those involving a proximal joint or requiring significant manipulation; abscess drainage, notably those which are large, complex, or in sensitive areas; cardioversion; placement of tube thoracostomy; debridement or suturing of a wound; lumbar puncture; foreign body removal; or painful examination. In some EDs, sedation of a patient in order to tolerate CT or MRI may also be within the scope of the emergency physician's practice.

Requirements of a Procedural Sedation Program

In the United States, the provision of anesthesia in hospitals is governed by regulation 482.52 set forth by the Centers for Medicare and Medicaid Services (CMS) within the Department of Health and Human Services (HHS). In 2010, CMS released a clarifying memo, in which deep sedation was classified as anesthesia, along with general and regional types.

This required the provider to be an anesthesiologist; certified registered nurse anesthetist (CRNA); anesthesia assistant; non-anesthesiologist MD or DO; or oral surgeon, dentist, or podiatrist qualified to administer anesthesia under state law. In January 2011, after nearly a year of discussion involving the American College of Emergency Physicians (ACEP), CMS revised its guidelines. Of great interest to the emergency medicine community was the affirmation that "emergency medicine-trained physicians have very specific skill sets to manage airways and ventilation that is necessary to provide patient rescue. Therefore, these practitioners are uniquely qualified to provide all levels of analgesia/sedation and anesthesia (moderate to deep to general)." They accepted the statements from both the Emergency Nurses Association and ACEP that "support the delivery of medications used for procedural sedation and analgesia by credentialed emergency nurses working under the direct supervision of an emergency physician. These agents include but are not limited to etomidate, propofol, ketamine, fentanyl, and midazolam." ACEP has interpreted this guidance to mean that procedural sedation of both moderate and deep degree falls within the purview of emergency medicine.

A good working relationship between the department of anesthesia and the ED is nevertheless of great importance in creating and maintaining a procedural sedation program. The representation of ED on a hospital sedation management committee will also ensure that issues unique to emergency medicine are raised regularly. Other specialties using procedural sedation have very different needs. Endoscopy, cardiac catheterization, transesophageal echocardiography, or dental procedures typically require a longer, but less profound, sedation than is required in an ED. Gaining approval for providing deep and dissociative sedation and using short-acting sedative agents, such as propofol and etomidate, can be of significant benefit for the care of the ED patient. Both moderate and deep sedation have been shown to be safe tools in the hands of emergency physicians [3–7]. These data can be used to reinforce the position of the ED regarding this issue.

Personnel requirements for moderate and deep sedation, as well as for the "dissociative" sedation obtained via ketamine, vary depending on the practice setting. A reasonable standard for most EDs in the United States, and one advocated in clinical practice guidelines, is to have a dedicated medical professional, usually a nurse, administer medications and monitor the patient for moderate or dissociative sedation [8]. The guidance of ACEP on the issue of the number of practitioners required to provide procedural sedation is that, when possible, two physicians should be present, one to provide the sedation and the other to perform the procedure. However, given limitations of the practice environment, there are circumstances in which the emergency nurse can monitor the patient, once stable sedation has been achieved, so that the emergency physician can perform the procedure.

Special Considerations for ED Patients

Two issues exist which set patients presenting to the ED apart from others requiring sedation. They are the variables of the last oral intake and the urgency of the required procedure. Striking a balance between safety and prompt treatment is a prime consideration for the emergency physician [9]. A 2020 consensus statement from the International Committee for the Advancement of Procedural Sedation highlights that clinically significant aspiration events are quite rare. Their recommendation is that urgent procedures should not be delayed on the basis of fasting time. Patients with elevated risk of aspiration should be considered for anesthesia care, or use of ketamine as the sedative agent [10].

The greatest aspiration risk factors in procedural sedation cases appear to be related to esophageal endoscopy, existing comorbid disease, and use of propofol as the sedative agent [11, 12].

Selection of Sedation Agents

Although many agents can be used to achieve either moderate or deep sedation in the ED, only a small number are in common use, either singly or in combination. The drug and dose should be primarily chosen as a function of the sedation assessment and procedural need (Figure 21.1). Given a choice between otherwise equivalent drugs, the recovery time is also an important factor. Regardless of the ultimate selection of agent, sedation in the ED has a very low incidence of significant complications. A meta-analysis of 9,652 sedations showed incidences of aspiration, laryngospasm, and need for endotracheal intubation to be 1.2/1,000, 1.6/1,000, and 4.2/1,000, respectively [13].

Midazolam–Fentanyl

This is a common pairing of an opioid and a benzodiazepine, to provide relief of pain and to cause sedation. Midazolam has a rapid onset of action, and a superior amnesic effect compared with other benzodiazepines [14]. Benefits of the use of midazolam include amnesia to the procedure and the ability to reverse its effects. However, longer procedural and recovery times are seen. A study comparing midazolam and etomidate at doses of 0.035 mg/kg and 0.10 mg/kg, respectively, showed a significantly longer time from initiation to recovery (16 vs. 32 minutes, $p < 0.001$) and a higher number of doses needed [15]. Regarding opioids, fentanyl is preferred for procedural sedation in the ED due to its rapid onset of action and short duration, as well as the relative lack of cardiovascular effect [16].

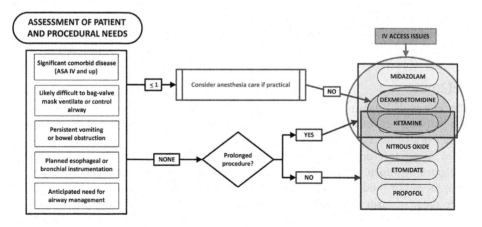

Figure 21.1 Patient factors and influences in procedural sedation.

Propofol

Propofol is close to an ideal agent for many procedural sedation needs in the ED. It produces even deep sedation reliably, with a very rapid onset and very short duration. It can cause airway compromise and hypoventilation, as well as hypotension from cardiovascular depression. For this reason, hypotensive patients or those at high risk of developing hypotension are likely not ideal candidates for this drug. Experience with its use by emergency physicians in thousands of cases shows that its safety profile in the hands of the emergency physician is as good as or better than that of other available agents. In one study, it was found to be as effective as midazolam without adverse effects. In the same study, the recovery time was 15 minutes for propofol, compared to 76 minutes for midazolam [17]. For a practice environment with limited time and resources, this represents a significant advantage. An evaluation of the cost-effectiveness of propofol relative to midazolam shows savings of time and cost [18]. A prospective study of 116 patients using propofol in the ED for procedural sedation showed it to be safe and well received by patients and physicians [19]. Compared to etomidate in a randomized controlled trial (RCT) of 214 patients, it was similar in adverse events and recovery time, but etomidate caused myoclonus in 20% of patients. Successful sedation was achieved in 97% of patients who received propofol, compared to 90% with etomidate [20]. A reasonable dosing strategy in healthy patients is to start with 0.5 to 1 mg/kg intravenous (IV) bolus and consider redosing with 0.25 mg/kg IV every 2 minutes until adequate sedation is achieved.

Etomidate

Etomidate has been used for years as an induction agent for endotracheal intubation. Its properties of rapid action, short duration, and cardiovascular stability also make it attractive for procedural sedation. In one study of 150 ED procedures performed with etomidate, five patients developed hypoxemia and required assisted ventilation. In 95% of cases, recovery to pre-procedure level of consciousness occurred within 30 minutes. Patient satisfaction was very high [21]. A double-blind RCT with 44 patients comparing etomidate against midazolam in fracture reduction showed a recovery time of 15 minutes and 32 minutes, respectively. Success of the procedure was 100% for the etomidate group, and 86% for the midazolam group. Side effects and adverse events were rare, but equal in the two groups. Given the frequency of myoclonus, reported to be as high as 80%, this might be a less optimal choice for reductions of fracture or dislocation.

Ketamine

The effects of ketamine do not easily fit into the previously discussed sedation scale. A significant benefit is the preservation of airway reflexes and respiratory drive, which makes it a better agent in cases where aspiration and hypoxemia are more significant risks. Respiratory depression has been described at the time of injection, which can be mitigated by infusing it over 1–2 minutes. Increases in blood pressure and heart rate are ubiquitous but mild, and easily controlled with sympatholytic agents. No reports have been made of cardiac ischemia resulting from ketamine administration. In a review of trials of ketamine, only one cardiorespiratory event with a poor outcome was identified in over 70,000 uses [22]. Ketamine alone has predictable and rapid effects when administered intramuscularly (IM). It is used commonly in children, and it is safe and effective to administer intranasally, which makes it an attractive option for the pediatric population [23] A phenomenon known as "emergence" in adults given ketamine causes discomfort in patients and physicians alike. There are a number of strategies that may be employed to counter this effect. A simple strategy some authors recommend is to coach patients that they can control or choose the dream they will have. A soothing atmosphere has been anecdotally seen to have beneficial effects, but may not be feasible in a busy ED. One study suggests that addition of midazolam 0.07 mg/kg IV at the time of ketamine administration decreases the incidence of this side effect from 50% to 7% [24]. This relatively high dose resulted in a few incidences of respiratory depression requiring transient ventilatory support. A more recent randomized, double-blind, placebo-controlled trial of midazolam 0.05 mg/kg or haloperidol 5 mg as premedication showed a reduction in relative risk for ketamine-induced agitation of 60.9% and 69.2%, respectively [25]. A smaller dose of benzodiazepine may be given either just before emergence, or on an as-needed basis. A large meta-analysis suggests that emergence dysphoria is present in only 1.4% of cases, although there is a wide variation in studies including adults [26]. Hypersalivation may also occur, which can be controlled by pretreatment with atropine 0.01 mg/kg IM or IV. The most feared complication, laryngospasm, occurs in 1.4% of cases [27]. Despite a number of studies, no clear risk factors have been identified in the ED sedation population. This complication can usually be managed with bag-valve mask ventilation, although rarely intubation is required.

Ketamine–Propofol

There is a robust body of literature describing the use of a mixture of ketamine and propofol ("ketofol") to provide procedural sedation. Mixtures between 1:1 and 4:1 have been studied, as have various administration sequences, from combined in the same syringe to sequentially and titrated. A 2015 meta-analysis of 6 RCTs showed a decrease in respiratory complications, but not a decrease in overall complication rate, compared to propofol alone [28]. A 2016 review and RCT meta-analysis found that the relative risks of hypotension, bradycardia, and respiratory complications were 0.11, 0.47, and 0.31 respectively, compared to propofol as monotherapy. They found no statistically significant increase in emergence reaction, muscular rigidity, or vomiting [29]. This conclusion is bolstered by a more recent systematic review and meta-analysis, which found a lower incidence of adverse respiratory events with ketofol compared to propofol alone, with no other significant differences in measures such as sedation time, cardiovascular effects, and patient satisfaction [30]. In children, similar results were found [31].

Ketamine–propofol offers another pharmacologic option that appears safe and effective, and may be of use in certain cases where there is concern for poor physiologic reserve, impaired cardiovascular function, or respiratory comorbidities.

Nitrous Oxide

Nitrous oxide (N_2O) is a colorless gas with a faint odor, which is heavier than air. It is not flammable, but serves as an oxidizing agent and should not be used near spark or flame. It has properties of sedation and analgesia that are useful in a number of settings. Although its exact mechanism in providing anesthesia is not known, it is a non-competitive inhibitor of *N*-methyl-D-aspartate (NMDA) receptors. By causing release of endogenous opioids in the brainstem, it also provides analgesia. It has a long history of use in both surgery and dentistry, and there is a more recent body of literature about its use in emergency procedural sedation, both in children and adults. It has a very rapid onset of action, and its effects are short-lived. It is typically delivered in a 30% to 50% concentration by mask, with the remainder of the gas mixture being oxygen. Its safety profile is excellent, with adverse effects of myelopathy, polyneuropathy, and seizures primarily associated with chronic abuse. Cardiac output and minute volume are unchanged. One hazard associated with its use is that, although it has a low solubility in the blood, it is much more soluble than nitrogen. Therefore, it diffuses into air-filled spaces in the body more rapidly than the nitrogen in those spaces can be absorbed. Expansion of pockets of gas is therefore a possibility, and its use in patients with "trapped air" in the body (e.g., pneumothorax) is contraindicated. Similarly, at the end of a procedural sedation, nitrous oxide can be rapidly cleared from the blood into the lung, displacing ambient air and causing hypoxia. For hospital staff exposed to nitrous oxide for prolonged periods, a theoretical concern is the inactivation of vitamin B12. If heavy use of this agent is expected, scavenger and ventilation systems are required.

For purposes of procedural sedation, the 50% concentration is superior to the 30%, without causing additional adverse effects. Nitrous oxide typically does not yield deeper levels of sedation, but could be used in cases where anxiolysis is the goal, or where adjunctive analgesia can be used, such as local anesthetic administration [32].

Dexmedetomidine

Dexmedetomidine is a highly selective alpha-2 adrenergic receptor agonist that provides sedation and anxiolysis by suppressing the release of excitatory neurotransmitters without causing significant respiratory depression. This makes it a potentially attractive option for procedural sedation in the ED, where rapid recovery and maintenance of ventilation are important. It has been increasingly used in other clinical settings. Its relatively slow onset of action relative to other agents suggests that it might not be a first choice for procedural sedation. There is a higher rate of hypotension and bradycardia, albeit transient, with the use of dexmedetomidine compared to other agents, in the ED literature. Although many uses have been suggested for dexmedetomidine in the emergency setting, the most promising based on current understanding is sedation to allow imaging of the pediatric patient [33]. However, better studies and familiarity with the drug will be necessary before widespread adoption can take place.

The medications available for procedural sedation, together with typical routes and dosage, are summarized in Table 21.1.

Special Populations

Elderly patients and those with significant systemic illnesses should have a more cautious sedation strategy, with initial doses on the lower end of the range, and repeated dosing if necessary to achieve the desired level of sedation.

Patients with obesity should have medication doses based on adjusted body weight to avoid oversedation or prolonged recovery.

Pregnant patients are at increased risk for hypoxemia, aspiration, and difficult intubation, especially after 16 weeks of pregnancy. Use of a promotility agent such as

Table 21.1 Medications for procedural sedation with typical routes and dosage.

Class	Medication	Typical Route and Dose				
		IV	IM	IN	INH	PO
Sedative	Propofol	0.5–1 mg/kg				
	Midazolam	0.05–1 mg/kg	0.1–0.15 mg/kg Max dose 10 mg	0.2–0.3 mg/kg Max dose 10 mg		0.25–0.5 mg/kg Max dose 20 mg
	Etomidate	0.1–0.2 mg/kg				
	Dexmedetomidine	0.5–1 mcg/kg bolus 0.2–1 mcg/kg/hr CI				
Analgesic	Fentanyl	0.5–1 mcg/kg bolus	0.5–1 mcg/kg	1–2 mcg/kg		
Mixed	Ketamine	1–2 mg/kg	4–5 mg/kg			
	Ketofol 1:1	0.5–1 mg/kg				
	Nitrous Oxide				30–50%	

metoclopramide and placement of the patient in left lateral decubitus position may reduce the likelihood of these events. There is very limited information on the safety of all the agents commonly used in procedural sedation. However, there are some data which suggest benzodiazepines may be teratogenic. This argues against the use of midazolam in this population.

Pediatric patients can benefit from non-pharmacologic techniques such as distraction and relaxation, which can at times even obviate the need for sedation. In a healthy child, sedation for CT imaging can be achieved with IV propofol, ketamine, etomidate, or dexmedetomidine. If IV access is an issue, midazolam, ketamine, and dexmedetomidine can be given by alternative routes. Sedation for MRI may be beyond the scope of practice of the emergency physician, given the long time required and the distance from the ED. For healthy children requiring sedation for a minimally painful procedure where some movement is tolerable, nitrous oxide or intranasal midazolam or dexmedetomidine are reasonable choices. For more painful procedures or those where movement is undesirable, ketamine, ketofol, or propofol with fentanyl are preferred over other agents.

Patients with kidney or liver dysfunction should be given lower starting doses of etomidate and midazolam, and patients with liver disease should be given lower starting doses of dexmedetomidine. No change needs to be made in dosing of propofol and ketamine.

A few representative cases describing procedural sedation management of patients in the ED setting follow.

Example Cases

Case 1

A 5-year-old girl arrives to the ED after a fall from a bicycle. Her physical examination and radiographic evaluation show an angulated fracture of the left radius and ulna. There is no tenting of the skin, and her neurovascular examination is normal distal to the injury. She has no other significant injury, and her medical history is unremarkable. The reduction and splinting of the fracture will require sedation. She weighs 20 kg. Her last meal was milk and cookies, ingested 2 hours before arrival.

In this circumstance, propofol with fentanyl is a reasonable choice, at a dose of 1–1.5 mg/kg IV. Alternatively, ketamine or ketofol could be used. If IV access cannot be obtained, ketamine is the only sedative agent that is reliable via the IM route, at a dose of 4–5 mg/kg. A benzodiazepine to moderate the emergence reaction can be considered as needed. Most patients do not require glycopyrrolate or atropine, unless the procedure is in the oropharynx.

Case 2

A 72-year-old woman comes to the ED with lightheadedness and palpitations. Her blood pressure is 64/36 and an electrocardiogram shows atrial fibrillation with a rapid ventricular rate of 140 beats per minute. ST segment depressions are seen inferiorly. The blood pressure does not respond to a bolus of normal saline. Given the patient's shock state and evidence of end-organ dysfunction, the decision is made to perform a synchronized cardioversion. She weighs 65 kg. Her last meal was beef stroganoff, consumed immediately before arrival.

In this instance, there are a few choices. Propofol might be a less attractive choice given the patient's hypotension. Alternatively, etomidate has good cardiovascular stability, although a longer duration of action. If this agent were selected, a dose on the lower side of the range 0.1–0.2 mg/kg should be selected. A reasonable amount would be 6 mg. Finally, given the significant concerns about worsening her hemodynamic status, ketamine could be used at a dose of 1–2 mg/kg. Assuming the cardioversion is successful, a dose of midazolam, ativan, or another benzodiazepine could be used to blunt the emergence reaction. Given the very short duration of the procedure, the risk–benefit equation of giving an adjunct opioid likely argues against its use.

Case 3

A 40-year-old man with a history of hypertension, opioid abuse, and renal insufficiency is brought to the ED after he notes his arm has been swollen at the antecubital area for the past 3 days. Physical evaluation augmented with ultrasound shows a large subcutaneous abscess with septations that will require a complicated drainage. He has normal vital signs with the exception of a blood pressure of 164/90, and there is no evidence of lymphangitic spread or surrounding cellulitis. He is just finishing up a sandwich as he is brought in for evaluation. Although he has no drug allergies, he does have a severe allergic reaction to eggs. His weight is 150 kg.

This patient has somewhat limited options. Local anesthesia will likely not be sufficient to permit a proper drainage. His egg allergy precludes the use of propofol. Ketamine could be used, but it could worsen his hypertension, and there is a risk of an uncomfortable and long recovery from the sedation. Etomidate, at a dose of 15 mg IV (0.1 mg/kg), remains a choice for this patient. Midazolam could also be used, but titration of the dose is often required and results in a longer recovery time than propofol or etomidate. For midazolam and etomidate, an adjunctive dose of an opioid analgesic would need to be given, such as fentanyl in doses of 50–100 μg IV, repeated as needed. His obesity is a moderate risk factor for adverse respiratory events. Anesthesia care could be considered. If this is not an option, ketamine would be the best choice of agent, in order to maintain airway and respiratory status.

Summary

Emergency physicians have the skills needed to safely administer moderate and deep procedural sedation. Representation on the hospital sedation committee is important in developing and maintaining an independent moderate and deep sedation practice. Brief deep sedation is more suited to the majority of ED cases. It is not generally necessary to delay sedation for urgent procedures due to recent oral intake.

References

1. Hockberger RS, Binder LS, Graber MA, et al. American College of Emergency Physicians Core Content Task Force II. The model of the clinical practice of emergency medicine. *Ann Emerg Med.* 2001;37:745–70.

2. Allison EJ, Aghababian RV, Barsan WG, et al. Core content for emergency medicine. Task Force on the Core Content for Emergency Medicine Revision. *Ann Emerg Med.* 1997;29:792–811.

3. Mallory MD, Baxter AL, Yanosky DJ, et al. Emergency physician-administered propofol sedation: a report on 25,433 sedations from the Pediatric Sedation Research Consortium. *Ann Emerg Med.* 2011;57:462–8.

4. Burton JH, Miner JR, Shipley ER, et al. Propofol for emergency department procedural sedation and analgesia: a tale

of three centers. *Acad Emerg Med.* 2006;13:24–30.

5. Green SM, Roback MG, Krauss B, et al. Predictors of airway and respiratory adverse events with ketamine sedation in the emergency department: an individual-patient data meta-analysis of 8,282 children. *Ann Emerg Med.* 2009;54:158–68.

6. Peña BMG, Krauss B. Adverse events of procedural sedation and analgesia in a pediatric emergency department. *Ann Emerg Med.* 1999;34:483–91.

7. Couloures KG, Beach M, Cravero JP, Monroe KK, Hertzog JH. Impact of provider specialty on pediatric procedural sedation complication rate. *Pediatrics.* 2011;127:e1154–60.

8. Godwin SA, Caro DA, Wolf SJ, et al. American College of Emergency Physicians. Clinical policy: procedural sedation and analgesia in the emergency department. *Ann Emerg Med.* 2005;45:177–96.

9. Green SM, Roback MG, Miner JR, Burton JH, Krauss B. Fasting and emergency department procedural sedation and analgesia: a consensus-based clinical practice advisory. *Ann Emerg Med.* 2007;49:454–61.

10. Green SM, Leroy PL, Roback MG, et al. An international multidisciplinary consensus statement on fasting before procedural sedation in adults and children. *Anaesthesia.* 2020;75:374–85.

11. Beach ML, Cohen DM, Gallagher SM, Cravero JP. Major adverse events and relationship to nil per os status in pediatric sedation/anesthesia outside the operating room: a report of the pediatric sedation research consortium. *Anesthesiology.* 2016;124:80–8.

12. Green SM, Mason KP, Krauss BS. Pulmonary aspiration during procedural sedation: a comprehensive systematic review. *Br J Anaesth.* 2017;118:344–54.

13. Bellolio MF, Gilani WI, et al. Incidence of adverse events in adults undergoing procedural sedation in the emergency department: a systematic review and meta-analysis. *Acad Emerg Med.* 2016;23:119–34.

14. Muse DA. Conscious and deep sedation. In Harwood-Nuss A, Wolfson AB, eds., *The Clinical Practice of Emergency Medicine*, 3rd ed. Philadelphia, PA: Lippincott Williams & Wilkins, 2001, 1761.

15. Hunt GS, Spencer MT, Hays DP. Etomidate and midazolam for procedural sedation: prospective, randomized trial. *Am J Emerg Med.* 2005;23:299–303.

16. Blackburn P, Vissers R. Pharmacology of emergency department pain management and conscious sedation. *Emerg Med Clin North Am.* 2000;18:803–27.

17. Havel CJ, Strait RT, Hennes H. A clinical trial of propofol vs. midazolam for procedural sedation in a pediatric emergency department. *Acad Emerg Med.* 1999;6:989–97.

18. Hohl CM, Nosyk B, Sadatsafavi M, Anis AH. A cost-effectiveness analysis of propofol versus midazolam for procedural sedation in the emergency department. *Acad Emerg Med.* 2008;15:32–9.

19. Zed PJ, Abu-Laban RB, Chan WW, Harrison DW. Efficacy, safety and patient satisfaction of propofol for procedural sedation and analgesia in the emergency department: a prospective study. *CJEM.* 2007;9:421–7.

20. Miner JR, Burton JH. Clinical practice advisory: emergency department procedural sedation with propofol. *Ann Emerg Med.* 2007;50:182–7.

21. Vinson DR, Bradbury DR. Etomidate for procedural sedation in emergency medicine. *Ann Emerg Med.* 2002;39:592–8.

22. Strayer RJ, Nelson LS. Adverse events associated with ketamine for procedural sedation in adults. *Am J Emerg Med.* 2008;26:985–1028.

23. Silva LO, Lee, JY, Bellilio F, Homme JL, Anderson JL. Intranasal ketamine for acute pain management in children: a systematic review. *Am J Emerg Med.* 2020;38(9):1860–6.

24. Sener S, Eken C, Schultz CH, Serinken M, Ozsarac M. Ketamine with and without midazolam for emergency department sedation in adults: a randomized controlled trial. *Ann Emerg Med.* 2011;57:109–14.

25. Aklaghi N, Payandemehr P, Yaseri M, Aklaghi AA, Abdolrazaghnejad A. Premedication with midazolam or halportidol to prevent recovery agitation in adults undergoing prodecural sedation with ketamine: a randomized double-blind clinical trial. *Ann Emerg Med.* 2019;73(5):462–9.

26. Green SM, Roback MG, Krauss B, et al. Predictors of emesis and recovery agitation with emergency department ketamine sedation: an individual-patient data meta-analysis of 8,282 children. *Ann Emerg Med.* 2009;54:171–80.

27. Green SM, Roback MG, Krauss B, et al. Predictors of airway and respiratory adverse events with ketamine sedation in the emergency department: an individual-patient data meta-analysis of 8,282 children. *Ann Emerg Med.* 2009;54:158–68.

28. Yan JW, McLeod SL, et al. Ketamine-propofol versus propofol alone for procedural sedation in the emergency department: a systematic review and meta-analysis. *Acad Emerg Med.* 2015;22:1003–13.

29. Jalili M, Bahreini M, et al. Ketamine-propofol combination (ketofol) vs propofol for procedural sedation and analgesia: systematic review and meta-analysis. *Am J Emerg Med.* 2016;34:558–69.

30. Ghojazadeh M, Sanaie S, Paknezhad SP, Faghih SS, Soleimanpour H. Using ketamine and propofol for procedural sedation of adults in the emergency department: a systematic review and meta-analysis. *Adv Pharm Bull.* 2019;9(1):5–11.

31. Foo TY, Norhyati MN, Yazid MB, et al. Ketamine–propofol (ketofol) for procedural sedation and analgesia in children: a systematic review and meta-analysis. *BMC Emerg Med.* 2020; 20(1):81.

32. Huang C, Johnson N. Nitrous oxide, from the operating room to the emergency department. *Curr Emerg Hosp Med Rep.* 2016;4:11–18.

33. Baumgartner K, Groff V, Yaeger LH, Fuller BM. The use of dexmedetomidine in the emergency department: a systematic review. *Acad Emerg Med.* 2022;00:1–13.

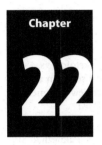

Chapter 22

Sedation in the Intensive Care Setting

Iaswarya Ganapathiraju and John P. Gaillard

Introduction

Critically ill patients in the intensive care unit (ICU) often require sedation and analgesia as part of a comprehensive care plan. Inappropriate sedation and analgesia (too little or too much) are known to lead to adverse outcomes in this patient population, including increasing the risk of delirium, worsening hemodynamics, or interrupting life-sustaining therapies, etc. [1]. In recent years, there has been a paradigm shift in providing sedation and analgesia to minimize physical discomfort and psycho-emotional stress while maintaining the patient's ability to interact with care providers. Balancing patient comfort and cognition with the need to provide appropriate care requires the critical care provider to have a comprehensive understanding of the pharmacodynamics of sedatives and analgesics, and to also to remain vigilant in evaluating ongoing needs for sedation and analgesia.

The goals of this chapter are to: (1) review the indications for sedation and analgesia in critically ill patients, (2) review commonly used sedation scales and methods used for patient monitoring, and (3) review specific medications and major side effects.

Indications

Historically, analgesia and sedation were considered one treatment, especially for patients on a mechanical ventilator. This thought process has changed with the release of practice guidelines for the management of pain, agitation, and delirium in 2013 [2]. Sedation and analgesia are now considered two separate treatment modalities.

Critically ill patients commonly experience pain. The etiology of pain in this patient population may be obvious, such as acute abdomen, kidney stones, trauma, and invasive procedures. However, there are more insidious causes that may be overlooked such as indwelling catheters and pressure injuries. In addition, there are several biochemical changes that occur locally at the site of injury or inflammation and at the level of central

> **Box 22.1** Common causes of encephalopathy in intensive care units
>
> Sepsis and systemic infections
> Metabolic derangements (e.g., hyponatremia, acidosis, uremia, hypoglycemia, hyperammonemia)
> Endocrine derangements (e.g., hypo- or hyperthyroidism, adrenal insufficiency)
> Medication-induced (side effects of prescribed medications, toxicities, and/or withdrawals)
> Structural abnormalities (e.g., ischemic or hemorrhagic stroke, seizures)

pain receptors, which lead to baseline hyperalgesia and allodynia in patients with critical illness [3, 4]. Regardless of the cause, the perception of pain is different for every patient.

Pain is often undertreated in the ICU for a variety of reasons: under-recognition by the caregiver, inability of the patient to express pain, renal or liver dysfunction, and unstable hemodynamics. It is imperative that the care team be diligent in treating pain, especially since inadequate pain control leads to anxiety or agitation, which subsequently begets the need for increased sedation. For this reason, an "analgesia-first" approach has come into favor in recent years, where the goal is to adequately treat pain first, then assess for further sedation needs.

Whereas the need for analgesia is determined by the patient and their clinical condition, the need for sedation is often determined by the care team. Historically, practice patterns favored deep sedation while patients were maintained on mechanical ventilation, often leading to a prolonged length of stay in the ICU. However, recent studies are showing that light or even no sedation may lead to similar outcomes while decreasing the risk of delirium. One such study randomized patients to no sedation versus light sedation with daily sedation interruptions and found no significant difference in 90-day mortality, ICU-free days, or ventilator-free days [5]. Though this may not indicate that no sedation is superior to light sedation, it shows that clinicians may be sedating patients more than necessary, possibly placing them at risk of unnecessary medication exposure, adverse reactions, critical illness-associated weakness, and delirium.

Nonetheless, critically ill patients may have various reasons to need sedation. Commonly, anxiety and agitation in critically ill patients can lead to disruption of important therapeutics and thus require administration of sedatives. However, providers should be aware that there are multiple causes of encephalopathy in the critically ill patient and evaluate the patient for potentially reversible causes. The most common of these causes are listed in Box 22.1.

Sedation Scales and Patient Monitoring

Critically ill patients are often unable to communicate concerns of pain or anxiety with care providers due to their medical condition or other confounding factors. Therefore, care providers need an objective and standardized way to assess the need for sedation. Frequent assessment of the patient's sedation level facilitates titration of the chosen agent(s) and minimizes the risk of under- or oversedation. Such an approach lowers cumulative sedative doses; limits duration of sedation therapy; and minimizes the development of agent-specific side effects, tolerance, or withdrawal. This led to the

Table 22.1 Richmond Agitation–Sedation Scale

Score	Description	
+4	Combative	Overly combative, violent, immediate danger to staff
+3	Very agitated	Pulls or removes tube(s) or catheter(s); aggressive
+2	Agitated	Frequent non-purposeful movement, fights ventilator
+1	Restless	Anxious but movements not aggressive or vigorous
0	Alert and calm	
−1	Drowsy	Not fully alert, but has sustained awakening to voice
−2	Light sedation	Briefly awakens with eye contact to voice
−3	Moderate sedation	Movement or eye opening to voice
−4	Deep sedation	No response to voice, but movement or eye opening to physical stimulation
−5	Unarousable	No response to voice or physical stimulation

development of sedation monitoring scales to standardize the administration of sedative medications to a predetermined end point.

The Richmond Agitation–Sedation Scale (RASS) is the most used of these scales in the ICU (Table 22.1). RASS has been validated in different ICU populations and shown to decrease the amount of sedation medicines used [6]. The goal for most patients is to maintain a RASS level of 0 or negative 1, which translates to the patient being alert and calm or drowsy but arousable, respectively. This approach optimizes the sedation level. However, this may be difficult to obtain in many critically ill patients. Some patients may need to be maintained at deeper sedation levels to facilitate synchronization with mechanical ventilation or to minimize the risk of dislodging invasive lines or drains. RASS goals should be personalized to each patient based on their critical illness and sedation needs.

Once a stable level of sedation is achieved, sedation should be discontinued at least once daily to allow spontaneous arousal in those ICU patients whose clinical condition is unlikely to deteriorate with scheduled sedation interruptions. This daily awakening has been shown to decrease the duration of mechanical ventilation and ICU length of stay, particularly when paired with spontaneous breathing trials [7].

Numerous cerebral function monitors (CFMs) have also been developed over the last decade that process raw cortical EEG signals and mathematically convert them to an analog numerical scale. The premise of CFMs is that consciousness translates to cortical electrical activity and that suppression of such activity can indicate progressive decreases in consciousness. CFMs are primarily utilized in the operating room to monitor anesthesia levels and minimize patient recall of unpleasant intraoperative events. In the ICU, CFMs are most used in patients receiving adjunctive neuromuscular blockade. There are limited data suggesting that CFMs can accurately assess consciousness in critically ill patients, and thus they have yet to be widely accepted for ICU sedation monitoring [8].

Given the close association between sedation and delirium, the Society of Critical Care Medicine recommends monitoring all ICU patients routinely for presence of delirium [9]. Several tools have been developed for the diagnosis of delirium in the intensive care unit. Among these, the Confusion Assessment Method for the ICU (CAM-ICU) is most commonly used. The assessment for delirium should first start with assessing wakefulness through the RASS, followed by a standardized delirium assessment scale in awake patients (RASS of –3 or higher). A patient is likely to have delirium per CAM-ICU if they display both feature 1 (acute change or fluctuating course of mental status) and feature 2 (inattention) plus either feature 3 (altered level of consciousness) or feature 4 (disorganized thinking) [6].

Specific Agents for Sedation and Analgesia

In this section, individual agents for sedation or analgesia are discussed, along with their common side effects. Although this list is not comprehensive, it will provide a basic understanding of each medication or medication class and alternative sedation/analgesia plans available. It is important to note that doses of these medications often need to be adjusted in critically ill patients for a variety of reasons (e.g., hemodynamic instability, renal or hepatic dysfunction, or age).

Most commonly, sedation and analgesia are administered via the intravenous (IV) route in the ICU setting for the sake of easy titration. However, in recent years, clinicians have begun to explore other modes of administration to minimize the risk of over-sedation as well as cost. Recent studies have evaluated the efficacy of enteral sedation along with IV sedation but have not shown benefit in terms of achieving RASS goals. Furthermore, one study showed that there was potential harm from an increased risk of adverse events such as self-extubation [10]. Further studies are needed to see if there is a role for enteral administration of sedation and analgesia in the ICU.

There are also several other options for alternative administrations to IV sedation: patient-controlled analgesia or sedation, enteral, transdermal, or directly via the central nervous system. These modalities will not be discussed in detail here, as their role in the ICU has not yet been fully elucidated. Clinicians should be aware that the risks and benefits of different medications, and modalities of administration should be constantly re-evaluated based on the evolution of a patient's critical illness.

The following agents are listed based on their frequency of use in the ICU. A summary of these agents and associated adverse effects is given in Table 22.2.

Opioids

Opioids represent the "gold standard" for analgesia in the ICU. There are three types of opioid receptors within the body (mu, gamma, and kappa). The mu receptors primarily mediate the analgesic effects. Mu receptors are found in the periphery and along the ascending and descending pain pathways of the spinal cord, brainstem, thalamus, and cortex. The benefits of these agents include analgesia, sedation (at higher doses), cough suppression, and quick reversibility with naloxone. Side effects include respiratory depression, impaired mentation, unreliable amnesia, nausea, vomiting, ileus, urinary retention, and dysphoria when given in the absence of pain. Specific opioid agents also produce pharmacologically active metabolites that can further potentiate analgesic and adverse effects in the setting of renal or hepatic dysfunction.

Table 22.2 Common agents used for sedation and analgesia in the intensive care units

Agent	Mechanism of action	Common side effects
Opioids	Mu opioid receptor agonists	Respiratory depression, impaired mentation, gastrointestinal upset, ileus, urinary retention, and dysphoria.
Benzodiazepines	GABA$_A$ receptor agonists	Respiratory depression, paradoxical agitation, delirium (particularly in elderly patients)
Propofol	GABA receptor upregulation	Hypotension, burning sensation at site of administration, hypertriglyceridemia, propofol-related infusion syndrome
Dexmedetomidine	Central alpha-2 agonist	Bradycardia, hypotension, adrenal suppression with bolus dosing
Ketamine	NMDA receptor antagonist	Can induce psychosis in patients with schizophrenia, hypertension

Abbreviations: GABA, gamma-aminobutyric acid; NMDA, N-methyl-D-aspartate.

Morphine is a naturally occurring opioid analgesic derived from poppy seeds and is the standard for comparison for other opioids. Its oral bioavailability varies between 35% and 75%, and its plasma half-life is approximately 2–3.5 hours. The analgesic effects of morphine can last up to 4–6 hours. Morphine is metabolized into morphine-6-glucuronide (M-6-G), which also carries analgesic effects but is eliminated by the kidney. M-6-G can accumulate in patients with renal insufficiency and potentiate adverse effects. Thus, it is reasonable to avoid morphine use in patients with renal insufficiency or failure. Additionally, morphine causes a decrease in sympathetic tone and increase in histamine release, which can result in hypotension, urticaria, or bronchospasm.

Fentanyl is a synthetic opioid that is approximately 100 times more potent than morphine. It is a highly lipophilic drug, allowing rapid onset of action within 30–60 seconds. This property also leads to redistribution of the drug into poorly perfused peripheral tissues, thus leading to a shorter duration of action of approximately 30–60 minutes. Fentanyl is available for administration through IV (most commonly used in the ICU setting), transdermal, and transbuccal routes. It is metabolized in the liver into inactive metabolites. It can rarely cause bradycardia (particularly at large doses) but does not stimulate histamine release. One rare complication of fentanyl administration is skeletal muscle rigidity (most common at high doses), which can potentially impair oxygenation and ventilation. Prolonged fentanyl IV administration can lead to accumulation at mu receptors and delayed onset of clinical effects (particularly respiratory depression) upon discontinuation. This effect is referred to as increased context-sensitive half-time.

Hydromorphone is a semi-synthetic opioid agonist and is preferred over morphine in patients with renal failure since it is metabolized in the liver into inactive metabolites, although animal models have shown dose-dependent risk of allodynia, myoclonus, and seizures. The onset of action of hydromorphone is approximately 30 minutes and duration of action is 4 hours. Hydromorphone does not stimulate histamine release [11].

In addition to the above agents, there are several others that can be used as enteral adjunctive therapy for analgesia, which will not be discussed in depth here since the role of enteral sedation and analgesia has not yet been studied in detail, as previously mentioned. Additionally, certain opioids may have indications for use in the ICU that are not related to analgesia. Meperidine, for example, is a synthetic opioid that has fallen out of favor for use for analgesia due to increased risk of myoclonus and seizure activity, particularly in the setting of renal dysfunction, but may benefit the patient undergoing targeted temperature management after cardiac arrest in inhibiting the shivering response.

It is also important for the clinician to be aware of opioid tolerance in critical illness. With long-term administration of opioids, biochemical changes to opioid receptors lead to upregulation of pro-nociceptive signaling pathways, as well as downregulation of opioid receptors, both of which lead to increased nociception and opioid tolerance. Downregulation of opioid receptors is notably more likely to happen with fentanyl and less so with morphine administration. The clinician may notice a trend towards escalating doses and frequency in patients on fentanyl therapy. In this situation, it may be reasonable to change therapy to another opioid for improved analgesic effects.

Another situation in which opioid tolerance may present challenges in the ICU is in the patient who is on chronic opioid therapy prior to critical illness. These patients are more likely to require higher doses of opioids and should be monitored carefully for adequate sedation and for adverse effects during therapy [3].

Benzodiazepines

Benzodiazepines were previously considered the cornerstone for sedation management in critically ill patients. They act on gamma-aminobutyric acid subtype A ($GABA_A$) receptors and lead to hyperpolarization of neuronal cells such that they reach a higher firing threshold. Benzodiazepines provide sedation, anxiolysis, anterograde amnesia, anticonvulsant effects, and lower intracranial pressures. The effects of benzodiazepines can also be reversed with the use of flumazenil, although *great caution* should be taken prior to administration of flumazenil to ensure the patient is not chronically on benzodiazepine therapy, as reversal in this patient population can lead to seizures that are difficult to control. Additionally, disadvantages of benzodiazepine use may include respiratory depression (though less so than opioids), lack of analgesia, paradoxical agitation, and development of delirium.

Several studies have evaluated the use of benzodiazepines versus other, newer sedative agents that are discussed in detail below. One study evaluated the use of propofol versus midazolam for sedation in the ICU. It showed reduced ICU length of stay and mechanical ventilation time in the propofol group [12]. Similarly, another study evaluated dexmedetomidine versus midazolam use. There was a lower prevalence of delirium and shorter duration of mechanical ventilation in the dexmedetomidine group [13]. Given the adverse effect profile of benzodiazepines and evidence for improved outcomes with use of other sedative agents, benzodiazepines are used with less frequency for sedation in the current ICU climate.

The most used benzodiazepine for sedation in the ICU setting is midazolam. It has a rapid onset of action (2–5 minutes) and relatively short duration (45–60 minutes). It is converted by the liver to the active metabolite alpha-hydroxymidazolam, which is subsequently excreted by the kidneys and can accumulate in patients with renal dysfunction. Midazolam should be used with caution in patients who require serial neurologic evaluations as it can take several hours for the effect of cumulative doses to wear off.

Lorazepam is a relatively insoluble benzodiazepine that must be commercially suspended with polyethylene glycol or propylene glycol for IV administration. This hyperosmolar preparation is irritating to the veins and can cause a high anion gap metabolic acidosis due to propylene glycol toxicity with long-term administration. For this reason, lorazepam infusions are no longer favored for sedation in the ICU setting. It is more common now to see lorazepam used only for the management of alcohol withdrawal.

Propofol

Propofol also exerts its sedative properties by upregulating GABA at $GABA_A$ receptors. It is a water-insoluble medication that is formulated in a lipid solution, which is available for administration only through the IV route. Its lipophilic nature allows for a rapid onset of action (within 30–60 seconds) and a short duration of action (5–10 minutes). This allows for rapid discontinuation of medication, which is particularly useful in the patient who is undergoing serial neurologic evaluations or spontaneous awakening/spontaneous breathing trials. Other advantages of propofol include anticonvulsant and antiemetic effects, decreased cerebral metabolic rate/intracranial pressure, and depression of airway reflexes. Propofol is metabolized in the liver into inactive metabolites, and its pharmacokinetics are unaltered by hepatic or renal disease.

The most common side effect of propofol is dose-dependent hypotension, which precludes its consistent use in many hemodynamically unstable ICU patients. It also has no analgesic properties and produces unreliable amnesia. Propofol can also be caustic to blood vessels upon administration. Given its emulsion in a soybean oil–glycerol–egg phosphatide solution, propofol accounts for 1.1 kcal/mL of energy, which must be accounted for in a patient's daily nutritional intake. This solution can also increase the risk of bacterial overgrowth when contaminated. To minimize this risk, propofol should be handled with strict antiseptic practices, and bottles/tubing should be changed out at least every 12 hours. Additionally, sodium metabisulfite is added to the preparation as a preservative but can result in allergic reactions in sulfite-sensitive patients.

Two more serious side effects of propofol are worth noting. The first is an elevation in triglyceride levels, which may induce pancreatitis. For this reason, best practice is to monitor triglyceride levels at least every 48–72 hours when administering propofol for a prolonged period of time and to discontinue or decrease propofol administration when levels reach more than 500 mg/dL. The second adverse reaction is a potentially fatal phenomenon known as propofol-related infusion syndrome, which presents as metabolic acidosis, rhabdomyolysis, hyperkalemia, and arrhythmia (especially bradycardia and pulseless electrical activity cardiac arrest). Treatment consists of stopping propofol and addressing clinical abnormalities. A rare side effect of propofol is green urine, which has no clinical consequence.

Dexmedetomidine

Dexmedetomidine is a centrally acting, pre-synaptic alpha-2 agonist that produces sedation via potassium and calcium channels located in the locus coeruleus of the brainstem to cause neuronal hyperpolarization, thereby decreasing the rate of central neuronal firing. It has a slightly longer onset of action (approximately 5 minutes) than the previous agents discussed. The peak action occurs at approximately 15 minutes from administration. It is metabolized in the liver into inactive metabolites.

Dexmedetomidine is unique from other agents discussed in that it has no effect on respiratory drive and can therefore be safely used for sedation in the non-intubated patient. It also has no minimal amnestic effects and preserves cognition throughout sedation. Other benefits include easy arousability to assess neurologic function, anxiolysis, and analgesic-sparing effects. It is commonly used as an adjunctive therapy in the patient undergoing alcohol withdrawal. It is important for the clinician to remember that, unlike propofol and benzodiazepines, dexmedetomidine has no antiepileptic properties and can mask the worsening of alcohol withdrawal symptoms [14].

Another noteworthy benefit of dexmedetomidine is its ability to induce a state close to physiologic stage 2 sleep. This has prompted interest in evaluating its use in the prevention of ICU delirium. A recent systematic review comparing dexmedetomidine with propofol showed a decreased incidence of ICU delirium in those receiving predominantly dexmedetomidine for sedation [15]. Another randomized, placebo-controlled trial evaluated the use of low-dose dexmedetomidine infusion at nighttime and showed decreased incidence of delirium in the study arm [16].

Dexmedetomidine also has significant side effects. It can cause a dose-dependent decrease in heart rate and can cause relative adrenal insufficiency by decreasing plasma noradrenaline or adrenaline levels. These effects are more pronounced when a loading dose is administered. Patients with volume depletion and high levels of underlying sympathetic tone are at increased risk of developing these side effects.

Ketamine

Ketamine is a competitive N-methyl-D-aspartate (NMDA) receptor antagonist originally derived from phencyclidine, which prevents glutamate-mediated neurotransmission. Ketamine also has activity against glutamate, nicotinic, and opioid receptors. It affects neurons in the somatosensory cortex in a way that prevents them from recognizing painful stimuli, producing a dissociative effect from sensory input. Thus, ketamine is known as a total IV anesthetic. Its onset of action is 30–60 seconds and duration of action is 15–20 minutes when given in bolus dosing. Once sedation is achieved with continuous infusion, increasing the dose will not achieve deeper sedation, but will prolong the duration of sedation.

Patients on ketamine seem awake and will continue to have laryngeal and corneal reflexes. They will also be able to swallow and protect their airway, making ketamine an excellent choice for sedation in procedural settings. Another benefit of ketamine over the agents discussed previously is that it inhibits the reuptake of endogenous catecholamines. Therefore, though it has a cardio-suppressive effect like other sedative agents, the increased availability of catecholamines leads to a neutral effect on hemodynamics. Caution should be used, however, in patients who have low catecholamine supplies (e.g., adrenal insufficiency) and those who cannot tolerate increased sympathetic tone (e.g., aortic dissection) [17].

Ketamine has purely analgesic effects at lower doses (1–5 µg/kg per minute) and has been studied as an adjunct to opioids to decrease opioid tolerance and use in the ICU setting. Though further studies need to be conducted to elucidate its exact role in this setting, low-dose ketamine infusion may be beneficial in patients who are opioid tolerant (taking naltrexone or buprenorphine, or on chronic opioid therapy), have refractory pain despite high-dose opioid administration, and are at risk of respiratory depression with escalating opioid therapy [18, 19] Ketamine may also have a role in the management of status epilepticus, status asthmaticus (due to bronchodilator properties), and alcohol withdrawal syndromes, but data for its use in these settings are limited.

Ketamine should be avoided in patients with schizophrenia as it can precipitate acute psychosis in this patient population. Historically, there was concern that ketamine led to elevated intracranial pressure, but this has since been disproven.

Other Adjunctive Analgesic Agents

Over recent years, clinicians have adapted a multimodal approach to the management of pain. Though the use of narcotics may, at times, be inevitable in patients in the ICU, consideration should be given to the addition of enteral and transdermal therapy that can reduce the need for opioids. The 2018 PADIS guidelines recommend using acetaminophen and neuropathic pain medication (such as gabapentin, carbamazepine, and pregabalin) as adjuncts to opioids in the ICU, with stronger evidence for gabapentin than for acetaminophen [9].

Other Adjunctive Sedative Agents

Haloperidol is a minimally sedating butyrophenone antipsychotic agent primarily administered in the ICU to treat delirium. It reliably maintains hemodynamic stability, has no respiratory depressant properties, demonstrates antiemetic activity, and has anxiolytic effects. Undesirable characteristics of haloperidol include lack of both analgesia and amnesia, lowering of the seizure threshold, and ventricular arrhythmias (including torsades de pointes) due to QT prolongation. Like other antipsychotics, haloperidol can cause akathisia (the inability to remain still) and dystonic extrapyramidal symptoms. Haloperidol is also associated with the development of neuroleptic malignant syndrome.

Clonidine is a pre-synaptic alpha-2 agonist, which is less selective for central receptors than dexmedetomidine. Its utility in sedation in the ICU setting has been studied previously with insufficient data to support its use. Notably, given its non-selective nature, clonidine has been shown to increase the risk of clinically significant hypotension in the ICU [20].

Guanfacine is another centrally acting alpha-2 agonist, similar to dexmedetomidine, which is given enterally. Guanfacine is more specific to central receptors, thereby minimizing the side effects of hemodynamic instability as may be seen with clonidine. There are limited data on its efficacy in the management of anxiety and agitation in the ICU setting (mostly in the form of case reports) [21]. However, it serves as a logical step-down, alternative, or adjunctive therapy with dexmedetomidine given its similar properties. Further studies need to be conducted to determine its role in sedation and anxiolysis in the critically ill patient.

Summary

Sedation and analgesia are crucial components of the care of a critically ill patient and should be approached as two separate entities of treatment. Analgesia should be prioritized first, as the critically ill patient is predisposed to increased painful stimuli and is also likely to develop hyperalgesia as a consequence of critical illness. Once appropriate analgesia has been achieved, sedation should be administered to achieve a predetermined RASS goal. The need for sedation and analgesia should be monitored regularly with the goal of minimizing unnecessary medication while optimizing patient care. Special attention should be given to the development of side effects of various agents being used. It is also important to be mindful of the development of delirium due to either over- or inadequate analgesia/sedation.

References

1. Pearson SD et al. Evolving targets for sedation during mechanical ventilation. *Curr Opin Crit Care.* 2020;26:47–52.

2. Barr J et al. Clinical practice guidelines for the management of pain, agitation, and delirium in adult patients in the intensive care unit. *Crit Care Med.* 2013;41:263–306.

3. Martyn JAJ et al. Opioid tolerance in critical illness. *N Engl J Med.* 2019;380:365–78.

4. Latremoliere A et al. Central sensitization: a generator of pain hypersensitivity by central neural plasticity. *J Pain.* 2009;10:895–926.

5. Olsen HT et al. Nonsedation or light sedation in critically ill, mechanically ventilated patients. *N Engl J Med.* 2020;382:1103–11.

6. Sessler CN et al. The Richmond Agitation–Sedation Scale: validity and reliability in adult intensive care unit patients. *Am J Respir Crit Care Med.* 2002;166:1338–44.

7. Girard TD et al. Efficacy and safety of a paired sedation and ventilator weaning protocol for mechanically ventilated patients in intensive care (Awake and Breathing Controlled trial): a randomized controlled trial. *Lancet.* 2008;371:126–34.

8. Shetty R et al. BIS monitoring versus clinical assessment for sedation in mechanically ventilated adults in the intensive care unit and its impact on clinical outcomes and resource utilization. *Cochrane Database Syst Rev.* 2018;2:CD011240.

9. Delvin JW et al. Clinical practice guidelines for the prevention and management of pain, agitation/sedation, delirium, immobility, and sleep disruption in adult patients in the ICU. *Crit Care Med.* 2018;46:825–73.

10. Cigada M et al. Sedation in the critically ill ventilated patient: possible role of enteral drugs. *Intensive Care Med.* 2005;31:482–6.

11. Datta S et al. Opioid pharmacology. *Pain Physician.* 2008;11:133–53.

12. Garcia R et al. A systematic review and meta-analysis of propofol versus midazolam sedation in adult intensive care (ICU) patients. *J Crit Care.* 2021;64:91–9.

13. Riker RR et al. Dexmedetomidine vs midazolam for sedation of critically ill patients: a randomized trial. *JAMA.* 2009;301:489–99.

14. Dixit D et al. Management of acute alcohol withdrawal syndrome in critically ill patients. *Pharmacotherapy.* 2016;36:797–822.

15. Pereira JV et al. Dexmedetomidine versus propofol sedation in reducing delirium among older adults in the ICU: a systematic review and meta-analysis. *Eur J Anesthesiol.* 2020;37:121–31.

16. Skrobik Y et al. Low-dose nocturnal dexmedetomidine prevents ICU delirium. *Am J Respir Crit Care Med.* 2018;197:1147–56.

17. Zanos P et al. Ketamine and ketamine metabolite pharmacology: insights into therapeutic mechanisms. *Pharmacol Rev.* 2018;70:621–60.

18. Buchheit JL et al. Impact of low-dose ketamine on the usage of continuous opioid infusion for the treatment of pain in adult mechanically ventilated patients in surgical intensive care units. *J Intensive Care Med.* 2019;34:646–51.

19. Guillou N et al. The effects of small-dose ketamine on morphine consumption in surgical intensive care unit patients after major abdominal surgery. *Anesth Analg.* 2003;97:843–7.

20. Wang JG et al. Clonidine for sedation in the critically ill: a systematic review and meta analysis. *Critical Care.* 2017;27:75.

21. Srour H et al. Enteral guanfacine to treat severe anxiety and agitation complicating critical care after cardiac surgery. *Semin Cardiothoracic Vasc Anesth.* 2018;22:403–6.

Additional Reading

Aitken LM et al. Protocol-directed sedation versus non-protocol-directed sedation to reduce duration of mechanical ventilation in mechanically ventilated intensive care patients. *Cochrane Database Syst. Rev.* 2015;1:CD009771.

Aitken LM et al. Sedation protocols to reduce duration of mechanical ventilation in the ICU: a Cochrane Systematic Review. *J. Adv. Nurs.* 2016;72:261–72.

Ely EW et al. Delirium in mechanically ventilated patients: validity and reliability of the confusion assessment method for the intensive care unit (CAM-ICU). *JAMA.* 2001;286:2703–10.

Slooter AJ et al. Delirium in critically ill patients. *Handb Clin Neurol.* 2017;141:449–66.

Chapter 23

Pediatric Sedation: Practical Considerations

Eshel A. Nir and Jue Teresa Wang

Introduction

The delivery of sedation to children presents a significant challenge to many clinicians from a variety of specialties on a daily basis [1]. While tremendous evidence exists to guide the clinician through the pharmacology, physiology, and medical issues involved, the final sedative regimen is most likely based on the specific training of the provider and the experience that the individual brings to the procedure [1]. Collectively, all providers tasked with providing sedation to children must acknowledge the inherent limitations of their experiences and training; only then can clinicians bring sober and intelligent judgment to this critical arena.

In this chapter we outlines the practical considerations entailed in sedating infants and children. The topics of oversight, safety, monitoring and outcomes are mentioned only briefly, as they are dealt with in depth in the following chapter. Similarly, we direct the interested reader to the relevant chapters regarding the pharmacology (Chapter 2) of the medications used and pain assessment in infants and children (Chapter 3). Dealing with emergencies in this population is described in Chapter 30). As always, clinicians have an obligation to understand the specific challenges of their environment and the patients in their care.

We discuss a general approach to pediatric sedation with attention to the unique variables that children bring to this clinical setting and the latest guidelines from different oversight authorities. The various relevant levels of sedation and their validated scales for pediatrics are considered. In focusing on the specific settings for pediatric sedation and the interplay of each setting on the sedation plan, we review the most recent recommendations for clinical preparation, and potential limitations or complications to be understood in these settings.

Pediatric Sedation Oversight

As stated previously, multiple specialties deliver pediatric procedural sedation in the inpatient and outpatient settings [1]. In 2018, the American Society of Anesthesiologists (ASA) joined forces with five other outpatient societies and updated their practice guidelines for moderate procedural sedation and analgesia [2]. These guidelines focus on moderate sedation administration for adults and children and replaced previous guidelines intended for non-anesthesiologists. A year later (2019), three important pediatric-specific guidelines followed: the conjoint American Academy of Pediatrics (AAP) and American Academy of Pediatric Dentistry updated guidelines for sedation for diagnostic and therapeutic procedures [3]; the European Society for Paediatric Anaesthesiology's safe pediatric procedural sedation and analgesia by anesthesiologists clinical practice statement [4]; and, in the realm of unscheduled procedural sedation, the American College of Emergency Physicians consensus practice guideline for both adults and children [5].

The development of a pediatric sedation program has historically occurred in response to clinical needs and often without institutional oversight. Current recommendations, however, include a mandate for an institutional oversight body with responsibility for setting credentialing requirements, a continuous quality improvement process, and other safety and clinical concerns. Current US Joint Commission policy requires this oversight be led by the department of anesthesiology in each facility. This is particularly important for pediatric patients.

At a minimum, any personnel responsible for provision of sedative drugs to children are expected to obtain credentialing through an institutional oversight committee [5]. It is typically required that such clinicians have advanced training in pediatric care and maintain current certification in pediatric advanced life support and also advanced cardiac life support if care is provided to adolescents [2, 3, 4]. Each institution should have a mechanism to recognize providers' deficiencies in sedation provision [6]. Once recognized, these should serve as an impetus for focused training to improve such skills. Each institution should develop a process to assist with such training and seek resources within and outside the institution to meet these needs [5]. A good example is the Society for Pediatric Sedation's formal sedation provider course [7], where excellent examples of systemic sedation credentialing are available.

Risks in Pediatric Sedation

In 2008, Bhatt et al., as part of a multidisciplinary pediatric emergency departments (EDs) consensus group (Pediatric Emergency Research Canada [PERC] and the Pediatric Emergency Care Applied Research Network [PECARN]), produced a set of definitions related to pediatric ED procedural sedation that seeks to recognize the requirement for clinical intervention as a critical element for an adverse event [8]; an adverse event is any clinical situation that prompts a specific intervention aimed at limiting a perceived threat to the patient's welfare. Other reports of adverse events have focused on specific clinical parameters to define these events, such as measured pulse oximetry, blood pressure, or clinical signs such as stridor or retractions. In 2012, Mason et al. suggested and validated an adverse event sedation reporting tool to standardize the international reporting and tracking of adverse events during procedural sedation [9]. In 2019, they published an account of almost 8,000 records from more than160,000 sedation encounters [10], using the aforementioned reporting tool in adults and children.

In a series of publications from 2007 to 2023, a similar initiative, the multicenter Pediatric Sedation Research Consortium (PSRC) tracked sedation practice in children outside the operating room in the United States over the course of years. The resulting database information showed, between 2007 and 2018, an overall adverse event rate of 1.35%, which increased to 1.75%. Airway obstruction was the most common adverse event, occurring in 1.55% of all sedation encounters. There were no deaths although 13 cardiac arrests occurred [1]. Important risk factors for adverse events that were recognized included asthma, cardiovascular diagnosis, ASA physical status score > III, developmental delay, transplant, metabolic or genetic syndrome [1], obstructive sleep apnea, obesity [11], prematurity and age younger than 3 months [12], and upper respiratory tract infections [13]. These data suggest that the critical nature of competent airway management skills is a foundation of all safe pediatric sedation programs [2, 3, 4] as well as adequate monitoring [3]; see also Chapter 24.

Unique Pediatric Anatomy and Physiology

The majority of children (~80%) present for sedation between the ages of 1 and 12 years [1, 10]. Knowledge of specific developmental issues (anatomical, physiological, behavioral) becomes a prerequisite before provision of sedative drugs.

As a child ages, the airway matures into the adult configuration at adolescence. Infants and toddlers have relatively large tongues and their larynx resides relatively higher in the neck and is anteriorly tilted [14]. Overall, children have more reactive airways; they are more likely to exhibit laryngospasm, or suffer more pronounced arterial desaturation should laryngospasm or bronchospasm occur. These facts make the sedated child more likely to experience an adverse airway event than an adult and lead to more pronounced desaturation. The clinician should consider the increased risks of airway-related events as being inversely related to age [15].

The small child's cardiovascular system tends toward higher vagal tone, leading to a bradycardic response with autonomic stimulation. For small infants, who rely on heart rate to increase cardiac output during times of stress, vagal discharge during airway manipulation, for example, can lead to decreased blood pressure or abnormal heart rhythms such as nodal bradycardia or junctional rhythms. Anticipation of this response during sedation and consideration of anticholinergic use (e.g., atropine or glycopyrrolate administration) is recommended.

Pulmonary function in the infant or small child is constrained by a small functional residual capacity, increasing the rapidity of oxygen depletion should apnea occur. Oxygen consumption is higher on a proportional basis compared with adults, but tidal volumes are relatively similar. Small children increase their respiratory rates to meet their increased oxygen requirements and, therefore, sedation-related decreases in respiratory rates combined with impaired pulmonary volumes of oxygen reserve can lead to an alarmingly rapid fall in oxygen saturation. Also, smaller children are much more prone to apnea with sedation compared to adults when drugs such as benzodiazepines, intravenous anesthetics such as propofol, and opiates are combined [16].

Behavioral Concerns

As children develop, the ability to communicate, understand, conceptualize, or manage shifts from simple responsiveness to environmental stimuli to complex reasoning and mature interaction with others. As children of all ages present for sedation, the provider must consider the developmental stage as well as behavioral and developmental pathologies to form an appropriate plan [17]. Small infants may be lulled by a cooperative and calm parent. Older children 2–8 years of age will exhibit a range of behaviors that must be considered. Use of immersive technologies (e.g., virtual reality) [18] or the services of child life specialists [19], should be considered, according to the child's developmental level. Refusal to take medications orally would prompt consideration of other routes: intranasal, intramuscular, subcutaneous, or rectal. Increased agitation may hinder the effect of sedatives, prompting additional doses that may cause an unexpected increase in sedation. Older children may accept intravenous lines, be more accepting of explanations, and transition more smoothly to the procedure area. They may, however, begin to perceive the clinical setting as a threat and refuse to cooperate. Most clinicians will start to respect a child's refusal for a procedure around age 11–12 years [20]. Most developmentally intact adolescents will exhibit behavior similar to adults. Although intellectually capable of understanding the complex connections between the need for a procedure and reassurance that sedation will reduce discomfort, an adolescent may still lack the emotional control to cooperate fully [20].

Pharmacology

Many drugs used for pediatric sedation have been in clinical use for decades and were released for use with minimal premarket safety trials in children and they have not been fully evaluated and approved by the Federal Drug Administration (FDA); hence "off-label" use is common. Current safety data are usually the result of retrospective analyses of rare events or comparative studies of specific regimens. Relevant pediatric pharmacologic data for typical sedatives has slowly emerged. For example, propofol has been FDA approved for induction down to 3 years of age and maintenance of anesthesia down to 2 months of age but not lower because its safety and effectiveness have not been established in those populations. Neither is it formally indicated for use in pediatric intensive care unit (ICU) sedation since the safety of this regimen has not been established. The safety and effectiveness of ketamine below the age 16 has not been established [21]. Tables 23.1–23.4 present the most commonly used drugs for procedural sedation and analgesia [22, 23], ranging from first-generation agents to the more recently developed generation 3.1 agents.

The pharmacology of sedative drugs in children is a complex field that must consider the child's age, renal function as a means for elimination of many drugs, liver function as a means of transformation of certain drugs to active forms and other drugs to inactive forms, and the interplay of total body water, protein synthesis, or distribution characteristics. Patience is required with certain medications as they may need to cross the blood–brain lipid barrier (e.g. benzodiazepines) and others may distribute rapidly to the muscles and delay onset or require additional boluses for effect (e.g., pentobarbital). Combining agents can improve clinical effect through synergism, but such synergism is responsible for the increased adverse events with specific combinations (e.g. propofol plus fentanyl) [1]. Therefore, most sedation protocols use a single agent with careful criteria and limited options for additional agents of another drug family; this is especially true for nursing sedation protocols where an additional agent can cause a child to quickly descend from light sedation to deep sedation or even general anesthesia [36].

Table 23.1 Drugs for pediatric procedural sedation: first-generation agents

Drug	Pediatric dosing	Onset (min)	Duration (min)	Comments
Chloral hydrate	*Oral:* 25–100 mg/kg, after 30 min can repeat 25–50 mg/kg (10–25% need redosing). *Maximum total dose:* 2 g or 100 mg/kg (whichever is less). Single use only in neonates.	*Oral:* 15–30	*Oral:* 60–120	Effects unreliable if age > 3 years; best if < 10 kg; terrible taste, unpredictable onset and duration; no longer recommended for sedation in children and is not available in many countries.
Pentobarbital	*Intravenous:* 1–6 mg/ kg, titrated in 1–2-mg/ kg increments every 2–5 min to desired effect, maximum 100 mg *Intramuscular:* 2–6 mg/kg maximum 100 mg *Oral or rectal* (< 4 years): 3–6 mg/kg, maximum 100 mg *Oral/rectal* (> 4 years): 1.5–3 mg/kg, maximum 100 mg	*Intravenous:* 3–5 *Intramuscular:* 10–15 *Oral or rectal:* 15–60	*Intravenous:* 15–90 *Intramuscular:* 60–120 *Oral or rectal:* 60–240	May produce paradoxical excitement in younger children. Adverse events are primarily respiratory depression with transient oxygen desaturation and apnea. May cause prolonged recovery times, delirium, sleepiness and ataxia. Avoid in patients with porphyria.
Methohexital	*Intravenous:* 0.5–1.0 mg/kg *Rectal:* 20-25 mg/kg	*Intravenous:* 1–2 *Rectal:* 10–15	*Intravenous:* 15–30 *Rectal:* 30-60	Avoid if temporal lobe epilepsy or porphyria.
Thiopental	*Rectal:* 25 mg/kg	*Rectal:* 10–15	*Rectal:* 60–120	Avoid in patients with porphyria.

Table 23.1 (cont.)

Drug	Pediatric dosing	Onset (min)	Duration (min)	Comments
Diazepam	*Intravenous:* Initial 0.05–0.1 mg/kg, then titrate slowly to maximum 0.25 mg/kg *Oral:* 0.2–0.5 mg/kg *Rectal:* 0.2–0.5 mg/kg	*Intravenous:* 4–5 *Oral:* 15–30 *Rectal:* 5–15	*Intravenous:* 60–120	Reduce dose when used in combination with opioids; Irritating to vein if given intravenously.
Morphine	*Intravenous:* Initial 0.05–0.15 mg/kg up to 3 mg/dose, may repeat every 5 min, titrate to effect.	*Intravenous:* 5–20	*Intravenous:* 120–240	Reduce dosing when combined with benzodiazepines.
Oral sucrose solution	*Oral:* 25% sucrose 2 mL, 1 mL per each cheek; can repeat, not to exceed 4 mL/h.	*Oral:* 0.5–2	*Oral:* 5–10	Oral sucrose has been shown to be most effective for procedural analgesia in neonates (< 30 days) and less in young infants (< 0.5 years).

Adapted from references [22, 23, 24, 25, 26, 27].

Alterations in dosing may be indicated depending on the clinical situation and the practitioner's experience with these drugs. Individual dosages may vary when used in combination with other drugs, especially when benzodiazepines are combined with opioids.

Table 23.2 Drugs for pediatric procedural sedation: second-generation and analgesic agents

Drug	Pediatric dosing	Onset (min)	Duration (min)	Comments
Midazolam	*Intravenous* (<5 years): Initial 0.05–0.1 mg/kg, then titrated to maximum 0.6 mg/kg *Intravenous* (>5 years): Initial 0.025–0.05 mg/kg, then titrated to maximum 0.4–0.5 mg/kg *Intramuscular:* 0.1–0.2 mg/kg *Oral:* 0.25–0.75 mg/kg, maximum 20 mg *Intranasal:* 0.2–0.5 mg/kg, maximum 10 mg *Rectal:* 0.25–0.5 mg/kg	*Intravenous:* 1–3 *Intramuscular:* 5–20 *Oral:* 15–30 *Intranasal:* 10–15 *Rectal:* 10–30	*Intravenous:* 45–60 *Intramuscular:* 60–120 *Oral:* 60–90 *Intranasal:* 15–60 *Rectal:* 60–90	Reduce dose when used in combination with opioids. May produce paradoxical excitement. Flumazenil can reverse effects; adverse events include respiratory depression, apnea, hyperactivity, aggressive behavior, and inconsolable crying. Pretreatment with lidocaine spray (10 mg/puff) 1 minute prior to intranasal midazolam decreases nasal mucosal irritation.
Fentanyl	*Intravenous:* Initial 1–2 µg/kg up to 50 µg/dose, may repeat 0.5–1 µg/kg every 3 min up to 25 µg/dose, titrate to effect *Intranasal:* 1.5–2 µg/kg maximum, 100 µg	*Intravenous:* 1–5 *Intranasal:* 5–10	*Intravenous:* 30–60 *Intranasal:* 45–60	Reduce dosing when combined with benzodiazepines, may cause respiratory depression and hypotension. May produce a state of general anesthesia, when combined sedation with propofol. Chest wall and glottic rigidity possible with intravenous push, especially in neonates.
Ketamine	*Intravenous:* 1–1.5 mg/kg slowly over 1 min; may repeat dose every 10 min as needed *Intramuscular:* 4–6 mg/kg, may repeat (2–4 mg/kg) after 10 min *Oral:* 5–10 mg/kg *Intranasal:* 1–10 mg/kg (usually 0.5–4 mg/kg)	*Intravenous:* 1–2 *Intramuscular:* 10–15 *Oral:* 15–30 *Intranasal:* 20	*Intravenous:* dissociation 15; recovery 60 *Intramuscular:* dissociation 15–40; recovery 90–150 *Oral:* 30–60 *Intranasal:* 35–70	Reduce dosing when combined with propofol. Relative contraindications: age <12 months, active pulmonary infections (including urinary infections), known or suspected cardiac disease, suspected increased intracranial pressure, glaucoma or acute eye injury (open globe), porphyria, thyroid disease, or seizures.

Table 23.2 (cont.)

Drug	Pediatric dosing	Onset (min)	Duration (min)	Comments
				Absolute contraindications: age < 3 months or patients with known or suspected psychosis.* Common adverse events include: unpleasant taste, dizziness, sleepiness, nausea and vomiting. Unpleasant dreams or hallucinations rare in children. Atropine or glycopyrrolate to counter hypersalivation should be discouraged, as no decrease in respiratory adverse events seen. Frequency of vomiting is reduced by premedication with ondansetron (0.08–0.15 mg/kg, typical dose 4 mg).
Nitrous oxide	*Inhalation:* Preset mixture with 50% (Entononx™, previously NitronOx™) or 70% nitrous oxide self-administered by demand valve mask (requires cooperative child). Continuous flow nasal mask in uncooperative child with close monitoring.	*Inhalation:* < 0.5	*Inhalation:* 3–5 following discontinuation	Requires specialized apparatus and gas scavenger capability. Several contraindications: absolute – conditions with trapped gas within body cavities (e.g., bowel obstruction, pneumothorax, middle ear infection); relative – nausea and vomiting. Adverse events: vomiting and dysphoria, occupational exposure and environmental concerns about nitrous oxide pollution.

Adapted from references [22, 23, 24, 25, 26, 27].

Alterations in dosing may be indicated depending on the clinical situation and the practitioner's experience with these drugs. Individual dosages may vary when used in combination with other drugs.

*Contraindications to ketamine use may include children younger than 3 months (higher risk of airway complications); procedures involving stimulation of posterior pharynx; history of tracheal surgery or stenosis; active pulmonary infection or disease (including upper respiratory infection); known or suspected cardiovascular disease; head injury associated with loss of consciousness; altered mental status; emesis; central nervous system masses, abnormalities, or hydrocephalus; glaucoma or acute globe injury; porphyria; thyroid disorder or thyroid medication.

Table 23.3 Drugs for pediatric procedural sedation: third-generation agents

Drug	Pediatric dosing	Onset (min)	Duration (min)	Comments
Etomidate	*Intravenous*: 0.1–0.3 mg/kg; repeat if inadequate response, 0.05 mg/kg every 5 min *Maximum total dose*: 0.6 mg/kg	*Intravenous*: < 0.5	*Intravenous*: 5–15	Adverse events include respiratory depression, myoclonus, nausea, and vomiting; causes pain during intravenous administration; avoid in severe illness, such as sepsis. Contraindicated in adrenal insufficiency.
Propofol	*Intravenous*: (0.5–2 years): 1–2 mg/kg, bolus(> 2 years): 0.5–1 mg/kg, bolus followed by 0.5 mg/kg every 3–5 min, up to 3 mg/kg *Intravenous infusion*: 50–200 µg/kg per min	*Intravenous*: < 0.5	*Intravenous*: 5–15	Frequent hypotension and respiratory depression, especially when combined with fentanyl. Reduce dosing when combined with ketamine. Peripheral injection-site pain. May (accidently) produce general anesthesia, especially with multiple bolus doses or high continuous infusion rate. Avoid in cardiorespiratory compromised patients and porphyria. In some institutions, propofol is approved for use by anesthesiologists only or others with specialized pediatric procedural sedation training, check local policies.
Dexmedetomidine	*Intravenous loading*: 1–3 µg/ kg for 10 min; then 0.5–2 µg/kg per hour *Intramuscular*: 1–3 µg/kg *Intranasal*: 1–3 µg/kg	*Intravenous*: 5–10 *Intramuscular*: 10–15 *Intranasal*: 10–30	*Intravenous*: 30–70 *Intramuscular*: 30–55 *Intranasal*: 30–90	Causes transient cardiac suppression (bradycardia and hypotension), with possible hypertension in high doses (3 µg/ kg), not described with intranasal use. Rarely causes upper airway obstruction, including laryngospasm. Absolute contraindications: metabolic, congenital or medications acting on the sinoatrial or atrioventricular node (e.g., digoxin, anti-cholinergic sialagogues, etc.).

Adapted from references [22, 23, 24, 25, 26, 27].
Alterations in dosing may be indicated depending on the clinical situation and the practitioner's experience with these drugs. Individual dosages may vary when used in combination with other drugs.

Table 23.4 Drugs for pediatric procedural sedation: generation 3.1 agents

Drug	Pediatric dosing	Onset (min)	Duration (min)	Comments
Ketamine–propofol (ketofol)	*Intravenous loading:* 0.5 mg/kg of ketamine followed by 0.5mg/kg Propofol (can be in 1 syringe, 1:1 ratio) or 0.5 mg/kg of ketamine followed by 1mg/kg propofol then 0.5–1mg/kg of either agent, as needed	*Intravenous:* 1–2 (similar to ketamine alone)	*Intravenous:* 30–45 (similar to ketamine alone)	The combination had not demonstrated superior clinical efficacy compared with propofol alone (and less hemodynamic stability yet less vomiting compared to ketamine alone).
Ketamine–dexmedetomidine (Ketodex)	*Intravenous loading:* 1 μg/kg of dexmedetomidine followed by 1–2 mg/kg of ketamine, *Intravenous infusion:* Dexmedetomidine 1–2 μg/kg per hour and bolus dosesas neede of ketamine (0.5–1 mg/kg)	*Intravenous:* 5–10 (for dexmedetomidine loading)	*Intravenous:* 27–45	Reduces/prevents tachycardia, hypertension, salivation, and emergence phenomena seen with ketamine and bradycardia and hypotension/hypertension seen with dexmedetomidine.
	Intranasal: 1 mg/kg of ketamine and 2 μg/kg of dexmedetomidine, preferably in a 1:2 syringe of 50 mg:100 μg/mL; needs 10 μL/kg of 1:2 solution in each nostril; may repeat 5 μL/kg of 1:2 solution in each nostril	*Intranasal:* 15	*Intranasal:* 55–70	See also references [28] (intravenous), [29] (intranasal) and [30] (intramuscular).
	Intramuscular: 2–3 mg/kg of ketamine and 0.75–1 μg/kg of dexmedetomidine	*Intramuscular:* 5	*Intramuscular:* unknown	
Sevoflurane	*Inhalation:* 0.3–0.6%	*Inhalation:* < 0.5	*Inhalation:* 3–5 following discontinuation	Requires specialized apparatus and gas scavenger capability. Contraindications – absolute: conditions with trapped gas within body cavities (e.g., bowel obstruction, pneumothorax, middle ear infection); relative: nausea and vomiting. Adverse events: vomiting and dysphoria, occupational exposure and environmental concerns about nitrous oxide pollution.

Drug	Administration	Onset (min)	Duration (min)	Notes
Methoxyflurane inhaler (Penthrox™, Penthrop™, Penthrane™)	*Inhalation:* Self-administered by a dedicated commercial inhaler (requires cooperative child). Preset 3mL liquid vial with 0.2–0.4%, rising to 0.5–0.7% with dilution-hole closed. *Maximum recommended dose:* 6 mL/24 h and 15 mL/7 d. Not to be used on consecutive days.	*Inhalation:* 0.5–5 (6–10 inhalations)	*Inhalation:* 20–25 (3 mL); 50–55 (6 mL); full consciousness regained within minutes following discontinuation	Deep sedation more common in patients < 5 years. Requires specialized apparatus and/or gas scavenger capability. Contraindicated in malignant hyperthermia, hepatic and renal dysfunction. No evidence of any renal toxicity when used short term (< 5 h), low-dose (< 1 minimum alveolar concentration agent. Currently licensed only in Australia, New Zealand, South Africa, Singapore, Saudi Arabia, and Europe (studies ongoing in the UK, Spain, Italy, Austria, Norway). Only transient adverse events noted: cough, dizziness, drowsiness, euphoria, disinhibition or hallucinations. See references [31] and [32].
Remimazolam (Byfavo™, CNS7056)	*Intravenous:* (Adults data only) 2.5–5mg bolus (0.1–0.2 µg/kg) then titrated to effect 1.25–2.5 mg every 2 min, to a maximum of 30mg *Intranasal:* (Adult data only) 10–40 mg powder or solution	*Intravenous:* 1–4 *Intranasal:* 10–20 (> 30 for 40 mg)	*Intravenous:* 10–40 *Intranasal:* Unknown	See references [33], [34] and [35]. Most common adverse events are blood pressure and heart rate changes (mild QT prolongation), nausea, and vomiting, headache, somnolence, and hypoxia. Has a lower abuse potential than that of midazolam. Severe pain and discomfort caused by intranasal route in adults.

Table 23.4 (cont.)

Drug	Pediatric dosing	Onset (min)	Duration (min)	Comments
				Currently licensed only in Japan (2020). Submitted for licensure in China (November 2018), the United States (undergoing phase 3 trial now, waiting for FDA approval), and Europe (November 2019). Not yet indicated for pediatric use, although there are several ongoing national clinical trials (NCTs) in children: NCT04720963 (intranasal); NCT04851717, and NCT04601350 (intravenous).

Adapted from references [22, 23, 24, 25, 26, 27] (unless otherwise stated).
Alterations in dosing may be indicated depending on the clinical situation and the practitioner's experience with these drugs. Individual dosages may vary when used in combination with other drugs, especially when benzodiazepines are combined with opioids.

Synergism between medications used for sedation and outpatient management of pediatric conditions can lead to erratic effects. For example, many medications used for the treatment of attention deficit disorder are stimulants and will lead to a relative tolerance to sedation [17]. Conversely, some antipsychotics increasingly prescribed to children for depression and bipolar disorder can augment the depressant effects of sedatives [37].

Clinical sedation for procedures is a dynamic process with a variable level of stimulation and invasiveness.

The ideal medication regimen optimizes the onset and potency of sedation in direct preparation and synchronization with the level of noxious stimulation

Comments on Specific Drugs

The following are generalized comments regarding the most frequently used sedatives with particular emphasis on unique characteristics of each generation nomenclature according to Krauss and Green [22].

First-Generation Agents

Although at one time considered "old gold," chloral hydrate, as well as other first-generation sedatives are out of fashion [23, 24]. Oral chloral hydrate was compared to intranasal midazolam, intranasal dexmedetomidine, and intranasal ketamine with all being superior in efficacy and safety [38, 39, 40]. Similar comparison studies were done for the barbiturate sedatives and they have been found to be less effective and less efficient, with a higher rate of adverse events, in particular vomiting, recovery agitation, longer recovery times, and higher rates of unplanned admission [24]. The only truly active first-generation sedative, mostly in neonates and young infants (< 6 months old) is oral sucrose solution [23, 25].

Second-Generation Agents

Ketamine

As a phencyclidine ("Angel Dust") derivative, ketamine is a second-generation agent that also has analgesic properties. Ketamine administration may induce concerning psycho-mimetic emergence delirium and agitation responses in children, though experience suggests that children are less prone (0.7% and 0.6-1.5%, more prominent in children under 3 years and those older than 13 years) to this phenomenon compared to adults [41, 42]. This has not been shown to be decreased with the coadministration of a benzodiazepine [23, 42] Sialorrhea may occur as well and increase the risk of a respiratory AE [23, 42]; anticholinergic coadministration does decrease the sialorrhea but does not decrease the risk of a respiratory adverse event [23, 42] . There is a relatively high risk for nausea and vomiting (8.4% and 1.2%, respectively) [41, 42]. The risk correlates with an intramuscular/intravenous loading dose > 2.5 mg/kg, and a total dose > 5 mg/kg [23, 41] may warrant prophylactic antiemetic therapy, most commonly with ondansteron (0.1 mg/kg) [23]. The risk of an adverse event increases with the use of multiple agents with ketamine, except benzodiazepines and dexmedetomedine [42], see also ketofol (ketamine–propofol) and ketodex (ketamine–dexmedetomidine); see generation 3.1 agents below.

Although controversial, intramuscular dosing of 4–5 mg per kg may be used for an uncooperative child, with onset of sedation typically within 5–15 minutes [17, 23]. After reaching a tranquil state, an intravenous line and a switch to another medication is possible. An oral dose of 5–10 mg/kg [24] or intranasal 1–10 mg/kg will typically sedate an uncooperative child at approximately the same time (~15–20 minutes) [43, 44], but with higher doses needed and less consistent results (48–85% sedation) [23, 44, 45]. A viable (and more consistent) alternative in these circumstances, tested recently is intranasal ketodex (see below) and an important adjunct for increased efficacy is the use of a mucosal atomizer device, as opposed to instilling droplets [46]. Ketamine is the only typical pediatric sedative drug with excellent analgesic properties and minimal respiratory depression.

Midazolam

Midazolam is a rapid and short-acting benzodiazepine that may be administered orally, rectally, intravenously, intramuscularly or nasally to achieve mild to moderate sedation [23, 26, 27]. It has good anxiolytic, amnestic and muscle relaxant properties [23]. Like all benzodiazepines, an excessive dose or adverse event synergism with opioids can induce general anesthesia and profound respiratory depression [22, 23, 24]. Atypical behavioral response may also occur when used as a single agent, resulting in dysphoria and paradoxical agitation [24, 23].

When given orally, a typical dose of 0.5 mg/kg will result in mild sedation after 15–20 minutes (see Table 23.2). The taste is bitter and is poorly tolerated unless masked in flavored syrup, which is the *raison d'être* to the invention of ADV6209 (gamma-cyclodextrin-midazolam Ozalin™; see below [47]). The duration of sedation can be erratic and may vary according to patient age and the administration route (see Table 23.2) [23] but usually lasts approximately 30–60 minutes. Of all the non-intravenous/intramuscular administration routes (rectal, oral, and intranasal) nasal administration has been the most consistent regarding rapid onset and short recovery [48, 23], especially when used for the uncooperative pediatric patient. Yet, nasal mucosal irritation (cough, gag, sore throat) causes distress in 40% [48] and therefore this route should be reserved for special circumstances only. Atomizing 10 mg per nostril of 4% lidocaine, 5 minutes prior [49] or coadministered with the midazolam [50] helps decrease this discomfort.

Nitrous Oxide

Recognized since the eighteenth century for its sedative and analgesic qualities, 50% nitrous oxide in oxygen provides excellent mild to moderate sedation for brief procedures or examinations. It is a rapidly acting agent (< 1 minute) and recovery from it is prompt and predictable; most patients will return to baseline level of consciousness within 5–10 minutes of discontinuation [22, 24] Excessive sedation or anesthesia may occur. It preserves spontaneous respiration, airway reflexes, and hemodynamic status [23]. The onset of sedation may be delayed depending on the child's minute ventilation, anxiety level, or other factors that cause decreased delivery of the gas. It has been shown to be safe for non-anesthesiologist-administered sedation in large studies [51] and with very few adverse events, mostly nausea, dysphoria, restlessness, and headache [22, 24]

Third-Generation Agents
Propofol

Propofol is an intravenous anesthetic agent that, when delivered at lower doses (0.5 mg/kg) or as an infusion (100–150 µg/kg per minute), can be used to induce various levels of sedation [23, 24]. At lower dose ranges, mild to moderate sedation can be obtained in children, though the lack of analgesia may cause erratic clinical effects during periods of stimulation. Propofol has the tendency to decrease respiratory effort in a dose-dependent way, especially when given as multiple boluses compared to continuous infusion [23]. Synergistic response for this adverse event with other sedatives can be profound with propofol [1]. Irritation at the site of injection or infusion is common [22, 23, 24] and sometimes results in unexpected patient movement that may dislodge an intravenous line or surprise the clinician. When it is used for sedation, small boluses (0.5 mg/kg) may be given every 3–5 minutes and the patient closely monitored for clinical effect. Over the course of a few minutes, if the desired effect is not achieved, additional small boluses may be given up to a maximum total dose of 3 mg/kg [23]. With patience and close monitoring, most children will respond successfully to the technique for all but the most stimulating procedures.

Clonidine and Dexmedetomidine

Alpha-2-adrenergic receptor agonists such as clonidine and dexmedetomidine are well known to cause sedation, anxiolysis, and hypnosis [24, 23]. Clonidine 2–4 µg/kg taken orally can produce effective sedation and analgesia, though onset times can be greater than 60–90 minutes. While clonidine is less specific for receptors in the central nervous system, dexmedetomidine exhibits highly selective preference for the receptors located in the locus ceruleus, the region responsible for producing sleep in humans [52]. For this reason, dexmedetomidine has emerged as a unique sedative drug capable of inducing a controlled state of moderate to deep sedation without depressing ventilation, blunting laryngeal reflexes, or significantly depressing cardiovascular parameters [53]. Administered as a bolus dose of 0.5–1 µg/kg over 10 minutes and followed by an infusion of 0.5–1 µg/kg per hour, most patients are moderately sedated with spontaneous ventilation and will tolerate endoscopy, examinations, minor surgical procedures, or mechanical ventilation [53]. Bradycardia and hypotension can occur, at around 1% of cases but with no major clinical implications [53].

Generation 3.1 Agents
Ketofol and Ketodex

Ketofol, a coadministration of ketamine and propofol, has gained popularity since 2007 from the belief that the combined product benefits from the positive traits of both medications while they annul each other's shortcomings [54]. They are usually constituted as a 1:1 mixture [55]. As both agents are short acting, recovery is rapid. The sympathomimetic effects of ketamine appear to counterbalance the respiratory depressing effects and hypotension of propofol. Propofol, in turn, decreases ketamine-induced nausea and vomiting and its recovery agitation [54, 55]. Sedation with both is additive (and possibly synergistic), allowing the use of lower doses of each drug. Ketamine adds an analgesic effect, with less pain on injection than with propofol. Ketofol sedation in the ED was reviewed in two important pro and con articles, updated in 2015 [54, 56]. A recent randomized control trial (RCT) of ketofol in children [57] compared it to ketamine alone for ED procedural sedation in children and found no significant differences in adverse events, although ketamine alone was more efficacious. Another recent study retrospectively reviewed the use of ketofol for botulinum toxin painful injections in children with cerebral palsy [58] and ascertained its safety in this population. Adverse events (10.1% of procedures) were mainly responsive hypoxemia (9.6%) and transient apnea (1.4%). A meta-analysis of the use of ketofol's in children in 2020 [59] surveyed 11 studies, 6 of which compared to other combined sedation regimens (ketodex, propodex, and opiates). It demonstrated low evidence for a decreased recovery time with ketofol and moderate evidence for reducing hypotension (but not bradycardia or respiratory depression). It also did not show any significant differences in clinician satisfaction, airway obstruction, apnea, desaturation, nausea, and vomiting. This meta-analysis is in striking contrast to a recent PSRC database study [42] where the coadministration of ketamine with propofol, an anticholinergic, or a barbiturate was associated with increased adverse events and serious adverse events. Future studies with better control comparisons will resolve this contradiction.

Ketodex, a coadministration of ketamine and dexmedetomidine, was introduced at a similar time to ketofol (in 2006) and has since been used both for intravenous [28, 60], intramuscular [30] and intranasal [29] procedural sedation. Complementing each other, when used together, dexmedetomidine may limit the tachycardia, hypertension, salivation, and emergence phenomena from ketamine; which in turn may prevent the bradycardia and hypotension from dexmedetomidine. Adding ketamine speeds the onset of sedation and eliminates the slow dexmedetomidine loading dose time [60].

Sevoflurane

Apart from its traditional role as a rapid induction and maintenance agent in pediatric anesthesia, sevoflurane has gained a respectable following since the late 1990s because of the possibility of its use as a sedation agent [61, 62], mostly for non-painful procedures, with a natural airway and a sealed face mask. Populations to be wary about are trisomy 21 patients with a predilection for bradycardia from sevoflurane and possible (rare) seizures from it. It is also contraindicated in malignant hyperthermia patients [63]. It was formally reintroduced for pediatric sedation in the paediatric intensive care unit (PICU) in a review of case reports by Tobias [63] and for mild to moderate pediatric sedation in the UK-based National Institute for Health and Care Excellence (NICE) 2010 guidelines [64, 65], as an alternative to chloral hydrate and midazolam (see Figure 23.1).

Overview of the Sedation Process and Medication Selection

The final planning of a safe and effective sedation regimen must account for many diverse factors, summarized in Figure 23.2 [22]. Pain management and sedation is most effective when clinicians are attentive to objective measures of patient distress [17, 20]. The topic of medication selection for pediatric sedation has been extensively reviewed [66]. There are multiple algorithms available, which should be selected according to the societal and geographical affiliations of the performing clinicians [67]. An important example is the NICE guidelines from 2010, quoted above regarding the reintroduction of volatiles (e.g., sevoflurane) for sedation [64]; see Figure 23.1.

Another important aspect of the sedation process is the ability to titrate the dosage to effect. A number of sedation scores to measure the effect have been devised and tested, some uniquely for children [68, 69, 70, 71] and some of these are considered below.

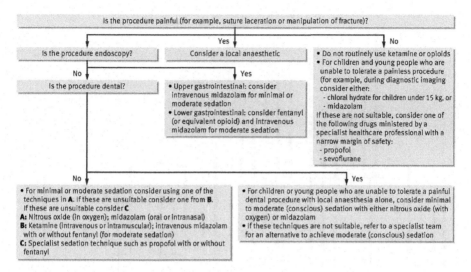

Figure 23.1 Strategy for choosing sedation from the NICE 2010 guidelines for sedation [65]. Reproduced with permission from the National Guideline Centre.

The Observer's Assessment of Alertness/Sedation Scale and Modified Observer's Assessment of Alertness/Sedation Scale

The Observer's Assessment of Alertness/Sedation (OAA/S) scale was initially developed by Chernik et al. in 1990 to measure the reversal of midazolam sedation by flumazenil in adults [72]. Consciousness level was assessed on multiple levels: responsiveness, speech, facial expression, and eyes (Table 23.5). Despite being extensively validated in adults, and its use in several sedation research studies in children [73, 74], the OAA/S scale has not been separately validated in children. However, it has been used in the validation of the University of Michigan Sedation Scale [75, see below] and in assessments of the reliability of the bispectral index (BIS) monitor in children [76].

By using only the "responsiveness" category of the OAA/S scale, Yuen et al. created the Modifed Observer Assessment of Alertness Sedation (mOAA/S) scale, in 2007 (Table 23.6) [77]. They validated it on 18 adults undergoing intranasal dexmedetomidine sedation. This was separately validated in the original Chernik study [72] but, as with the OAA/S scale, has not been separately validated in children, although it was tested in recent sedation research studies in children [78].

University of Michigan Sedation Scale

Developed in 2002 by Malviya et al., the University of Michigan Sedation Scale (UMSS) is an assessment tool that has been shown to be valid when compared to the OAA/S and other scales of sedation [75]. Similar to OAA/S scale, it is a responsiveness (or consciousness) scale (Table 23.7) to speech or sound that was validated on 32 children sedated on oral chloral hydrate for CT imaging. The UMSS was shown to be both rapid to administer and repeatable. Inter- and intra-observer reliability was very good, although poorly

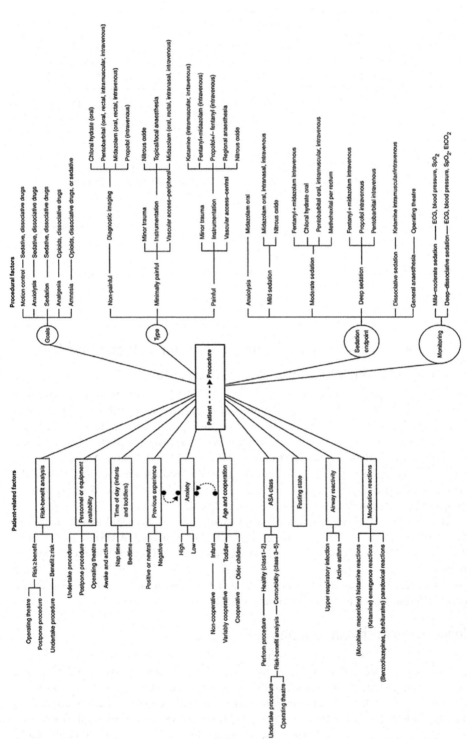

Figure 23.2 Factors determining medication choices and sedation endpoints. SpO₂= oxygen saturation. EtCO₂= end-tidal carbon dioxide. Reprinted with permission from Krauss and Green. *Lancet* 2006;367:770.

Table 23.5 The Observer's Assessment of Alertness/Sedation (OAA/S) scale

Level of responsiveness	Speech	Facial expression	Eyes	Score
Responds readily to name spoken in normal tone	Normal	Normal	Clear, No ptosis	5
Lethargic responses to name spoken in normal tone	Mild slowing or thickening	Mild relaxation	Glazed or mild ptosis (less than half the eye)	4
Responds only after name is called loudly and/or repeatedly	Slurring or prominent slowing	Marked relaxation (slack jaw)	Glazed and marked ptosis (half the eye or more)	3

Reproduced from Chernik et al. [72] and Yuen et al. [77] with permission from Wolters Kluwer Health, Inc.

Table 23.6 Modifed Observer's Assessment of Alertness/Sedation scale (mOAA/S)

MOAA/S Scale	Scale	ASA classification
Responds readily to name spoken in normal tone	5	Minimal
Lethargic response to name spoken in normal tone	4	Moderate
Responds only after name is called loudly and/or repeatedly	3	Moderate
Responds only after mild prodding or shaking	2	Moderate
Responds only after painful trapezius squeeze	1	Deep
Does not respond to painful trapezius squeeze	0	Deep/general anesthesia

Table 23.7 University of Michigan Sedation Scale (UMSS)

0	Awake and alert
1	Minimally sedated: tired/sleepy, appropriate response to verbal conversation and/for sound
2	Moderately sedated: somnolent/sleeping, easily aroused with light tactile stimulation or a simple verbal command
3	Deeply sedated: deep sleep, arousable only with significant physical stimulation
4	Unarousable

Reproduced from Malviya et al. [75] with permission from Elsevier.

correlated with the BIS [79]. That study was conducted on first- and second-generation agents (oral chloral hydrate, oral midazolam with intravenous phenobarbital and intravenous midazolam with intravenous meperidine. Since then, in the last decade, several recent pediatric sedation studies used it as a reference target, especially for more novel agents, such as intravenous/intranasal dexmedetomidine for ICU and EEG sedation [80, 81], intranasal fentanyl with nitrous oxide in the ED [82], intranasal midazolam volume for ED laceration repair [83], and propofol gradual induction in the operating room [84]. The latter study, which was done in Seoul in 2021, comes to be the closest to a validation study of UMSS in the pediatric population. And, coming full circle, the antiquated 1974 Ramsay sedation scale (validated only for adults) [68] was validated in 2021 for children when compared to the UMSS [85].

Children's Hospital of Wisconsin Sedation Scale

In the same year as the UMSS, the Children's Hospital of Wisconsin Sedation Scale (CHWSS) was developed by Hoffman et al. (Table 23.8). This is a Ramsay scale of sedation, modified by simplification for the lighter sedation continuum needed for pediatric procedural sedation [86]. From level 0 (unresponsive to painful stimulus) to level 6 (anxious, agitated, or in pain) its seven-point scale has been used to assess propofol EEG and BIS spectrums in infants and children [87] as well as to investigate ketamine procedural sedation in the ED [88].

Dartmouth Operative Conditions Scale

Whenever there are multiple solutions in science and in medicine, by parsimony it means there is no good solution. A repeating problem in the above scales (mOAA/S, UMSS, CHWSS) is the need to touch the patient; this is most likely impossible during a procedure such as a prolonged imaging or therapeutic scan. It is also highly undesirable, arousing the patient and thus interfering with the procedure for which they were sedated in the first place. To solve this conundrum, a team of pediatrician and anesthesiologists joined forces and refined a scale in order to optimize procedural sedation conditions across provider and interventions [89]. They did so by recording children undergoing 12 common procedures (CT and MRI scans, voiding cystourethrograms, bone marrow biopsies, cardiac catheterizations, and fracture reductions). The scale enables comparisons of pain or stress, movement, consciousness, and side effects that occur during the procedure and is easily assessed at frequent intervals. It was the first to comprehensively look at sedation behavior and quantify it. It was dubbed the Dartmouth Operative Conditions Scale (DOCS), which then was validated by reviewing videos from 95 procedures with sedation provided by various providers with different and techniques.

Table 23.8 Children's Hospital of Wisconsin Sedation Scale (CHWSS)

6	Anxious, agitated, has pain
5	Spontaneously awake without stimulation
4	Sleepy, eyes open or can be awakened easily with audible stimulation
3	Can be awakened with loud sound and light tactile stimulation
2	Can be awakened slowly (with difficulty) with constant painful stimulation
1	Sleepy and unresponsive to painful stimulation
0	Completely unresponsive to painful stimulation

Reproduced from Hoffman et al. [86] with permission from the American Academy of Pediatrics Publications.

Table 23.9 Dartmouth Operative Conditions Scale (DOCS)

Patient state		Observed behaviors		
Pain/stress	(0) Eyes closed or calm expression	(1) Grimace or frown	(2) Crying, sobbing, or screaming	
Movement	(0) Still	(1) Random little movement	(2) Major purposeful movement	(3) Thrashing, kicking, or biting
Consciousness	(0) Eyes open	(−1) Ptosis, uncoordinated, or "drowsy"	(−2) Eyes closed	
Sedation side effects	(−0) Spo$_2$ <92%	(−1) Noise with respiration	(−1) Respiratory pauses >10 s	(−1) BP decrease of >50% from baseline

Reproduced from Cravero et al. [89] with permission from Wolters Kluwer Health, Inc.

Inter- and intra-observer correlation, construct, and criterion validity were all very good [89]. The DOCS was later used for comparison of provider/technique in adult endoscopic ultrasound [90] in the same hospital, and recently adapted for pediatric esophagogastroduodenoscopy, with less success [91]. See Table 23.9.

Pediatric Sedation State Scale

To simplify and linearize the DOCS, the Pediatric Sedation State Scale (PSSS) was developed and validated through a Delphi process by experts in pediatric sedation, and guidelines were published on the topic in 2017 [92]. It was tested on 20 sedation providers to assess interrater reliability and, 6 months later (on a subgroup), to confirm intrarater reliability. The PSSS includes six sedation states associated with adequate sedation and also describes adverse events associated with excessive sedation. It recognizes behaviors associated with an inadequate sedation state, such as purposeful movements, crying or shouting, thrashing, and expressions of pain or anxiety (Table 23.10). It was validated by comparing it with a pediatric validated observational distress scale in 96 children undergoing laceration repair under three different doses of intranasal midazolam.

The PSSS has also been recently included as a primary outcome measure in two studies: a multicenter (400 pediatric procedural sedations) and a single-center (150 sedations) study, to end in 2024, and 2022, respectively. The former study [ketodex, NCT04195256] tests, with a Bayesian dose-finding protocol, three different doses of intranasal ketodex for this purpose [93]. The latter [Tsze et al., NCT04586504] tests four different doses of intranasal midazolam for this purpose, a change of practice from the team previously using the UMSS [83] for a similar study.

Sedation in pediatric intensive care has a different targets/goals, namely the "Goldilocks zone" of being awake and able to calm [94], not too deep or light thus

Table 23.10 Pediatric Sedation State Scale (PSSS)

State	Behavior
5	Patient is moving (purposefully or nonpurposefully) in a manner that impedes the proceduralist and requires forceful immobilization This includes crying or shouting during the procedure, but vocalization is not required. Score is based on movement.
4	Moving during the procedure (awake or sedated) that requires gentle immobilization for positioning. May verbalize some discomfort or stress, but there is no crying or shouting that expresses stress or objection.
3	Expression of pain or anxiety on face (may verbalize discomfort), but not moving or impeding completion of the procedure. May require help positioning (as with a lumbar puncture) but does not require restraint to stop movement during the procedure.
2	Quiet (asleep or awake), not moving during procedure, and no frown (or brow furrow) indicating pain or anxiety. No verbalization of any complaint..
1	Deeply asleep with normal vital signs, but requiring airway intervention and/or assistance (eg, central or obstructive apnea, etc).
0	Sedation associated with abnormal physiologic parameters that require acute intervention (ie, oxygen saturation <90%, blood pressure is 30% lower than baseline, bradycardia receiving therapy).

Reproduced from Cravero et al. [92] with permission from the American Academy of Pediatrics Publications.

preventing unintended line dislodging, bucking on endotracheal tubing, as well as extubation failure and hemodynamic instability [70]. This is enabled by the use of standardized sedation scoring systems on mechanically ventilated pediatric patients, at regular intervals. These scoring systems (the COMFORT scale, COMFORT-B scale, State Behavioral Scale (SBS), Richmond Agitation–Sedation Scale) have been validated and used in the PICU, and extensively reviewed elsewhere [69, 70]. An important consideration for depth of sedation evaluation in this population, during prolonged mechanical ventilation is the use of muscle relaxants and/or hemodynamically reactive medications. In these cases, the BIS monitor has been shown to have acceptable correlation with the Ramsay or COMFORT scores [69, 70], although the SNAP-II™ modified BIS algorithm did not show a good correlation with the SBS [95]. This is important, as the SBS has recently (February 2022) been endorsed by the Society of Critical Care Medicine (SCCM), together with the COMFORT-B scale, to assess the level of sedation in mechanically ventilated pediatric patients, with a strong recommendation from moderate evidence in their clinical practice guidelines [96].

Common Pediatric Sedation Scenarios

Imaging Studies

Imaging studies are mostly painless and short, and they are the most common indication for procedural sedation in children [1]. Yet failure to obtain an image entails possible harm by multiple exposures (to ionizing radiation) or the risk of adverse events (by multiple sedation encounters) [97, 98]. Success may be improved by evaluation of the child's state before starting the sedation to assess their anxiety and maturity, parental anxiety, and the ability for the sedation provider to assuage and pacify the child. Often, a radiograph can be obtained with distraction or pretend play measures alone [99], with the aid of child life specialists [19] or virtual reality generators, before [18] or during [100] a procedure. For longer scans such as CT to be completed more extensive pharmacological intervention may be needed. These have been reviewed by Slovis [101] and Berkenbosch [102], with propofol, etomidate, and dexmedetomidine found to be most successful agents with ketamine as a good runner up. Low-dose intravenous dexmedetomidine loading doses (0.5–1 µg/kg bolus in 1 minute) with one more bolus later on, or a 0.5–1 µg/kg per hour infusion were the original norm for radiology imaging [102]. These were later enhanced by fewer failure rates with higher (2–3 µg/kg) loading doses [102]; and with needleless (intranasal) administration routes both as a premedication [103] and peri-procedure sedation [104, 105]. Surprisingly, a recent database (Pediatric Health Information System) study found that the sedatives most commonly used in children to obtain head CT images in the ED were opioids (~40–53%) and benzodiazpenes (~32–53%) [106]. Ketofol has also shown promise in a recent audit [107]. Lengthier studies such as MRI are poorly tolerated by most children and require more extensive measures. Not all MRI studies are created equal (length of protocol, inherent aspiration risk, functional MRI, diffusion MRI, magnetic resonance angiography/venography with contrast, MRI enterography) and a detailed discussion with the radiology team is paramount [108] It is a very hazardous environment as well and a thorough knowledge of the additional risks (temperature maintenance, noise exposure, ferromagnetic projectiles), needed adaptations, and implicit limitations of such an environment is mandated [108, 109]. For non-pharmacological intervention options for pediatric comfort, the Belgian "submarine" protocol [110] and the Cornell "MRI-am-a-Hero" [111] have shown reduction of sedation use in 5–6 and 4–7 year olds, respectively. Similar programs (Try Without) at Boston Children's and Mass General Hospital, have utilized music, videos and child life specialists for sedation reduction [112]. Pharmacological options are divided according to intravenous access. If present, a high-dose dexmedetomidine loading dose and drip have been perfected [113, 114, 115, 116], propofol drips utilized [117] and compared to ketofol [118], as well as more recent ketodex regimens [102]. When intravenous access is absent, the use of either intranasal dexmedetomidine on its own [119, 120] or with intranasal midazolam [121] has been shown to be effective, as was intranasal ketamine [122] and intramuscular dexmedetomidine [123]. Other non-painful imaging procedures are pediatric transthoracic echocardiography studies, for which both intranasal dexmedetomidine [124] and intranasal ketamine and intranasal midazolam [38] were shown to be good options, in lieu of chloral hydrate. It has also been demonstrated that the painless auditory brainstem response testing can be done on a 3–4 µg/kg intranasal dose of dexemedetomidine on its own [125] or with buccal midazolam [39] with high rates of success; as was the use of intravenous propofol [126, 127] and ketofol [128]. Surprisingly, oral chloral hydrate fared better than intranasal midazolam, for this indication [129]. Less chartered waters are the effect sedation has on the ability to adequately accomplish a voiding cystoureterogram (VCUG). Previous reports were contradictory as to the retentive effect both propofol [130] and nitrous oxide [131] may have. A recent systematic review found that only oral midazolam (0.5 mg/kg) was effective for VCUG distress alleviation, whereas fentanyl or chloral hydrate were not [132]. Nitrous oxide 50% was cited as an alternative, but its side effects may hinder its use.

Hemato-Oncology-Related Procedures

As the second most common indication for pediatric procedural sedation (13.5–21.5% of all cases) in the last decade (according to the PSRC) [1], pediatric hemato-oncology includes some of the trickiest of procedural sedations on some of the sickest children: bone marrow aspirations, Ommaya reservoir taps or medication installation and/or biopsy, lumbar puncture and/or intrathecal medication administration, nuclear medicine procedures, peripherally inserted central catheter placement, renal/liver biopsies, surgical procedures, dental examination and/or treatment, and other procedures. Some of these are mostly painful procedures (lumbar punctures, bone marrow aspirations, biopsies) and this pain overshadows the patient's oncological pain [133]. In a now more than 20-year-old systematic review, Murat et al. focused on the pain alleviation analgosedation protocols from the turn of the millennium [133]. These included ketamine versus midazolam, fentanyl, and meperidine. Since then, both a self-administered nitrous oxide service for lumbar puncture sedation with local anesthetic [134] as well as a benzodiazepine–nitrous oxide-based sedation with topical local anesthetic [135] were described. For external beam radiation therapy, non-anesthesiologist midazolam administration was preferred, but also propofol, dexmedetomidine, and ketamine protocols have been described [136]. Proton beam radiation therapy should ideally be managed under propofol [137]. These are mainly painless interventions but the sedation is mostly targeting anxiolysis. Similar studies were done with intravenous dexmedetomidine for nuclear medicine imaging [138], as well as ketofol [128]. In a guideline published in 2003, the Society of Nuclear Medicine and Molecular Imaging reviewed the possible regimens for procedural sedation in nuclear medicine, including most, if not all, possible medications at the time (i.e., ketamine, opiates, benzodiazepines, phenothiazines, barbiturates and chloral hydrate) [139]. For biopsies, both nursing-administered ketamine–midazolam sedation [140] as well as ketodex for anterior mediastinal biopsies on spontaneous breathing have been deemed safe [60].

Gastroentorology Procedures

Endoscopy (Esophagogastroduodenoscopy and Colonoscopy)

Gastroenterology has been the third most common indication for pediatric procedural sedation (8.5–9.5% of all cases) in the last decade (according to the PSRC) [1], and includes a very wide range of procedures: upper endoscopy, gastrostomy tube placement and/or change, percutaneous endoscopic gastrostomy, cecostomy tube change and/or placement, and liver biopsies. These procedures have been shown to entail a risk of severe adverse events (mostly respiratory), which have reduced considerably in the three epochs described in the PSRC study [1]. These sedation practices were originally mapped in the North American Society of Pediatric Gastroenterology Hepatology and Nutrition (NASPHAGAN) survey in 2007 [141]. In the NASPHAGAN study it was ascertained that 23% of the respondents never used general anesthesia (whereas 10% always did), neither inhalational nor total intravenous anesthesia (mostly propofol). However, the different sedation regimens used at the time were not described. From the PSRC data, Biber et al. managed to conclude these were mostly intensivist-driven propofol regimens, with additional fentanyl or midazolam, if needed [142]. These authors noted a 4.8% adverse event rate, mostly respiratory (4%). These practices were also elucidated in a systematic review of 11 RCTs and 15 non-RCTs, which showed that propofol-based procedural sedation was the best practice for gastrointestinal endoscopy in children. It was as safe as opioid–benzodiazepine combination regimens, yet it could be safely administered by specifically trained non-anesthesiologists [143]. There were not enough data on midazolam-, ketamine-, and sevoflurane-based sedations. A study a year later showed that the use of intravenous ketodex (ketamine 2 mg/kg and dexemeetomidine 1 µg/kg, bolused over 5 minutes) enabled good conditions for upper gastrointestinal endoscopies in 89% of pediatric cases [28]. Similar conclusions to the systematic review were reached in a large retrospective study on the use of propofol (by anesthesiologists) versus fentanyl/midazolam (by pediatricians) for colonoscopy in a tertiary center [144], which showed a better success rate with this regimen. Another large study showed similar success rates using a combined propofol and fentanyl with or without midazolam regimen for both upper and lower gastrointestinal procedures in a large tertiary center [145]. In 2014, the American Society for Gastrointestinal Endoscopy (ASGE) came out with their guidelines on modifications in endoscopic practice for pediatric patients, which stated "Propofol and general anesthesia as "commonly used (regimens) for pediatric endoscopy, usually based on age or anticipated patient intolerance of the procedure" [146]. In their updated (2018) general guidelines for sedation and anesthesia in gastrointestinal endoscopy, they focus on adults and mention both the use of opioids and benzodiazepines, patient-controlled sedation, as well as non-anesthesiologist propofol sedation and state that the services of an anesthesiologist are most cost efficient with "complex endoscopic procedures or patients with multiple medical comorbidities or at risk for airway compromise" [147]. An interesting recent RCT found that the use of carbon dioxide insufflation (instead of room air) by the gastroenterologist for a colonoscopy reduced abdominal bloating and the need for post-procedure opiate use in children [148]. This insufflation and bloating is the essence of the feared aspiration risk and the tendency to manage the child's airway with an endotracheal tube for these procedures. The jury is still out on the topic as both increased respiratory adverse events without improved efficiency [149, 150] as well as no increase in adverse events [151] have been witnessed. Esophagogastroduodenoscopy procedures have also been managed successfully with laryngeal mask airways in children [152]. In a recent large retrospective chart review, Hartjes et al. noticed that only 19% of gastrointestinal endoscopy patients, overseen by anesthesiologists, underwent endotracheal intubation, mostly for esophagogastroduodenoscopy. Their sedation regimens included between one and six different medications, mostly propofol and midazolam [153]. For a comprehensive recent overview on the history and future of pediatric sedation for endoscopy, see Cox et al. [154].

MRI Enterography

MRI enterography is a novel imaging technique, utilizing oral contrast fluids to examine the small intestines to the ileocecal valve for inflammatory bowel disease (IBD) diagnosis in children. Appropriate timing of oral contrast administration is crucial (20 mL/kg, < 2 hours prior to the scan) for bowel demonstration and study success, followed by an additional glass of water [155]. As the age of diagnosis of IBD is decreasing, younger and younger patients may undergo this procedure and, accordingly, need sedation to enable it [155]. Because of the inherent aspiration risk (post procedure vomiting of 8%), a general anesthetic by anesthesiologists with endotracheal intubation and oral gastric tube insertion and suctioning is the preferred method of sedation [156].

Emergency Department

The topic of pediatric ED sedation has been a subject for extensive reviews in the last decade [24, 27]. A whole set of research consortia (e.g., PERC, PECARN, PSRC) [8] have arisen to answer the question of what works and what's safe in pediatric emergency procedural sedation [157] and what are risk factors for adverse events in these sedations [158, 159]. Preference was noted to single-agent ketamine and forgoing premedication with opiates, and fasting status was not shown to be an independent predictor for aspiration risk [160]. In a recent thorough review of practices across 35 pediatric EDs, both indications and medications have undergone major changes [161]. A similar picture is seen across pediatric EDs in Europe [162]. The most useful addition in recent years are multiple studies on intranasal administration of sedative and analgesic drugs in pediatric EDs (reviewed in Pansini et al. [26])

Pediatric sedation in the midst of a critical event such as trauma, fractures, or acute illness requires a dedicated team approach. It is unlikely that a single agent will permit procedural sedation and residual sedative effects can complicate evaluation of the child's mental status. The ideal regimen will have prompt onset and offset, minimally affect the vital signs, provide potent analgesia for painful interventions, and not obtund the respiratory drive.

Ketamine is advantageous in many settings as it exhibits many features of an ideal agent. It has a prompt onset, potent analgesia and amnestic effects, and relatively short effective duration. It can be administered orally, rectally, or by intravenous or intramuscular injection. Ketamine has the undesirable tendency to cause salivation and the additional secretions are thought by some to increase the risk of coughing or laryngospasm. An anticholinergic agent such as glycopyrrolate or atropine can be coadministered. Lastly, there continues to be significant concern regarding the propensity for ketamine to cause an agitated dysphoric state typically referred to as dissociation, where the patient experiences negative psychic phenomena. This is pharmacologically related to ketamine's similarity to phencyclidine (aka: the street drug Angel Dust). In children, such negative experiences are less significant than in adults and, as such, ketamine remains a reasonable and frequently deployed sedative agent in EDs in the United States.

Considerable debate continues over the use of propofol by non-anesthesiologists. Propofol infusions may provide hypnosis, amnesia, and anesthesia but no analgesia. Careful clinical monitoring is needed to detect apnea or airway obstruction. It can be difficult to maintain adequate sedation if stimulation occurs or a painful procedure is attempted. The addition of a potent analgesic can improve sedation for painful procedures but concomitantly increases the risk of apnea and airway compromise.

Pediatric Intensive Care Units

Critically ill children present an exceptionally significant set of challenges. Sedation must be considered in the context of the child's immediate clinical state, the level of sedation considered necessary, the potential risks of any administered sedative drugs, and the familiarity with sedation techniques of the staff providing care. These have been extensively reviewed in recent literature [69, 70, 163]. In February 2022, clinical practice guidelines were formulated by the SCCM [96] on the use of protocolized sedation in all critically ill pediatric patients requiring sedation and/or analgesia during mechanical ventilation. They strongly recommended that dexmedetomidine be considered as a primary agent for sedation (moderate level of evidence) and suggest that a continuous propofol sedation (< 48 hours; at doses less than 4 mg/kg per hour for prevention of propofol infusion syndrome) may be a useful adjunct during the peri-extubation period to facilitate weaning of other analgosedative agents prior to extubation. They also suggest consideration of adjunct sedation with ketamine in patients who are not otherwise at an optimal sedation depth target (gauged by the SBS and/or the COMFORT-B scale, see above). They recommended minimizing benzodiazepine-based sedation when feasible in critically ill pediatric patients to decrease the incidence and/or duration or severity of delirium and iatrogenic withdrawal syndrome (IWS). They similarly suggest monitoring for IWS with opioid-based sedation protocols. Thereare good trial data that demonstrate the role of dexmedetomidine in decreasing the need of any other sedative agents in the PICU whilst decreasing sedation scores [164] and its role in alleviating benzodiazepine/opioid IWS in the PICU [165]. A retrospective review was done on 60 PICU patients in one center, maintained on a prolonged ketamine drip. Indications varied but, in all cases, both opioid sparing and sedation targets in difficult-to-sedate patients were achieved with minimal side effects [166]. Recently, there has been a resurgence in the use of volatiles as sedation for PICU patients [69]. This has come about by using syringe pumps to deliver the volatiles in fluid form and the anesthetic conserving device (AnaConDa®) to help evaporate it and conserve it in the closed circuits of the ventilator. In a study on 23 critically ill children, these have been used to deliver sevoflurane, for a median of 5 days at a concentration of 0.8%. Only 30% showed hypotension and a third had withdrawal [167]. The same system was tested previously for isoflurane in the long-term sedation of 15 critically ill children [168], with none showing hypotension.

Neonatal [169] and pediatric cardiac ICUs [170] face challenges that are even more rigorous. Prolonged ventilation of premature infants with profound systemic morbidities is often required.

Apart from the agents suggested for neonates in the AAP guideline quoted above [169], there has been a 50-fold increase in the use of dexmedetomidine in neonates, although up to now there is no formal FDA indication [171]. Another recent innovation is the use of intranasal administration of sedatives in neonates, mainly for procedural sedation [172]. Table 23.11 lists dosing suggestions for sedatives in neonates, from a thorough summary of the literature [173]. Note the limited formal information on dosing of propofol, ketamine and dexmedetomidine in neonates.

Summary

Practical pediatric sedation remains a considerable challenge for many clinicians. The many factors that inherently affect pediatric physiology, pharmacology, and behavior must be recognized by all clinicians attempting to sedate children. Institutional oversight must seek to balance the needs of their patients with the risks of sedation. Individual clinicians should seek continuous improvement of personal training and experience to further their ability to care for sedated children.

Acknowledgments

The authors wish to thank Dr. Corey E. Collins, the author of this chapter in the previous two editions of the manual.

Table 23.11 Drugs for procedural sedation and analgesia in the neonatal intensive care unit

Topical/local anesthetics	EMLA: 0.5–1 g, one application daily
Propofol	*Intubation*: 1–3 mg/kg, intravenous bolus *Continuous*: manual dosing regimen has been suggested, but has not yet been validated
Ketamine	Still limited data, commonly part of multimodal analgosedation
Remifentanil	*Intubation*: 1–3 µg/kg, commonly part of multimodal analgosedation *Continuous*: 0.1–2 µg/kg per minute during procedure
Chloral hydrate	25–75 mg/kg per dose, oral or rectal
Morphine	*Intermittent*: 50–200 µg/kg per dose, intravenous/intramuscular/subcutaneous, every 4 hours *Continuous*: loading 50–100 µg/kg over 1 hour, followed by 5–20 µg/kg per hour
Fentanyl	*Intermittent*: 0.5–4 µg/kg, intravenous slow push, as required (every 2–4 hours) *Continuous*: 0.5–3 µg/kg per hour
Midazolam	*Intermittent*: 0.05–0.15 mg/kg over at least 5 minutes, (every 2–4 hours) *Continuous*: 0.01–0.06 mg/kg per hour
Dexmedetomidine	*No firm dosing advice available, practices vary* Loading dose 1 µg/kg within 10 minutes, followed by 0.5–0.8 µg/kg per hour
Acetaminophen	*Intravenous*: loading dose 20 mg/kg, maintenance 10 mg/kg per dose *Oral*: loading dose 20–25 mg/kg, maintenance 12–15 mg/kg/dose *Rectal*: loading dose 30 mg/kg, maintenance 12–18 mg/kg per dose *Maintenance intervals*: every 6 hours (term), every 8 hours (32–36 weeks), every 12 hours (< 32 weeks)

Dosing suggestions, reflecting the overall limited information on dosing in neonates.
Reproduced from Allegaert and van den Anker [174] with permission from Springer Nature.

References

1. Kamat PP, McCracken CE, Simon HK, et al. Trends in outpatient procedural sedation: 2007–2018. *Pediatrics*. 2020;145 (5):e20193559; PMID:32332053

2. Practice Guidelines for Moderate Procedural Sedation and Analgesia 2018: A report by the American Society of Anesthesiologists Task Force on Moderate Procedural Sedation and Analgesia, the American Association of Oral and Maxillofacial Surgeons, American College of Radiology, American Dental Association, American Society of Dentist Anesthesiologists, and Society of Interventional Radiology. *Anesthesiology*. 2018;128(3):437–79. PMID:29334501

3. Coté CJ, Wilson S, American Academy of Pediatrics. Guidelines for monitoring and management of pediatric patients before, during, and after sedation for diagnostic and therapeutic procedures. *Pediatrics*. 2019;143(6):e20191000. PMID: 31138666.

4. Zielinska M, Bartkowska-Sniatkowska A, Becke K, et al. Safe pediatric procedural

sedation and analgesia by anesthesiologists for elective procedures: a clinical practice statement from the European Society for Paediatric Anaesthesiology. *Paediatr Anaesth.* 2019;29(6):583–90. PMID:30793427

5. Green SM, Roback MG, Krauss BS, et al. Unscheduled procedural sedation: a multidisciplinary consensus practice guideline. *Ann Emerg Med.* 2019;73(5): e51–65. PMID:31029297

6. Blike GT, Christoffersen K, Cravero JP, Andeweg SK, Jensen J. A method for measuring system safety and latent errors associated with pediatric procedural sedation. *Anesth Analg.* 2005;101(1):48-58. PMID: 15976205

7. Society for Pediatric Sedation. Sedation provider course. https://pedsedation.org/offerings/sedation-provider-course (accessed May 2024)

8. Bhatt M, Kennedy RM, Osmond MH, et al. Consensus Panel on Sedation Research of Pediatric Emergency Research Canada (PERC) and the Pediatric Emergency Care Applied Research Network (PECARN). Consensus-based recommendations for standardizing terminology and reporting adverse events for emergency department procedural sedation and analgesia in children. *Ann Emerg Med.* 2009;53 (4):426–35.e4. doi:10.1016/j. annemergmed.2008.09.030; PMID: 19026467

9. Mason KP, Green SM, Piacevoli Q, International Sedation Task Force. Adverse event reporting tool to standardize the reporting and tracking of adverse events during procedural sedation: a consensus document from the World SIVA International Sedation Task Force. *Br J Anaesth.* 2012;108(1):13-20. doi:10.1093/bja/aer407; PMID:22157446

10. Mason KP, Roback MG, Chrisp D, et al. Results from the Adverse Event Sedation Reporting Tool: a global anthology of 7952 records derived from >160,000 procedural sedation encounters. *J Clin Med.* 2019;8(12):2087. doi:10.3390/jcm8122087; PMID:31805686

11. Scherrer PD, Mallory MD, Cravero JP, et al. The impact of obesity on pediatric procedural sedation-related outcomes: results from the Pediatric Sedation Research Consortium. *Paediatr Anaesth.* 2015;25(7):689–97. doi:10.1111/pan.12627; PMID:25817924

12. Havidich JE, Beach M, Dierdorf SF, et al. Preterm versus term children: analysis of sedation/anesthesia adverse events and longitudinal risk. *Pediatrics.* 2016;137(3): e20150463. doi:10.1542/peds.2015-0463; PMID:26917674

13. Mallory MD, Travers C, McCracken CE, Hertzog J, Cravero JP. Upper respiratory infections and airway adverse events in pediatric procedural sedation. *Pediatrics.* 2017;140(1):e20170009. doi:10.1542/peds.2017-0009; PMID:28759404

14. Harless J, Ramaiah R, Bhananker SM. Pediatric airway management. *Int J Crit Illn Inj Sci.* 2014;4(1):65–70. doi:10.4103/2229-5151.128015; PMID:24741500

15. Ferrari LR. The pediatric airway: anatomy, challenges, and solutions. In Mason KP, ed., *Pediatric Sedation Outside of the Operating Room.* Cham: Springer, 2021, 125–39. https://doi.org/10.1007/978-3-030-58406-1_8

16. Andropoulos, DB. Pediatric physiology: how does it differ from adults? Mason KP, ed., *Pediatric Sedation Outside of the Operating Room.* Cham: Springer, 2021, 141–54. https://doi.org/10.1007/978-3-030-58406-1_9

17. Reddy SK, Deutsch N. Behavioral and emotional disorders in children and their anesthetic implications. *Children (Basel).* 2020;7(12):253. doi:10.3390/children7120253; PMID:33255535

18. Han SH, Park JW, Choi SI, et al. Effect of immersive virtual reality education before chest radiography on anxiety and distress among pediatric patients: a randomized clinical trial. *JAMA Pediatr.* 2019 1;173 (11):1026–31. doi:10.1001/jamapediatrics.2019.3000; PMID:31498380

19. Tyson ME, Bohl DD, Blickman JG. A randomized controlled trial: child life

services in pediatric imaging. *Pediatr Radiol.* 2014;44(11):1426–32. doi:10.1007/s00247-014-3005-1; PMID:24801818

20. Bryant BE, Adler AC, Mann DG, Malek J. "You can't make me!" Managing adolescent dissent to anesthesia. *Paediatr Anaesth.* 2021;31(4):397–403. doi:10.1111/pan.14119; PMID:33386692

21. Bollinger, L.L., Yao, L.P. (2021). Pediatric sedatives and the Food and Drug Administration (FDA): challenges, limitations, and drugs in development. Mason KP, ed., *Pediatric Sedation Outside of the Operating Room.* Cham: Springer, 2021, 647–56. https://doi.org/10.1007/978-3-030-58406-1_32

22. Krauss B, Green SM. Procedural sedation and analgesia in children. *Lancet.* 2006;367(9512):766–80. doi:10.1016/S0140-6736(06)68230-5; PMID: 16517277

23. Cravero JP, Roback MG. Pediatric procedural sedation: pharmacologic agents. Topic 82857 Version 28.0 In *UpToDate*, Stack AM, Randolph AG, eds. www.uptodate.com/contents/procedural-sedation-in-children-selection-of-medications (accessed April 27, 2022)

24. Kost S, Roy A. Procedural sedation and analgesia in the pediatric emergency department: a review of sedative pharmacology. *Clin Pediatr Emerg Med.* 2010;11(4):233–43.

25. Meesters N, Simons S, van Rosmalen J, et al. Waiting 2 minutes after sucrose administration-unnecessary? *Arch Dis Child Fetal Neonatal Ed.* 2017;102(2):F167–9. doi:10.1136/archdischild-2016-310841; PMID:28157669PMCID

26. Pansini V, Curatola A, Gatto A, Intranasal drugs for analgesia and sedation in children admitted to pediatric emergency department: a narrative review. *Ann Transl Med.* 2021;9(2):189. doi:10.21037/atm-20-5177; PMID:33569491

27. Kennedy RM (2021). Sedation in the emergency department: a complex and multifactorial challenge. In Mason KP,

ed., *Pediatric Sedation Outside of the Operating Room.* Cham: Springer, 2021, 413–73 https://doi.org/10.1007/978-3-030-58406-1_22

28. Goyal R, Singh S, Shukla RN, Patra AK, Bhargava DV. Ketodex, a combination of dexmedetomidine and ketamine for upper gastrointestinal endoscopy in children: a preliminary report. *J Anesth.* 2013;27(3):461–3. doi:10.1007/s00540-012-1538-8; PMID:23223916

29. Yang F, Liu Y, Yu Q, Analysis of 17 948 pediatric patients undergoing procedural sedation with a combination of intranasal dexmedetomidine and ketamine. *Paediatr Anaesth.* 2019;29 (1):85–91. doi:10.1111/pan.13526; PMID:30484930

30. Guthrie DB, Boorin MR, Sisti AR, et al. Retrospective comparison of intramuscular admixtures of ketamine and dexmedetomidine versus ketamine and midazolam for preoperative sedation. *Anesth Prog.* 2021;68(1):3-9. doi:10.2344/anpr-67-04-02; PMID:33827122

31. Hartshorn S, Middleton PM. Efficacy and safety of inhaled low-dose methoxyflurane for acute paediatric pain: a systematic review. *Trauma.* 2019;21 (2):94–102. doi:10.1177/1460408618798391

32. Jephcott C, Grummet J, Nguyen N, Spruyt O. A review of the safety and efficacy of inhaled methoxyflurane as an analgesic for outpatient procedures. *Br J Anaesth.* 2018;120(5):1040–8. doi:10.1016/j.bja.2018.01.011; PMID:29661381

33. Prescribing information for BIFAVO. https://bynder.acaciapharma.com/m/403e8c343b2922de/original/Byfavo-PI.pdf

34. Kim KM. Remimazolam: pharmacological characteristics and clinical applications in anesthesiology. *Anesth Pain Med (Seoul).* 2022;17(1): 1–11. doi:10.17085/apm.21115; PMID: 35139608

35. Pesic M, Schippers F, Saunders R, Webster L, Donsbach M, Stoehr T.

Pharmacokinetics and pharmacodynamics of intranasal remimazolam: a randomized controlled clinical trial. *Eur J Clin Pharmacol.* 2020;76(11):1505–16. doi: 10.1007/s00228-020-02984-z; PMID:32886178

36. Shildt N, Traube C, Dealmeida M, "Difficult to sedate": successful implementation of a benzodiazepine-sparing analgosedation protocol in mechanically ventilated children. *Children (Basel).* 2021; 28;8(5):348. doi:10.3390/children8050348; PMID:33924822

37. Liu XI, Schuette P, Burckart GJ, et al. A comparison of pediatric and adult safety studies for antipsychotic and antidepressant drugs submitted to the United States food and drug administration. *J Pediatr.* 2019;208:236–42.e3. doi:10.1016/j.jpeds.2018.12.033; PMID:30679050

38. Alp H, Elmacı AM, Alp EK, Say B. Comparison of intranasal midazolam, intranasal ketamine, and oral chloral hydrate for conscious sedation during paediatric echocardiography: results of a prospective randomised study. *Cardiol Young.* 2019;29(9):1189–95. doi:10.1017/S1047951119001835; PMID:31451130

39. Li BL, Yuen VM, Zhou JL, et al. A randomized controlled trial of oral chloral hydrate vs intranasal dexmedetomidine plus buccal midazolam for auditory brainstem response testing in children. *Paediatr Anaesth.* 2018;28 (11):1022–8. doi:10.1111/pan.13498; PMID: 30281180

40. Fong CY, Lim WK, Li L, Lai NM. Chloral hydrate as a sedating agent for neurodiagnostic procedures in children. *Cochrane Database Syst Rev.* 2021;8(8): CD011786. doi:10.1002/14651858. CD011786.pub3; PMID:34397100

41. Green SM, Roback MG, Krauss B, et al. Emergency Department Ketamine Meta-Analysis Study Group. Predictors of emesis and recovery agitation with emergency department ketamine sedation: an individual-patient data meta-analysis of 8,282 children. *Ann Emerg Med.* 2009;54(2):171–80.e1–4. doi:10.1016/j.annemergmed.2009.04.004; PMID:19501426

42. Grunwell JR, Travers C, McCracken CE, Procedural sedation outside of the operating room using ketamine in 22,645 children: a report from the Pediatric Sedation Research Consortium. *Pediatr Crit Care Med.* 2016;17(12):1109-1116. doi:10.1097/PCC.0000000000000920; PMID:27505716

43. Tsze DS, Steele DW, Machan JT, Akhlaghi F, Linakis JG. Intranasal ketamine for procedural sedation in pediatric laceration repair: a preliminary report. *Pediatr Emerg Care.* 2012;28 (8):767–70. doi:10.1097/PEC.0b013e3182624935; PMID:22858745

44. Oliveira J E Silva L, Lee JY, Bellolio F, Homme JL, Anderson JL. Intranasal ketamine for acute pain management in children: A systematic review and meta-analysis. *Am J Emerg Med.* 2020;38 (9):1860–6. doi:10.1016/j.ajem.2020.05.094; PMID:32739857

45. Poonai N, Canton K, Ali S, et al. Intranasal ketamine for procedural sedation and analgesia in children: a systematic review. *PLoS ONE.* 2017;12(3): e0173253. doi:10.1371/journal.pone.0173253; PMID:28319161

46. Pandey RK, Bahetwar SK, Saksena AK, Chandra G. A comparative evaluation of drops versus atomized administration of intranasal ketamine for the procedural sedation of young uncooperative pediatric dental patients: a prospective crossover trial. *J Clin Pediatr Dent.* 2011;36(1):79–84. doi:10.17796/jcpd.36.1.1774746504g28656; PMID:22900449

47. Marçon F, Guittet C, Manso MA, et al. Population pharmacokinetic evaluation of ADV6209, an innovative oral solution of midazolam containing cyclodextrin. *Eur J Pharm Sci.* 2018;114:46–54. doi:10.1016/j.ejps.2017.11.030. PMID: 29203151

48. Klein EJ, Brown JC, Kobayashi A, Osincup D, Seidel K. A randomized clinical trial comparing oral, aerosolized

intranasal, and aerosolized buccal midazolam. *Ann Emerg Med.* 2011;58 (4):323–9. doi:10.1016/j. annemergmed.2011.05.016; PMID:21689865

49. Smith D, Cheek H, Denson B, Pruitt CM. Lidocaine pretreatment reduces the discomfort of intranasal midazolam administration: a randomized, double-blind, placebo-controlled trial. *Acad Emerg Med.* 2017;24(2):161–7. doi:10.1111/acem.13115; PMID:27739142

50. O'Connell NC, Woodward HA, Flores-Sanchez PL, et al. Comparison of preadministered and coadministered lidocaine for treating pain and distress associated with intranasal midazolam administration in children: a randomized clinical trial. *J Am Coll Emerg Physicians Open.* 2020 26;1(6):1562–70. doi:10.1002/emp2.12227; PMID:33392564

51. Tsze DS, Mallory MD, Cravero JP. Practice patterns and adverse events of nitrous oxide sedation and analgesia: a report from the pediatric sedation research consortium. *J Pediatr.* 2016;169:260-5.e2. doi:10.1016/j.jpeds.2015.10.019; PMID: 26547401

52. Veselis, R.A., Arslan-Carlon, V., (2021). Sedation: is it sleep, is it amnesia, what's the difference? In Mason KP, ed., *Pediatric Sedation Outside of the Operating Room.* Cham: Springer, 2021, 223–45. https://doi.org/10.1007/978-3-030-58406-1_14

53. Sulton C, McCracken C, Simon HK, et al. Pediatric procedural sedation using dexmedetomidine: a report from the Pediatric Sedation Research Consortium. *Hosp Pediatr.* 2016;6(9):536–44. doi:10.1542/hpeds.2015-0280; PMID:27516413

54. Green SM, Andolfatto G, Krauss B. Ketofol for procedural sedation? Pro and con. *Ann Emerg Med.* 2011;57(5):444–8. doi:10.1016/j.annemergmed.2010.12.009; PMID:21237532

55. Prescilla RP (2021). Clinical pharmacology of sedatives, reversal agents, and adjuncts. In Mason KP, ed., *Pediatric Sedation Outside of the Operating Room.* Cham: Springer, 2021, 171–97. https://doi.org/10.1007/978-3-030-58406-1_11

56. Green SM, Andolfatto G, Krauss BS. Ketofol for procedural sedation revisited: pro and con. *Ann Emerg Med.* 2015;65(5):489–91. doi:10.1016/j.annemergmed.2014.12.002; PMID:25544732

57. Weisz K, Bajaj L, Deakyne SJ, et al. Adverse events during a randomized trial of ketamine versus co-administration of ketamine and propofol for procedural sedation in a pediatric emergency department. *J Emerg Med.* 2017;53 (1):1–9. doi:10.1016/j.jemermed.2017.03.024; PMID:28433211

58. Louer R, McKinney RC, Abu-Sultaneh S, Lutfi R, Abulebda K. Safety and efficacy of a propofol and ketamine based procedural sedation protocol in children with cerebral palsy undergoing botulinum toxin injections. PM R. 2019;11(12):1320–1325. doi:10.1002/pmrj.12146; PMID:30761757

59. Foo TY, Mohd Noor N, Yazid MB, et al. Ketamine–propofol (ketofol) for procedural sedation and analgesia in children: a systematic review and meta-analysis. *BMC Emerg Med.* 2020;20(1):81. doi:10.1186/s12873-020-00373-4; PMID:33032544

60. Tobias JD. Dexmedetomidine and ketamine: an effective alternative for procedural sedation? *Pediatr Crit Care Med.* 2012;13(4):423–7. doi:10.1097/PCC.0b013e318238b81c; PMID:22067985

61. Galinkin JL, Janiszewski D, Young CJ, et al. Subjective, psychomotor, cognitive, and analgesic effects of subanesthetic concentrations of sevoflurane and nitrous oxide. *Anesthesiology.* 1997;87(5):1082–8. doi:10.1097/00000542-199711000-00012; PMID:9366460

62. Janiszewski DJ, Galinkin JL, Klock PA, et al. The effects of subanesthetic concentrations of sevoflurane and nitrous oxide, alone and in combination, on analgesia, mood, and psychomotor performance in healthy volunteers. *Anesth Analg.* 1999;88(5):1149–54.

doi:10.1097/00000539-199905000-00034; PMID: 10320186

63. Tobias JD. Therapeutic applications and uses of inhalational anesthesia in the pediatric intensive care unit. *Pediatr Crit Care Med.* 2008;9(2):169–79. doi:10.1097/PCC.0b013e31816688ef; PMID:18477930

64. Sury M, Bullock I, Rabar S, Demott K, Guideline Development Group. Sedation for diagnostic and therapeutic procedures in children and young people: summary of NICE guidance. *BMJ.* 2010;341:c6819. doi:10.1136/bmj.c6819; PMID:21163835

65. National Institute for Health and Care Excellence. Sedation in under 19s: using sedation for diagnostic and therapeutic procedures, 2010. www.nice.org.uk/guidance/cg112.

66. Cravero JP, Roback MG. Selection of medications for pediatric procedural sedation outside of the operating room. Topic 85542 Version 32.0. In *UpToDate*, Stack AM, Randolph AG, eds. www.uptodate.com/contents/selection-of-medications-for-pediatric-procedural-sedation-outside-of-the-operating-room (accessed June 2, 2022)

67. Cravero JP, Roback MG. Selection of medications for pediatric procedural sedation outside of the operating room. Society guideline links: procedural sedation in children. Topic 126190, Version 12.0. In *UpToDate*, Stack AM, Randolph AG, eds. www.uptodate.com/contents/selection-of-medications-for-pediatric-procedural-sedation-outside-of-the-operating-room (accessed June 2, 2022)

68. Andropoulos DB. Sedation scales and discharge criteria: how do they differ? Which one to choose? Do they really apply to sedation? In Mason KP, ed., *Pediatric Sedation Outside of the Operating Room.* Cham: Springer, 2021, 83–94. https://doi.org/10.1007/978-3-030-58406-1_5

69. Kamat P, Tobias JD. Sedation in the pediatric intensive care unit: challenges, outcomes, and future strategies in the United States. In Mason, KP, ed., *Pediatric Sedation Outside of the Operating Room.* Cham: Springer, 2021, 345–72. https://doi.org/10.1007/978-3-030-58406-1_19

70. Egbuta C, Mason KP. Current state of analgesia and sedation in the pediatric intensive care unit. *J Clin Med.* 2021;10 (9):1847. doi:10.3390/jcm10091847; PMID:33922824

71. Sury MR, Bould MD. Defining awakening from anesthesia in infants: a narrative review of published descriptions and scales of behavior. *Paediatr Anaesth.* 2011;21(4):364–72. doi: 10.1111/j.1460-9592.2011.03538.x; PMID:21324047

72. Chernik DA, Gillings D, Laine H. Validity and reliability of the Observer's Assessment of Alertness/Sedation Scale: study with intravenous midazolam. *J Clin Psychopharmacol.* 1990;10(4):244–51. PMID:2286697

73. Shannon M, Albers G, Burkhart K, et al. Safety and efficacy of flumazenil in the reversal of benzodiazepine-induced conscious sedation. The Flumazenil Pediatric Study Group. *J Pediatr.* 1997;131(4):582–6. doi:10.1016/s0022-3476(97)70066-0; PMID:9386663

74. Madan R, Kapoor I, Balachander S, Kathirvel S, Kaul HL. Propofol as a sole agent for paediatric day care diagnostic ophthalmic procedures: comparison with halothane anaesthesia. *Paediatr Anaesth.* 2001;11(6):671–7. doi:10.1046/j.1460-9592.2001.00741.x; PMID:11696142

75. Malviya S, Voepel-Lewis T, Tait AR, et al. Depth of sedation in children undergoing computed tomography: validity and reliability of the University of Michigan Sedation Scale (UMSS). *Br J Anaesth.* 2002;88(2):241–5. doi:10.1093/bja/88.2.241; PMID:11878656

76. Sadhasivam S, Ganesh A, Robison A, Kaye R, Watcha MF. Validation of the bispectral index monitor for measuring the depth of sedation in children. *Anesth Analg.* 2006;102(2):383–8. doi:10.1213/01.ANE.0000184115.57837.30. PMID:16428529

77. Yuen VM, Irwin MG, Hui TW, Yuen MK, Lee LH. A double-blind, crossover assessment of the sedative and analgesic

effects of intranasal dexmedetomidine. *Anesth Analg.* 2007;105(2):374-80. doi:10.1213/01.ane.0000269488.06546.7c; PMID:17646493

78. Liu Y, Yu Q, Sun M, Median effective dose of intranasal dexmedetomidine sedation for transthoracic echocardiography examination in postcardiac surgery and normal children: an up-and-down sequential allocation trial. *Eur J Anaesthesiol.* 2018;35(1):43–8. doi:10.1097/EJA.0000000000000724; PMID:28937531

79. Shields CH, Styadi-Park G, McCown MY, Creamer KM. Clinical utility of the bispectral index score when compared to the University of Michigan Sedation Scale in assessing the depth of outpatient pediatric sedation. *Clin Pediatr (Phila).* 2005;44(3):229–36. doi:10.1177/000992280504400306; PMID:15821847

80. Su F, Nicolson SC, Zuppa AF. A dose-response study of dexmedetomidine administered as the primary sedative in infants following open heart surgery. *Pediatr Crit Care Med.* 2013;14(5):499–507. doi:10.1097/PCC.0b013e31828a8800; PMID:23628837

81. Kaplan E, Shifeldrim A, Kraus D, et al. Intranasal dexmedetomidine vs oral triclofos sodium for sedation of children with autism undergoing electroencephalograms. *Eur J Paediatr Neurol.* 2022;37:19–24. doi:10.1016/j.ejpn.2022.01.005; PMID:35016051

82. Hoeffe J, Doyon Trottier E, Bailey B, et al. Intranasal fentanyl and inhaled nitrous oxide for fracture reduction: the FAN observational study. *Am J Emerg Med.* 2017;35(5):710–15. doi:10.1016/j.ajem.2017.01.004; PMID:28190665

83. Tsze DS, Ieni M, Fenster DB, et al. Optimal volume of administration of intranasal midazolam in children: a randomized clinical trial. *Ann Emerg Med.* 2017;69(5):600–9. doi:10.1016/j.annemergmed.2016.08.450. PMID:27823876

84. Jang YE, Ji SH, Lee JH, et al. The relationship between the effect-site concentration of propofol and sedation scale in children: a pharmacodynamic modeling study. *BMC Anesthesiol.* 2021;21(1):222. doi:10.1186/s12871-021-01446-y; PMID:34503455

85. Lozano-Díaz D, Valdivielso Serna A, Garrido Palomo R, et al. Validation of the Ramsay scale for invasive procedures under deep sedation in pediatrics. *Paediatr Anaesth.* 2021;31(10):1097–104. doi:10.1111/pan.14248; PMID:34173295

86. Hoffman GM, Nowakowski R, Troshynski TJ, Berens RJ, Weisman SJ. Risk reduction in pediatric procedural sedation by application of an American Academy of Pediatrics/American Society of Anesthesiologists process model. *Pediatrics.* 2002;109(2):236–43. doi:10.1542/peds.109.2.236; PMID:11826201

87. Jeleazcov C, Schmidt J, Schmitz B, Becke K, Albrecht S. EEG variables as measures of arousal during propofol anaesthesia for general surgery in children: rational selection and age dependence. *Br J Anaesth.* 2007;99(6):845–54. doi:10.1093/bja/aem275; PMID:17965418

88. Herd DW, Anderson BJ, Keene NA, Holford NH. Investigating the pharmacodynamics of ketamine in children. *Paediatr Anaesth.* 2008;18(1):36–42. doi:10.1111/j.1460-9592.2007.02384.x; PMID:18095964

89. Cravero JP, Blike GT, Surgenor SD, Jensen J. Development and validation of the Dartmouth Operative Conditions Scale. *Anesth Analg.* 2005;100(6):1614–21. doi:10.1213/01.ANE.0000150605.43251.84; PMID:15920183

90. Trummel JM, Surgenor SD, Cravero JP, Gordon SR, Blike GT. Comparison of differing sedation practice for upper endoscopic ultrasound using expert observational analysis of the procedural sedation. *J Patient Saf.* 2009;5(3):153–9. doi:10.1097/PTS.0b013e3181b53f80; PMID:19927048

91. Chandran V, Jagadisan B, Ganth B. Validation of Adapted Dartmouth Operative Conditions Scale for sedation during pediatric

esophagogastroduodenoscopy. *Paediatr Anaesth.* 2017;27(6):621–8. doi:10.1111/pan.13127; PMID:28370856

92. Cravero JP, Askins N, Sriswasdi P, Validation of the Pediatric Sedation State Scale. *Pediatrics.* 2017;139(5):e20162897. doi:10.1542/peds.2016-2897; PMID:28557732

93. Poonai N, Coriolano K, Klassen T, et al. Adaptive randomised controlled non-inferiority multicentre trial (the Ketodex Trial) on intranasal dexmedetomidine plus ketamine for procedural sedation in children: study protocol. *BMJ Open.* 2020;10(12):e041319. doi:10.1136/bmjopen-2020-041319; PMID:33303457

94. Vet NJ, Kleiber N, Ista E, de Hoog M, de Wildt SN. Sedation in critically ill children with respiratory failure. *Front Pediatr.* 2016;4:89. doi:10.3389/fped.2016.00089; PMID:27606309

95. Thompson C, Shabanova V, Giuliano JS Jr. The SNAP index does not correlate with the State Behavioral Scale in intubated and sedated children. *Paediatr Anaesth.* 2013;23(12):1174–9. doi:10.1111/pan.12258; PMID:24103039

96. Smith HAB, Besunder JB, Betters KA, 2022 Society of Critical Care Medicine clinical practice guidelines on prevention and management of pain, agitation, neuromuscular blockade, and delirium in critically ill pediatric patients with consideration of the ICU environment and early mobility. *Pediatr Crit Care Med.* 2022;23(2):e74–110. doi:10.1097/PCC.0000000000002873; PMID:35119438

97. Emrath ET, Stockwell JA, McCracken CE, Simon HK, Kamat PP. Provision of deep procedural sedation by a pediatric sedation team at a freestanding imaging center. *Pediatr Radiol.* 2014;44(8):1020–5. doi:10.1007/s00247-014-2942-z; PMID:24859263

98. Callahan MJ, Cravero JP. Should I irradiate with computed tomography or sedate for magnetic resonance imaging? *Pediatr Radiol.* 2022;52(2):340–4. doi:10.1007/s00247-021-04984-2; PMID:33710404

99. Etzel-Hardman D, Kapsin K, Jones S, Churilla H. Sedation reduction in a pediatric radiology department. *J Healthc Qual.* 2009;31(4):34–9. doi:10.1111/j.1945-1474.2009.00035.x; PMID:19753806

100. Wang E, Thomas JJ, Rodriguez ST, Kennedy KM, Caruso TJ. Virtual reality for pediatric periprocedural care. *Curr Opin Anaesthesiol.* 2021;34(3):284–91. doi:10.1097/ACO.0000000000000983; PMID: 33935176

101. Slovis TL. Sedation and anesthesia issues in pediatric imaging. *Pediatr Radiol.* 2011;41(Suppl 2):514–6. doi:10.1007/s00247-011-2115-2; PMID:21847732

102. Berkenbosch JW. Options and considerations for procedural sedation in pediatric imaging. *Paediatr Drugs.* 2015;17(5):385–99. doi:10.1007/s40272-015-0140-6; PMID:26156106

103. Ghai B, Jain K, Saxena AK, Bhatia N, Sodhi KS. Comparison of oral midazolam with intranasal dexmedetomidine premedication for children undergoing CT imaging: a randomized, double-blind, and controlled study. *Paediatr Anaesth.* 2017;27(1):37–44. doi:10.1111/pan.13010; PMID: 27734549

104. Mekitarian Filho E, Robinson F, de Carvalho WB, Gilio AE, Mason KP. Intranasal dexmedetomidine for sedation for pediatric computed tomography imaging. *J Pediatr.* 2015;166(5):1313–15. e1. doi:10.1016/j.jpeds.2015.01.036; PMID:25748567

105. Azizkhani R, Heydari F, Ghazavi M, et al. Comparing sedative effect of dexmedetomidine versus midazolam for sedation of children while undergoing computerized tomography imaging. *J Pediatr Neurosci.* 2020;15(3):245–51. doi:10.4103/jpn.JPN_107_19; PMID:33531939

106. Burger RK, Figueroa J, McCracken C, Mallory MD, Kamat PP. Sedatives used in children to obtain head CT in the emergency department. *Am J Emerg Med.* 2021;44:198–202. doi:10.1016/j.ajem.2020.02.035; PMID:32107128

107. Gupta A, Sen I, Bhardwaj N, et al. Prospective audit of sedation/anesthesia practices for children undergoing computerized tomography in a tertiary care institute. *J Anaesthesiol Clin Pharmacol.* 2020;36(2):156–61. doi:10.4103/joacp.JOACP_16_19; PMID:33013027

108. Practice advisory on anesthetic care for magnetic resonance imaging: an updated report by the American Society of Anesthesiologists Task Force on Anesthetic Care for magnetic resonance imaging. *Anesthesiology.* 2015;122 (3):495–520. doi:10.1097/ALN.0000000000000458; PMID: 25383571

109. Gorlin A, Hoxworth JM, Mueller J. Occupational hazards of exposure to magnetic resonance imaging. *Anesthesiology.* 2015;123(4):976–7. doi:10.1097/ALN.0000000000000826; PMID:26372135

110. Theys C, Wouters J, Ghesquière P. Diffusion tensor imaging and resting-state functional MRI-scanning in 5- and 6-year-old children: training protocol and motion assessment. *PLoS ONE.* 2014;9(4): e94019. doi:10.1371/journal.pone.0094019; PMID:24718364

111. Xu HS, Cavaliere RM, Min RJ. Transforming the imaging experience while decreasing sedation rates. *J Am Coll Radiol.* 2020;17(1 Pt A):46–52. doi:10.1016/j.jacr.2019.08.005; PMID:31570312

112. Jaimes C, Gee MS. Strategies to minimize sedation in pediatric body magnetic resonance imaging. *Pediatr Radiol.* 2016;46(6):916–27. doi:10.1007/s00247-016-3613-z; PMID:27229508

113. Berkenbosch JW, Wankum PC, Tobias JD. Prospective evaluation of dexmedetomidine for noninvasive procedural sedation in children. *Pediatr Crit Care Med.* 2005 ;6(4):435–9; quiz 440. doi:10.1097/01.PCC.0000163680.50087.93; PMID:15982430

114. Mason KP, Zurakowski D, Zgleszewski SE, et al. High dose dexmedetomidine as the sole sedative for pediatric MRI. *Paediatr Anaesth.* 2008;18(5):403–11. doi:10.1111/j.1460-9592.2008.02468.x; PMID:18363626

115. Siddappa R, Riggins J, Kariyanna S, Calkins P, Rotta AT. High-dose dexmedetomidine sedation for pediatric MRI. *Paediatr Anaesth.* 2011;21(2):153–8. doi:10.1111/j.1460-9592.2010.03502.x; PMID:21210884

116. Mason KP, Fontaine PJ, Robinson F, Zgleszewski S. Pediatric sedation in a community hospital-based outpatient MRI center. *AJR Am J Roentgenol.* 2012;198(2):448–52. doi:10.2214/AJR.11.7346; PMID:22268192.

117. Veselis R, Kelhoffer E, Mehta M, et al. Propofol sedation in children: sleep trumps amnesia. *Sleep Med.* 2016;27–28:115–20. doi:10.1016/j.sleep.2016.10.002; PMID: 27938911

118. Schmitz A, Weiss M, Kellenberger C, et al. Sedation for magnetic resonance imaging using propofol with or without ketamine at induction in pediatrics: a prospective randomized double-blinded study. *Paediatr Anaesth.* 2018;28 (3):264–74. doi:10.1111/pan.13315; PMID:29377404

119. Tug A, Hanci A, Turk HS, et al. Comparison of two different intranasal doses of dexmedetomidine in children for magnetic resonance imaging sedation. *Paediatr Drugs.* 2015;17(6):479–85. doi:10.1007/s40272-015-0145-1; PMID:26323489

120. Olgun G, Ali MH. Use of intranasal dexmedetomidine as a solo sedative for MRI of infants. *Hosp Pediatr.* 2018; hpeds.2017-0120. doi: 10.1542/hpeds.2017-0120; PMID: 29363517

121. Sulton C, Kamat P, Mallory M, Reynolds J. The use of intranasal dexmedetomidine and midazolam for sedated magnetic resonance imaging in children: a report from the Pediatric Sedation Research Consortium. *Pediatr Emerg Care.* 2020;36 (3):138–42. doi:10.1097/PEC.0000000000001199; PMID: 28609332

122. Gyanesh P, Haldar R, Srivastava D, et al. Comparison between intranasal dexmedetomidine and intranasal ketamine as premedication for procedural sedation in children undergoing MRI: a double-blind, randomized, placebo-controlled trial. *J Anesth.* 2014;28 (1):12–18. doi:10.1007/s00540-013-1657-x; PMID:23800984

123. Mason KP, Lubisch NB, Robinson F, Roskos R. Intramuscular dexmedetomidine sedation for pediatric MRI and CT. *AJR Am J Roentgenol.* 2011;197(3):720–5. doi:10.2214/AJR.10.6134; PMID:21862817

124. Miller J, Xue B, Hossain M, et al. Comparison of dexmedetomidine and chloral hydrate sedation for transthoracic echocardiography in infants and toddlers: a randomized clinical trial. *Paediatr Anaesth.* 2016;26(3):266–72. doi:10.1111/pan.12819; PMID:26616644

125. Reynolds J, Rogers A, Medellin E, Guzman JA, Watcha MF. A prospective, randomized, double-blind trial of intranasal dexmedetomidine and oral chloral hydrate for sedated auditory brainstem response (ABR) testing. *Paediatr Anaesth.* 2016;26(3):286–93. doi:10.1111/pan.12854; PMID: 26814038

126. Levit Y, Mandel D, Matot I. Frequency-specific auditory brainstem response testing with age-appropriate sedation. *Int J Pediatr Otorhinolaryngol.* 2018;108:73–9. doi:10.1016/j.ijporl.2018.02.028; PMID:29605369

127. Kandil AI, Ok MS, Baroch KA et al. Why a propofol infusion should be the anesthetic of choice for auditory brainstem response testing in children. *Anesth Analg.* 2022;134(4):802–9. doi:10.1213/ANE.0000000000005693; PMID:35113042.

128. Ahmed SS, Hicks S, Slaven JE, Nitu M. Intermittent bolus versus continuous infusion of propofol for deep sedation during ABR/nuclear medicine studies. *J Pediatr Intensive Care.* 2017;6 (3):176–81. doi:10.1055/s-0036-1597628; PMID:31073444

129. Stephen MC, Mathew J, Varghese AM, Kurien M, Mathew GA. A randomized controlled trial comparing intranasal midazolam and chloral hydrate for procedural sedation in children. *Otolaryngol Head Neck Surg.* 2015;153 (6):1042–50. doi:10.1177/0194599815599381; PMID:26286872

130. Merguerian PA, Corbett ST, Cravero J. Voiding ability using propofol sedation in children undergoing voiding cystourethrograms: a retrospective analysis. *J Urol.* 2006;176(1):299–302. doi:10.1016/S0022-5347(06)00584-2; PMID:16753428

131. Alizadeh A, Naseri M, Ravanshad Y, et al. Use of sedative drugs at reducing the side effects of voiding cystourethrography in children. *J Res Med Sci.* 2017;22:42. doi:10.4103/1735-1995.202139; PMID:28465701

132. Rao J, Kennedy SE, Cohen S, Rosenberg AR. A systematic review of interventions for reducing pain and distress in children undergoing voiding cystourethrography. *Acta Paediatr.* 2012;101(3):224–9. doi:10.1111/j.1651-2227.2011.02482.x; PMID:21981332

133. Murat I, Gall O, Tourniaire B. Procedural pain in children: evidence-based best practice and guidelines. *Reg Anesth Pain Med.* 2003;28(6):561–72. doi:10.1016/j.rapm.2003.08.023; PMID:14634949

134. Livingston M, Lawell M, McAllister N. Successful use of nitrous oxide during lumbar punctures: a call for nitrous oxide in pediatric oncology clinics. *Pediatr Blood Cancer.* 2017;64(11). doi:10.1002/pbc.26610; PMID:28475231

135. Goldman RD. Analgesia for lumbar puncture in infants and children. *Can Fam Physician.* 2019;65(3):192–4. PMID:30867175

136. Harris EA. Sedation and anesthesia options for pediatric patients in the radiation oncology suite. *Int J Pediatr.* 2010;2010:870921. doi:10.1155/2010/870921; PMID:20490268

137. Frei-Welte M, Weiss M, Neuhaus D, Ares C, Mauch J. Kinderanästhesie zur

Protonenbestrahlung: Medizin fern ab der Klinik [Pediatric anesthesia for proton radiotherapy: medicine remote from the medical centre]. *Anaesthesist.* 2012;61(10):906–14 (in German). doi:10.1007/s00101-012-2085-2; PMID:23053305

138. Mason KP, Robinson F, Fontaine P, Prescilla R. Dexmedetomidine offers an option for safe and effective sedation for nuclear medicine imaging in children. *Radiology.* 2013;267(3):911–7. doi: 10.1148/radiol.13121232; PMID: 23449958.

139. Mandell GA, Shalaby-Rana E, Gordon I. Society of Nuclear Medicine procedure guideline for pediatric sedation in nuclear medicine. January 5, 2003. http://s3 .amazonaws.com/rdcms-snmmi/files/ production/public/pg_ch31_0703.pdf.

140. Mason KP, Padua H, Fontaine PJ, Zurakowski D. Radiologist-supervised ketamine sedation for solid organ biopsies in children and adolescents. *AJR Am J Roentgenol.* 2009;192(5):1261–5. doi:10.2214/AJR.08.1743; PMID:19380549

141. Lightdale JR, Mahoney LB, Schwarz SM, Liacouras CA. Methods of sedation in pediatric endoscopy: a survey of NASPGHAN members. J Pediatr Gastroenterol Nutr. 2007;45(4):500–2. doi:10.1097/MPG.0b013e3180691168; PMID:18030225

142. Biber JL, Allareddy V, Allareddy V, Prevalence and predictors of adverse events during procedural sedation anesthesia-outside the operating room for esophagogastroduodenoscopy and colonoscopy in children: age is an independent predictor of outcomes. *Pediatr Crit Care Med.* 2015;16(8): e251–9. doi:10.1097/ PCC.0000000000000504; PMID:26218257

143. van Beek EJ, Leroy PL. Safe and effective procedural sedation for gastrointestinal endoscopy in children. *J Pediatr Gastroenterol Nutr.* 2012;54(2):171–85. doi:10.1097/MPG.0b013e31823a2985; PMID: 21975965

144. Cohen S, Glatstein MM, Scolnik D, et al. Propofol for pediatric colonoscopy: the experience of a large, tertiary care pediatric hospital. *Am J Ther.* 2014;21 (6):509–11. doi:10.1097/ MJT.0b013e31826a94e9; PMID:23567786

145. Amornyotin S, Aanpreung P, Prakarnrattana U, et al. Experience of intravenous sedation for pediatric gastrointestinal endoscopy in a large tertiary referral center in a developing country. *Paediatr Anaesth.* 2009;19 (8):784–91. doi:10.1111/j.1460-9592.2009.03063.x; PMID:19624366

146. ASGE Standards of Practice Committee, Lightdale JR, Acosta R, et al. Modifications in endoscopic practice for pediatric patients. *Gastrointest Endosc.* 2014;79(5):699–710. doi:10.1016/ j.gie.2013.08.014; PMID:24593951

147. ASGE Standards of Practice Committee, Early DS, Lightdale JR, et al. Guidelines for sedation and anesthesia in GI endoscopy. *Gastrointest Endosc.* 2018;87 (2):327–37. doi:10.1016/j.gie.2017.07.018; PMID:29306520

148. Kresz A, Mayer B, Zernickel M, Posovszky C. Carbon dioxide versus room air for colonoscopy in deeply sedated pediatric patients: a randomized controlled trial. *Endosc Int Open.* 2019;7 (2):E290–7. doi:10.1055/a-0806-7060; PMID:30705964

149. Hoffmann CO, Samuels PJ, Beckman E, et al. Insufflation vs intubation during esophagogastroduodenoscopy in children. *Paediatr Anaesth.* 2010;20 (9):821–30. doi:10.1111/j.1460-9592.2010.03357.x; PMID:20716074

150. Patino M, Glynn S, Soberano M, et al. Comparison of different anesthesia techniques during esophagogastroduedenoscopy in children: a randomized trial. *Paediatr Anaesth.* 2015;25(10):1013–9. doi:10.1111/ pan.12717; PMID:26184697

151. Rajasekaran S, Hackbarth RM, Davis AT, et al. The safety of propofol sedation for elective nonintubated esophagogastroduodenoscopy in pediatric patients. *Pediatr Crit Care Med.*

2014;15(6):e261–9. doi:10.1097/
PCC.0000000000000147;
PMID:24849145

152. Acquaviva MA, Horn ND, Gupta SK. Endotracheal intubation versus laryngeal mask airway for esophagogastroduodenoscopy in children. *J Pediatr Gastroenterol Nutr.* 2014;59(1):54–6. doi:10.1097/ MPG.0000000000000348; PMID:24637966

153. Hartjes KT, Dafonte TM, Lee AF, Lightdale JR. Variation in pediatric anesthesiologist sedation practices for pediatric gastrointestinal endoscopy. *Front Pediatr.* 2021;9:709433. doi:10.3389/fped.2021.709433; PMID:34458212

154. Cox CB, Laborda T, Kynes JM, Hiremath G. Evolution in the practice of pediatric endoscopy and sedation. *Front Pediatr.* 2021 14;9:687635. doi:10.3389/ fped.2021.687635; PMID:34336742

155. Ngamprasertwong P, Mahmoud M. Anesthesia for MRI enterography in children. *J Clin Anesth.* 2014;26(3):249. doi:10.1016/j.jclinane.2013.11.013; PMID:24806075

156. Mollard BJ, Smith EA, Lai ME, et al. MR enterography under the age of 10 years: a single institutional experience. *Pediatr Radiol.* 2016;46(1):43–9. doi:10.1007/ s00247-015-3431-8; PMID:26224108

157. Hartling L, Milne A, Foisy M, et al. What works and what's safe in pediatric emergency procedural sedation: an overview of reviews. *Acad Emerg Med.* 2016;23(5):519–30. doi:10.1111/ acem.12938; PMID:26858095

158. Bellolio MF, Puls HA, Anderson JL, et al. Incidence of adverse events in paediatric procedural sedation in the emergency department: a systematic review and meta-analysis. *BMJ Open.* 2016;6(6): e011384. doi:10.1136/bmjopen-2016- 011384; PMID:27311910

159. Bhatt M, Johnson DW, Chan J, et al. Risk factors for adverse events in emergency department procedural sedation for children. *JAMA Pediatr.* 2017;171

(10):957–64. doi:10.1001/ jamapediatrics.2017.2135; PMID:28828486

160. Bhatt M, Johnson DW, Taljaard M, et al. Association of preprocedural fasting with outcomes of emergency department sedation in children. *JAMA Pediatr.* 2018;172(7):678–85. doi:10.1001/ jamapediatrics.2018.0830. Erratum in *JAMA Pediatr.* 2018;172(8):787; PMID:29800944

161. Miller AF, Monuteaux MC, Bourgeois FT, Fleegler EW. Variation in pediatric procedural sedations across children's hospital emergency departments. *Hosp Pediatr.* 2018;8(1):36–43. doi: 10.1542/ hpeds.2017-0045; PMID:29233853

162. Sahyoun C, Cantais A, Gervaix A, et al. Pediatric Emergency Medicine Comfort and Analgesia Research in Europe (PemCARE) group of the Research in European Pediatric Emergency Medicine. Pediatric procedural sedation and analgesia in the emergency department: surveying the current European practice. *Eur J Pediatr.* 2021;180(6):1799–813. doi:10.1007/s00431-021-03930-6. Erratum in *Eur J Pediatr.* 2021 Feb 13; PMID:33511466

163. Poh YN, Poh PF, Buang SN, Lee JH. Sedation guidelines, protocols, and algorithms in PICUs: a systematic review. *Pediatr Crit Care Med.* 2014;15 (9):885–92. doi: 10.1097/ PCC.0000000000000255; PMID:25230314

164. Sperotto F, Mondardini MC, Dell'Oste C, et al. Pediatric Neurological Protection and Drugs (PeNPAD) Study Group of the Italian Society of Neonatal and Pediatric Anesthesia and Intensive Care (SARNePI). Efficacy and safety of dexmedetomidine for prolonged sedation in the PICU: a prospective multicenter study (PROSDEX). *Pediatr Crit Care Med.* 2020;21(7):625–36. doi:10.1097/ PCC.0000000000002350; PMID:32224830

165. Mondardini MC, Daverio M, Caramelli F, et al. Dexmedetomidine for prevention of opioid/benzodiazepine withdrawal

syndrome in pediatric intensive care unit: Interim analysis of a randomized controlled trial. *Pharmacotherapy.* 2022;42(2):145–53. doi:10.1002/phar.2654; PMID:34882826

166. Sperotto F, Giaretta I, Mondardini MC, et al. Ketamine prolonged infusions in the pediatric intensive care unit: a tertiary-care single-center analysis. *J Pediatr Pharmacol Ther.* 2021;26(1):73–80. doi:10.5863/1551-6776-26.1.73; PMID: 33424503

167. Mencía S, Palacios A, García M, et al. An exploratory study of sevoflurane as an alternative for difficult sedation in critically ill children. *Pediatr Crit Care Med.* 2018;19(7):e335–41. doi:10.1097/PCC.0000000000001538; PMID: 29557840

168. Eifinger F, Hünseler C, Roth B, et al. Observations on the effects of inhaled isoflurane in long-term sedation of critically ill children using a modified AnaConDa© system. *Klin Padiatr.* 2013;225(4):206–11. doi:10.1055/s-0033-1345173; PMID:23797368

169. Committee on Fetus and Newborn and Section on Anesthesiology and Pain Medicine. Prevention and management of procedural pain in the neonate: an update. *Pediatrics.* 2016;137(2): e20154271. doi:10.1542/peds.2015-4271; PMID: 26810788

170. Nasr VG, DiNardo JA. Sedation and analgesia in pediatric cardiac critical care. *Pediatr Crit Care Med.* 2016;17(8 Suppl 1):S225–31. doi:10.1097/PCC.0000000000000756; PMID:27490604

171. Stark A, Smith PB, Hornik CP, et al. Medication use in the neonatal intensive care unit and changes from 2010 to 2018. *J Pediatr.* 2022;240:66–71.e4. doi:10.1016/j.jpeds.2021.08.075; PMID:34481808

172. Snyers D, Tribolet S, Rigo V. Intranasal analgosedation for infants in the neonatal intensive care unit: a systematic review. *Neonatology.* 2022;119(3):273–84. doi:10.1159/000521949;PMID:35231912

173. Allegaert K, van den Anker J. Sedation in the neonatal intensive care unit: international practice. In Mason KP, ed., *Pediatric Sedation Outside of the Operating Room.* Cham: Springer, 2021, 305–43. https://doi.org/10.1007/978-3-030-58406-1_18

Additional Reading

Mason KP (ed.). *Pediatric Sedation Outside of the Operating Room: A Multispecialty International Collaboration.* Springer Nature, Switzerland, 3rd Ed. 2021. ISBN-9783030584061. 910 pp. https://doi.org/10.1007/978-3-030-58406-1

Tobias JD, Cravero JP, eds. *Procedural Sedation for Infants, Children, and Adolescents.* Elk Grove Village, IL: American Academy of Pediatrics, 2016.

Society for Pediatric Sedation (SPS) Podcast, accessible at: https://sps-podcast.captivate.fm/listen

Safety and Outcomes in Pediatric Sedation

Lisa Lee and Joel Stockman

Introduction

The need for pediatric sedation services has been increasing, as much as 10% per year [1]. In order to meet this need, there will be an increasing number of providers of various backgrounds who will be administering sedation in a non-operating room environment in the future. It is therefore necessary to adhere to standard guidelines for the safe administration of sedation to this special population. Compared to adults, the care of the pediatric patient is often complicated by the need for deeper levels of sedation to achieve therapeutic goals, and the physiologic and anatomic differences that make them more vulnerable to hypoxemia and respiratory arrest that could lead to subsequent cardiac arrest. The requirements for safe sedation have been well summarized by Coté [2]: There is a need for informed consent, a complete medical history, formal evaluation of the airway to anticipate any possible issues, review of fasting status, sufficient physiologic monitoring and staffing by providers who are not involved with the performance of the procedure and who are adequately trained to provided resuscitation if necessary.

The emphasis of this chapter is on safety, with a review of fasting, monitoring, and equipment guidelines set forth by various medical organizations with a vested interest in pediatrics. We also discuss outcomes of various studies on the administration of sedation in the pediatric patient and present some of the outcome data from the Pediatric Sedation Research Consortium. In addition, we address concerns regarding neurotoxicity of medications administered, pediatric syndromes that are of special concern in sedation, and common syndromes that are associated with airway compromise. Details on the pharmacology of specific drugs used in sedation and pediatric resuscitation protocols have been reviewed elsewhere in this book.

Monitoring Recommendations in Pediatric Sedation

While different specialties have set forth guidelines regarding monitoring requirements during sedation, fundamentally all have the common goal of detecting physiologic changes and alerting the provider to action to avoid possible adverse events (Table 24.1). All of these guidelines have a minimum requirement for the monitoring of heart rate and adequacy of respirations and gas exchange during the administration of sedation. These requirements can be met with some combination of ECG, pulse oximetry, non-invasive blood pressure cuff, and end-tidal carbon dioxide monitoring.

Both the American Academy of Pediatrics/American Academy of Pediatric Dentistry (AAP/AAPD) [3] and American College of Emergency Physicians (ACEP) [4] guidelines state that there had not been an established standard for the frequency of documentation of vital signs. The American Society of Anesthesiologists (ASA) [5] suggests that vital signs should be recorded every 5 minutes, so that the person administering the sedation is aware of acute changes or trends in the patient's status.

Interestingly, in a 2012 study on data collected by the Pediatric Sedation Research Consortium [6] on the frequency of use of various physiologic monitoring modalities showed a large degree of variation in the monitoring practices of pediatric sedation providers. In only 52% of cases were guidelines from one of these four societies adhered to. Most often (86% of cases) pulse oximetry measuring SpO_2 and blood pressure monitoring were used. The next most commonly used combination was SpO_2, blood pressure, and ECG which were used in 63% of pediatric sedation. This variation in practice may have been due to the practitioner's perceived level of risk based on the pharmacologic agent being used or the expected level of sedation to be achieved. Also, monitoring may have been limited to what equipment was readily available to the practitioner at the time. This study highlights the need for more consistent practice in monitoring.

In addition to the use of monitoring equipment, it is also highly recommended that necessary resuscitation equipment be readily available in case there are perturbations in the patient's physiologic status that require intervention. At minimum, there should be a method for administering supplemental oxygen via positive pressure available, such as an appropriate-sized self-inflating bag-valve mask device, suction, emergency resuscitation drugs (atropine, epinephrine, succinylcholine), equipment for establishing an airway (laryngoscope, endotracheal tube, laryngeal mask airway), equipment for establishing intravenous or intraosseous access and advanced cardiovascular life support- or pediatric advanced life support-trained personnel immediately available who have the skill with pediatric airways to perform interventions, should the patient become over-sedated, have an allergic reaction, or have respiratory or cardiac arrest.

Recommendations on Fasting Times in Pediatric Sedation

With regards to fasting status, both the AAP/AAPD and ACEP guidelines state that there have not been published guidelines on required fasting prior to the administration of sedation and available studies have been underpowered or otherwise limited. Since the majority of studies on aspiration risk have been based on studies involving general anesthesia, the AAP/AAPD recommends following the same fasting guidelines as those used for general anesthesia while the ACEP guidelines do not make any specific recommendations in regards to a required time. However, the AAP/AAPD, ASA, and ACEP all

Table 24.1 Monitoring guidelines

	Level of conscious ness	Respiratory rate	Oxygen saturation	Exhaled carbon dioxide	Heart rate	Blood pressure	Cardiac rhythm
AAP/ AAPD joint guidelines	Intermittent respiratory rate	Continuous pulse oximetry	End-tidal carbon dioxide monitor	Continuous pulse oximetry	Intermittent recording of blood pressure	+/− ECG depending on whether or not patient has cardiac disease
ACEP guidelines	Patient response	Capnometry	Pulse oximetry	Capnometry	Pulse oximetry	Recording of blood pressure	
ASA guidelines	Patient response	Observation or auscultation	Continuous pulse oximetry	+/− End-tidal capnography for moderate sedation, definite for deep sedation	By ECG or pulse oximetry	Intermittent recording of blood pressure	Continuous ECG

agree that the risk of aspiration, with consideration of the depth of sedation anticipated, needs to be balanced with the risk of not proceeding with an urgent/emergent procedure.

In a prospective observation study [7] of 107,947 pediatric patients with known nothing by mouth (nil per os; NPO) status who received sedation for a procedure or radiologic study, there was no demonstrable difference in rates of aspiration between those patients who were NPO compared to those who were not (odds ratio [OR], 0.81; 95% confidence interval [CI], 0.08 to 4.08). It was noted that infants with ASA physical status III or IV and those who had a gastroenterology diagnosis, airway, or gastrointestinal procedure were at a higher risk for a major complication such as cardiac arrest, aspiration, and unplanned admission. After adjusting for age, ASA physical status, propofol use, sedation provider, and emergent status, there was still no increased incidence of major complications associated with NPO status (OR, 0.75; 95% CI, 0.40 to 1.39). The incidence of aspiration in this study was low at about one aspiration in 10,000 cases, so this study was not powered to definitely state that NPO status was not associated with aspiration risk. However, it is the largest study available to date on this subject. As stated in the AAP/AAPD, ASA, and ACEP guidelines, the sedation provider should still weigh up the risks and benefits of administering sedation in children who do not meet the stricter NPO guidelines suggested for general anesthesia, keeping in mind that, for behavioral reasons, pediatric patients often require moderate to deep sedation in order to undergo a procedure or radiologic study.

Other Outcomes from the Pediatric Sedation Research Consortium Database

It has been suggested that pediatric sedation can be safely administered by anesthesiologists and non-anesthesiologists alike [1]. However, there are some considerations with patient selection where certain patient factors may necessitate general anesthesia and intubation to ensure safe administration of sedation. In a study published in 2011 [8], the Pediatric Sedation Research Consortium performed a multivariable logistic regression on data collected from 2004 to 2008 to determine risk factors associated with adverse events during propofol sedation. They found that the risk of a serious adverse event (e.g., airway obstruction, desaturation, apnea, laryngospasm, aspiration, unplanned admission, cardiac arrest, emergency anesthesia consult, unplanned intubation, or death) was associated with substantial underlying illness classified as ASA physical status greater than II, patients weighing less than 5 kg, use of anticholinergics, upper airway disease, history of prematurity, and concurrent administration of benzodiazepines, ketamine, and opioids. These findings highlight the need for caution with the use of multiple sedation medications at the same time and the need for careful selection of appropriate candidates for sedation. The ACEP guidelines suggest that reversal agents should be readily available if opioids and or benzodiazepines are used. Location also appears to play a role in the occurrence of adverse events, with dental suites and the cardiac catheterization laboratories having the highest risk [9]. Upper airway disorders with regards to sedation are discussed later in this chapter.

Neurotoxicity Concerns in Pediatric Sedation

A common parental concern regarding sedation, particularly if repeated episodes of sedation are necessary (i.e., burn dressing changes), is that the medications given may affect the long-term neurodevelopment of the child. In the late 1990s to early 2000s, a number of *in vitro* and *in vivo* animal studies suggested that the use of common anesthetic agents could cause neurotoxicity and therefore behavioral and cognitive changes affecting development. Nearly every agent used in sedation has been implicated, including ketamine [10, 11, 12], midazolam [13], propofol [14], and inhaled anesthetic agents [13, 15, 16]. The sole exception so far has been dexemedetomidine, which is an alpha-2 agonist that may be neuroprotective [17, 18]. Extrapolation of animal study data to human outcomes has been difficult because the vulnerable period, comparable length of exposure, and dose necessary to produce the same effects in children are not known. A number of retrospective cohort studies in children have been performed [19–25], but the conclusions on whether or not these agents influence neurodevelopment in young children are mixed and are confounded by the presence of other factors such as surgery or illness that may have contributed to changes in neurodevelopment.

So far, two recent prospective, randomized, controlled trials have not shown a difference in cognitive or behavioral changes at a later time in children exposed to an anesthetic agent at a young age versus those who were not (the GAS trial 2019 [26] and PANDA 2016 study [27]), but studies with longer-term follow-up and of those patients with repeated exposures are necessary to fully delineate the risk. The most recent consensus statement by Smart Tots [28] states that, "because most anesthetic drugs have been shown to cause injury in animal experiments, no specific medications or technique can be chosen that are safer than any other" and "decisions regarding the timing of a procedure requiring anesthesia should be discussed with all members of the care team as well as the family or caregiver before proceeding. The benefits of an elective procedure should always be weighed against all of the risks associated with anesthesia and surgery." The risk of exposure can also be minimized by timing and completing the procedure or study in a manner where the child is under sedation for the minimal amount of time that would be safe.

Pediatric Syndromes of Special Concern for Procedural Sedation

Obesity

Obesity is a widespread problem in the United States for both the young and old. According to the Centers for Disease Control and Prevention (CDC), pediatric obesity is defined as a body mass index greater than the 95th percentile for a given age and gender. As of a 2018 survey, 19.3% of children aged 2 to 19 years met the CDC definition of obesity, affecting 14.4 million children and adolescents [29]. Globally, 39 million children under the age of 5 were overweight or obese in 2020 [30]. Multiple studies show that obese children receiving general anesthesia are at greater risk for airway complications. Complications include difficulty with mask ventilation and laryngoscopy, as well as a greater likelihood for airway obstruction and desaturation throughout the intraoperative and postoperative period [31, 32, 33]. Scherrer et al. analyzed 28,792 children aged 24 months to 18 years within the Pediatric Sedation Research Consortium database and found that obese children are at a greater risk for sedation-related adverse events, such as airway obstruction, oxygen desaturation, increased secretions, and laryngospasm. Thus, airway intervention was utilized to a greater degree: manipulation to relieve obstruction, airway suctioning, and mask ventilation. Recovery from sedation tended to be longer. The authors also determined that obese children were more likely to have their procedures cancelled due to sedation-related complications [34]. Although obesity may be the child's only known health issue, obese children may have undiagnosed comorbidities such as hypertension, sleep apnea, type 2 diabetes, and asthma. Obese children may warrant further screening tests prior to their procedure including arterial blood pressure, ECG, a formal sleep study, respiratory function testing, and blood glucose measurement [35, 36].

Optimal drug dosing in this population is unclear. Burke et al. presented a retrospective study involving 10,498 overweight or obese children. They found that obese patients may have received a relative overdose if actual rather than lean body mass was used to determine drug dosing [37]. Few dosing strategies exist for obese children based on limited studies. Assumptions can be made based on adult data, for which lean body weight appears to be the optimal scaler for most anesthetics and opioid medications [38, 39].

Obstructive Sleep Apnea

The prevalence of childhood obstructive sleep apnea (OSA) is high, estimated between 1% and 6%, with a peak incidence occurring between 2 and 8 years of age. There is a second peak in adolescence, which is associated with obesity. The prevalence of OSA tends to be higher in obese children, and the severity parallels the degree of obesity [40, 41, 42]. OSA is defined as sleep-disordered breathing characterized by prolonged partial upper airway obstruction and/or intermittent complete obstruction that disturbs normal sleep patterns and leads to abnormal ventilation during sleep [43]. Children will experience fragmented sleep and recurrent hypoxemia and hypercarbia associated with episodic apnea. The severity of OSA is marked during polysomnography with the apnea/hypopnea index (AHI). Apnea is defined as the cessation of breathing, despite effort, for 10 seconds. Hypopnea occurs when there is a 50% reduction in airflow, which is associated with a 3% drop in oxygen saturation. Pediatric OSA is categorized as mild (AHI 1–5), moderate (AHI 6–10), or severe (AHI >10). Although polysomnography remains the gold standard for OSA detection, its use is prohibited by cost, availability, and reliability. McKenzie et al. found that 95% of obese children with significant OSA will be identified if they report apnea or restless sleep, or if there is significant tonsillar hypertrophy present on physical examination [44]. Obesity, craniofacial abnormalities affecting the airway, and tonsillar hypertrophy predispose children to OSA. Children affected by OSA may experience night terrors, new-onset enuresis, restless sleep, increased respiratory effort during sleep, or intermittent vocalization during sleep. The child may be difficult to arouse in the morning, unusually tired during the day, and may fall asleep in non-stimulating environments despite getting a full night's sleep. Furthermore, the child may be irritable, aggressive, or have difficulty maintaining concentration [41].

As in normal sleep, sedation will promote the collapse of the upper airway. Children with OSA are especially at risk for sedative and opioid-induced upper-airway obstruction and respiratory depression. If subjected to moderate sedation, ventilation should be continuously monitored with capnography. Deep sedation should be avoided, especially with regard to procedures near the airway. Added awareness should continue into the immediate post-procedure period.

Common Syndromes Associated with Airway Compromise

Clinicians rarely encounter difficult airways in children. The limited studies regarding this topic focus on findings occurring during the induction of general anesthesia. The difficult airway can be divided into two categories: (1) unexpected difficult face-mask ventilation with an incidence of approximately 6.6% (determined by the presence of at least two factors - the use of continuous positive airway pressure ≥ 5 cmH$_2$O, an oral airway, two-handed ventilation, desaturation $< 95\%$, or an unexpected increase in fraction of inspired oxygen requirement); and (2) unexpected difficult intubation (as characterized by a Cormack and Lehane grade III or IV laryngeal view) with an incidence of approximately 1.2% [45, 46]. In a study of 77,272 pediatric general anesthesia cases carried out with a supraglottic airway device, Jagannathan et al. found that the incidence of an expected difficult airway was 0.6% when the difficult airway marker was based on the International Statistical Classification of Diseases and Related Health Problems (ICD)-9 designation of diagnoses with diseases associated with a difficult airway (e.g., Pierre Robin, Treacher Collins, Goldenhar syndromes, etc.) [47].

Syndromes associated with craniofacial abnormalities can pose serious risks with sedation, as these patients may experience difficult mask ventilation, difficult tracheal intubation, or both. Beyond the routine preoperative evaluation, assessment of a syndromic child should focus on the predictors of expected difficult airway: head and facial abnormalities (e.g., large or misshapen head, facial asymmetry, overbite, small mouth, reduced mouth opening, and large tongue), neck mobility (e.g., reduced movement or instability), or masses (of the neck or oral cavity). Any abnormal features of the head and neck may also contribute to the presence of OSA, which is common in conjunction with certain syndromes [48]. A few relatively common syndromes are discussed here, and broken down by anatomical issue related to the airway. Syndromes associated with the neck include trisomy 21 and Klippel–Feil syndrome. Trisomy 21 (or Down syndrome) is known for atlanto-occipital joint instability, as well as an enlarged tongue. Children with Klippel–Feil syndrome have a stiff cervical spine, which impairs mobility during patient positioning. Syndromes featuring mandibular hypoplasia include Goldenhar, Pierre Robin, and Treacher Collins syndromes. Midface hypoplasia is seen in Crouzon syndrome and Apert syndrome. Children with mucopolysaccharidoses, which are infiltrative disorders such as Hunter syndrome and Hurler syndrome, are associated with a high prevalence of airway obstruction, restrictive pulmonary disease, and cardiovascular manifestations that predispose these patients to higher anesthetic risk [49, 50, 51]. Sedation for high-risk individuals should be undertaken in a setting with access to advanced airway equipment under the care of a pediatric anesthesiologist. Therefore, advanced screening is important to identify and transfer a patient with an expected difficult airway to a tertiary care center if the need for sedation is anticipated.

Summary

Pediatric sedation services have been steadily increasing in the past few years. With this increase comes a need for cohesive guidelines to insure safe sedation administration. Monitoring guidelines all share the common goal of detecting physiologic changes to quickly alert the provider to take action as soon as possible to avoid an adverse event. Fasting guidelines exist to decrease the risk of aspiration, which typically follow the guidelines proposed for general anesthesia. Obesity and OSA are common in the pediatric population and put these children at increased risk for airway obstruction and subsequent desaturation while under sedation, requiring greater vigilance during the entire perioperative period. Procedures on children with syndromes associated with craniofacial abnormalities pose a great risk, and should be undertaken by experienced practitioners in a setting with access to advanced airway equipment.

References

1. Couloures, KG, Beach M, Cravero JP, Monroe KK, Hertzog JH. Impact of provider specialty on pediatric procedural sedation complication rates. *Pediatrics.* 2011;127:e1154

2. Coté CJ. Round and round we go: sedation – what is it, who does it and have we made things safer for children? *Pediatr Anesthes.* 2008;18:3–8.

3. American Academy of Pediatrics, American Academy of Pediatric Dentistry, Coté CJ, Wilson S. Guidelines for monitoring and management of pediatric patients during and after sedation for diagnostic and therapeutic procedures: an update. *Pediatrics.* 2006;118(6):2587–602. Reaffirmed January 2015.

4. Godwin SA, Caro DA, Wolf SJ, et al. Clinical policy: procedural sedation and analgesia in the emergency department. *Ann Emerg Med.* 2005;45(2):177–96.

5. American Society of Anesthesiologists Task Force on Sedation and Analgesia by Non-Anesthesiologists. Practice guidelines for sedation and analgesia by non-anesthesiologists. *Anesthesiology.* 2002;96(4):1004–17.

6. Langhan ML, Mallory M, Hertzog J, et al. Physiologic monitoring practices during pediatric procedural sedation: a report from the Pediatric Sedation Research Consortium. *Arch Pediatr Adolesc Med.* 2012;166(11):990–8. doi:10.1001/archpediatrics.2012.1023

7. Beach ML, Cohen DM, Gallagher SM, Cravero JP. Major adverse events and relationship to nil per os status in pediatric sedation/anesthesia outside the operating room: a report of the Pediatric Sedation Research Consortium. Anesthesiology. 2016;124(1):80–8.

8. Mallory MD, Baxter AL, Yanosky DJ, Cravero JP, Pediatric Sedation Research Consortium. Emergency physician-administered propofol sedation: a report on 25,433 sedations from the pediatric sedation research consortium. *Ann Emerg Med.* 2011;57(5):462–8.e1. doi:10.1016/j.annemergmed.2011.03.008

9. Grunwell JR, Travers C, Stormorken AG, et al. Pediatric procedural sedation using the combination of ketamine and propofol outside of the emergency department: a report from the Pediatric Sedation Research Consortium. *Pediatr Crit Care Med.* 2017;18(8):e356–63. doi:10.1097/PCC.0000000000001246; PMID:28650904

10. Ikonomidou C, Bosch F, Miksa M, et al. Blockade of NMDA receptors and apoptotic neurodegeneration in the developing brain. *Science.* 1999;283(5398):70–4.

11. Paule MG, Li M, Allen RR, et al. Ketamine anesthesia during the first week of life can cause long-lasting cognitive deficits in rhesus monkeys. *Neurotoxicol Teratol.* 2011;33(2):220–30.

12. Slikker W Jr, Zou X, Hotchkiss CE, et al. Ketamine-induced neuronal cell death in the perinatal rhesus monkey. *Toxicol Sci.* 2007;98(1):145–58.

13. Jevtovic-Todorovic V, Hartman RE, Izumi Y, et al. Early exposure to common anesthetic agents causes widespread neurodegeneration in the developing rat brain and persistent learning deficits. *J Neurosci.* 2003;23(3):876–82.

14. Briner A, Nikonenko I, De Roo M, et al. Developmental stage-dependent persistent impact of propofol anesthesia on dendritic spines in the rat medial prefrontal cortex. *Anesthesiology.* 2011;115(2):282–93.

15. Sanchez V, Feinstein SD, Lunardi N, et al. General anesthesia causes long-term impairment of mitochondrial morphogenesis and synaptic transmission in developing rat brain. *Anesthesiology.* 2011;115(5):992–1002.

16. Istaphanous GK, Ward CG, Nan X, et al. Characterization and quantification of isoflurane-induced developmental apoptotic cell death in mouse cerebral cortex. *Anesth Analg.* 2013;116(4):845–54.

17. Duan X, Li Y, Zhou C, Huang L, Dong Z. Dexmedetomidine provides neuroprotection: impact on ketamine-induced neuroapoptosis in the developing rat brain. *Acta Anaesthesiol Scand.* 2014;58(9):1121–6.

18. Sifringer M, von Haefen C, Krain M, et al. Neuroprotective effect of dexmedetomidine on hyperoxia-induced toxicity in the neonatal rat brain. *Oxid Med Cell Longev.* 2015;2015:530371.

19. Wilder RT, Flick RP, Sprung J, et al. Early exposure to anesthesia and learning disabilities in a population-based birth cohort. *Anesthesiology.* 2009;110(4):796–804.

20. Sprung J, Flick RP, Katusic SK, et al. Attention-deficit/hyperactivity disorder after early exposure to procedures requiring general anesthesia. Mayo Clinic Proceedings. 2012;87(2):120–9.

21. DiMaggio C, Sun LS, Li G. Early childhood exposure to anesthesia and risk of developmental and behavioral disorders in a sibling birth cohort. *Anesth Analg.* 2011;113(5):1143–51.

22. Hansen TG, Pedersen JK, Henneberg SW, et al. Academic performance in adolescence after inguinal hernia repair in infancy: a nationwide cohort study. *Anesthesiology.* 2011;114(5):1076–85.

23. Bartels M, Althoff RR, Boomsma DI. Anesthesia and cognitive performance in children: no evidence for a causal relationship. *Twin Res Hum Genet.* 2009;12(3):246–53.

24. Ing C, DiMaggio C, Whitehouse A, et al. Long-term differences in language and cognitive function after childhood exposure to anesthesia. *Pediatrics.* 2012;130(3):e476–85.

25. Ing CH, DiMaggio CJ, Malacova E, et al. Comparative analysis of outcome measures used in examining neurodevelopmental effects of early childhood anesthesia exposure. *Anesthesiology.* 2014;120(6):1319–32.

26. McCann ME, de Graaff JC, Dorris L, et al. Neurodevelopmental outcome at 5 years of age after general anaesthesia or awake-regional anaesthesia in infancy (GAS): an international, multicentre, randomised, controlled equivalence trial. *Lancet.* 2019;393(10172):664–677. doi:10.1016/S0140-6736(18)32485-1. Erratum in *Lancet.* 2019;394(10199):638. PMID: 30782342

27. Sun LS, Li G, Miller TL, et al. Association between a single general anesthesia exposure before age 36 months and neurocognitive outcomes in later childhood. *JAMA.* 2016;315(21):2312–20.

28. Smart Tots. Consensus statement on the use of anesthetic and sedative drugs in infants and toddlers (2015, October). https://smarttots.org/wp-content/uploads/2015/10/ConsensusStatementV910.5.2015.pdf

29. Centers for Disease Control and Prevention. Childhood obesity facts. www.cdc.gov/obesity/data/childhood.html (accessed January 9, 2022).

30. World Health Organization. Obesity and overweight. www.who.int/news-room/fact-sheets/detail/obesity-and-overweight (accessed January 9, 2022)

31. van Hoff SL, O'Neill ES, Cohen LC, Collins BA. Does a prophylactic dose of propofol reduce emergence agitation in children receiving anesthesia? A systematic review and meta-analysis. *Paediatr Anaesth.* 2015;25(7):689–97.

32. Nafiu OO, Green GE, Walton S, et al. Obesity and risk of peri-operative complications in children presenting for adenotonsillectomy. *Int J Pediatr Otorhinolaryngol.* 2009;73(1):89–95.

33. Nafiu OO, Reynolds PI, Bamgbade OA, et al. Childhood body mass index and

perioperative complications. *Paediatr Anaesth.* 2007:17(5): 426–30.

34. Scherrer PD, Mallory MD, Cravero JP, et al. The impact of obesity on pediatric procedural sedation-related outcomes: results from the Pediatric Sedation Research Consortium. *Paediatr Anaesh.* 2015;25(7):689–97.

35. Tait AR, Voepel-Lewis T, Burke C, et al. Incidence and risk factors for perioperative adverse respiratory events in children who are obese. *Anesthesiology.* 2008;108(3):375–80.

36. Owen J, John R. Childhood obesity and the anaesthetist. *Contin Educ Anaesth Crit Care Pain.* 2012;12(4):169–75.

37. Burke CN, Voepel-Lewis T, Wagner D. A retrospective description of anesthetic medication dosing in overweight and obese children. *Paediatr Anaesth.* 2014;24(8):857–62.

38. Ingrande J, Lemmens HJM. Dose adjustment of anaesthetics in the morbidly obese. *Br. J. Anaesth.* 2010;105 (Suppl 1):i16–23.

39. Kendrick JG, Carr RR, Ensom MHH. Pharmacokinetics and drug dosing in obese children. *J Pediatr Pharmacol Ther.* 2010;15(2):94–109.

40. Marcus C, Brooks L, et al. Diagnosis and management of childhood obstructive sleep apnea syndrome. *Pediatrics.* 2012;130(3);e714–55.

41. Practice guidelines for the perioperative management of patients with obstructive sleep apnea. *Anesthesiology.* 2014;120(2):1–19.

42. Patino M, Sadhasivam S, Mahmoud M. Obstructive sleep apnoea in children: perioperative considerations. *Brit J Anaesthia.* 2013;111(51):i83–95.

43. Kirk V, Kahn A, Brouillette RT. Diagnostic approach to obstructive sleep apnea in children. *Sleep Med Rev.* 1998;2(4):255–69.

44. McKenzie SA, Bhattacharya A, Sureshkumar R, et al. Which obese children should have a sleep study? *Respir Med.* 2008;102(11):1581–5.

45. Valois-Gomez T, Oofuvong M, Auer G, et al. Incidence of difficult bag-mask ventilation in children: a prospective observational study. *Paediatr Anaesth.* 2013;23(10):920–6.

46. Russo SG, Becke K. Expected difficult airway in children. *Curr Opin Anesthesiol.* 2015;28(3):321–6.

47. Jagannathan N, Sequera-Ramos L, Sohn L. Elective use of supraglottic airway for primary airway management in children with difficult airways. *Br. J. Anaesth.* 2013;112(4):742–8.

48. Mick NW. The difficult pediatric airway. www.uptodate.com.

49. Walker R, Balani KG, Bruce IA, et al. Anaesthesia and airway management in mucopolysaccharidosis. *J Inherit Metab Dis.* 2013;36(2):211–9.

50. Infisino A. Pediatric upper airway and congenital anomalies. *Anesthesiology Clin N Am.* 2002;20:747–66.

51. Raj D, Luginbuehl I. Managing the difficult airway in the syndromic child. *Contin Educ Anaesth Crit Care Pain.* 2014;15(1):1–7.

Chapter 25

Sedation in the Office and Other Outpatient Settings

Emily Goldenberg and Debra E. Morrison

Introduction

The office or outpatient setting as a site for procedures is, metaphorically, a small lifeboat (not a pirate ship!) on the high seas away from port and the mothership, far from immediate aid. Whether the site is a detached procedural area on the campus of a large medical center, or a procedure room in a physician's office, the metaphor is appropriate. The lifeboat and her crew must be capable and equipped to handle emergencies without immediate help from the outside. At a medical center, even a detached outpatient procedural area may have access to a rapid response team with rescue capabilities. However, such advanced emergency support teams will not be as close as they would be if the procedure were taking place in the main hospital. Help may be even more distant when working at a freestanding outpatient surgical suite or a physician's office, when the municipal emergency response system (911) must be activated. Therefore, the crew of the lifeboat must be prepared to perform the primary resuscitation as they are the first responders.

A shared culture of safety is essential to successful sedation in the office or outpatient setting. A standard policy and procedure document should be developed, followed, re-examined, and revised as needed. Whether the location or its parent organization undergoes official accreditation, the policy and procedure should align with national patient safety guidelines.

Patients and procedures should be appropriately selected for the specific setting where the procedure is to occur. Similarly, the plan for sedation should be appropriate to the patient, the procedure, and the setting. A pre-procedure safety checklist (time-out) should be developed and used consistently. Routine debriefings after each procedure allow for improvements to process, efficiency, and safety to be made.

The Team

The procedural team functioning independently must be highly skilled and experienced. In his book. *The Checklist Manifesto* [1], Dr. Atul Gawande discusses the importance of the team in healthcare, rather than the individuals who comprise it. The book's message is as much about teamwork as it is about checklists. Dr. Gawande explains, "In a world in which success now requires large enterprises, teams of clinicians, high-risk technologies, and knowledge that outstrips any one person's abilities, individual autonomy hardly seems the ideal we should aim for."

In many private offices, physicians perform procedures with the help of medical assistants. This is an adequate approach for procedures performed under local anesthesia. If minimal or moderate sedation is being used, however, a registered nurse (RN) or team of RNs with sedation education and experience is needed. The RN must be adequately equipped with medications for sedation (intravenous and oral), reversal agents, emergency medications, monitoring equipment, and equipment for immediate resuscitation. Both the RN and the physician should have current basic life support and advanced cardiac life support certification. There is no substitute for preparedness and experience, both of which allow the team to recognize potential problems early and prepare to intervene. Ideally, the RN administering sedation should be confident to command the attention of the physician in order to "stop the assembly line" and focus all care on the patient when necessary.

The RN must be aware of the details of each procedure in order to anticipate challenges or problems, while reading cues from both the physician and the patient in order to administer sedation safely. When the sedation nurse is involved with the preprocedural patient evaluation, they are familiar with and may develop rapport with the patient, and are able to advocate for them. The nurse who is administering sedation and monitoring the patient should not be responsible for assisting with the procedure to the degree that they are distracted from caring for the patient.

The physician should form a partnership with the nurse and lead the team in respect for the nurse, especially if they express concerns. A nurse who fears derision or dismissal may hesitate to speak up with concerns for the patient or may worry silently, potentially delaying successful intervention should a problem arise. The procedural physician may enter "the zone" while performing a procedure but should maintain a "third ear" open to communication from the RN administering sedation and monitoring the patient. Even at a critical period during the procedure, the physician should be able to acknowledge any communication from the nurse. The physician should plan well and anticipate necessary equipment and contingencies in advance, so that the procedure runs smoothly and in a timely manner.

Medical assistants, schedulers, and surgical technologists are integral members of the team. Their perceptions, impressions, patient interactions, and helping hands allow the process to proceed smoothly, safely, and successfully.

The procedural physician should take the lead to encourage team members to speak up and ensure that the environment is one of safe communication and not intimidation. Care revolves around the patient, not the procedure.

The Setting

The setting for any sedation procedure must be fully equipped and staffed with everything needed for the planned procedure, sedation, and immediate rescue and resuscitation.

If sedation procedures are infrequent in the outpatient setting, it is helpful to have easily accessible safety plans and reference guides to help with preparation. Important steps are more likely to be omitted without frequent practice. These plans list all equipment and medications needed as well as the emergency supplies that should be readily available. It is frustrating, inconvenient, and potentially dangerous to discover, when the procedure is underway, that a needed piece of equipment or medication cannot be obtained. Such delay may negatively influence team morale and may harm the patient. Remember, the more remote the location, the more diligent the preparation must be, since there are few or no immediate emergency resources.

Policy and Procedure

An appropriate policy and procedure should be developed, based on National Patient Safety Goals [2] and the Association of PeriOperative Registered Nurses (AORN) recommendations [3, 4].

Safety standards should be consistent with National Patient Safety Goals as outlined by the Joint Commission and the American Society of Anesthesiologists [2, 5, 6].

Procedure Selection

The procedural physician's scope of practice and the office's physical capabilities determine the range of procedures possible in a given setting. The physician should pare the list to include only those procedures that are appropriate for the office or outpatient setting. Complex procedures or those that require longer recovery time or delayed discharge are better suited for a different location.

Criteria for Selection

- Consider the length of each procedure and schedule only those that can be completed and fully recovered from in the period of a working day.
- If a procedure involves blood loss, schedule it in a facility where transfusion is an option.
- Procedures should be amenable to local anesthesia with minimal or moderate sedation. Procedures that require deeper sedation or anesthesia should be scheduled when and where anesthesia care can be provided.

Patient Selection

A patient's height, weight, medical and surgical diagnoses, and prescribed medications should be considered in patient selection, as well as the patient's comfort level with undergoing a procedure while awake. Avoid complications and sedation failure by selecting patients who are amenable to safe sedation in an office-based setting. Consider scheduling patients with the following characteristics for anesthesia care rather than sedation:

- obesity
- known difficult airway or significant craniofacial abnormalities
- obstructive sleep apnea
- coagulopathy
- heart or lung disease that is a threat to life

- significant neurologic disease
- history of anesthesia/sedation complications or sedation failure
- intolerance of medications routinely used for sedation
- routine medications or drugs that may react with sedation agents
- chronic pain or anxiety with a baseline need for analgesics or anxiolytics
- pediatric patients may not cooperate

Sedation Plan

The plan for sedation should be made according to the type and length of the procedure, using rapid-onset and short-acting agents. It is advisable in the outpatient setting to use agents such as fentanyl and midazolam that have readily available reversal agents. A relatively short-acting oral benzodiazepine such as alprazolam might be included as premedication. Diphenhydramine and ondansetron are helpful adjuncts for treating side effects of opioids. It is important that the physician and the nurse administering the sedation be familiar with the contraindications, actions, and adverse effects of all medications used, as well as with the reversal agents.

Reversal agent doses for each patient should be predetermined so that these medications may be administered quickly and accurately if needed. A hurried intravenous push of an incorrect dose may produce an adverse event in itself. Drug dosing calculators are available on the internet and in many electronic medical record systems. These calculators are commonly used for pediatric patients, but they are useful for all patients, saving time and preventing errors.

Many patients express the desire to be "knocked out" for a procedure. If this is the patient's expectation and the procedure is amenable to local anesthesia with minimal or moderate sedation, it is important to address the intended degree of sedation honestly, rather than misleading the patient. Some patients insist that they were unconscious during a similar procedure because they were not awake or do not recall being awake during the procedure. Evaluation, planning, discussion, and informed consent can take time but it is important to clarify expectations in advance.

Sometimes a short, relatively painless procedure can be done with local anesthetic alone. Anxiety may be treated with one dose of oral or intravenous medication, in addition to the local anesthetic. This would be considered minimal sedation. Music (with headphones if appropriate), virtual-reality glasses (if appropriate), and pleasant conversation ("verbal valium") are wonderful and safe adjuncts to pharmacologic sedation.

A patient may not want any sedation. In this case, the nurse may stand by to offer comfort, conversation, and reassurance that action will be taken if the patient needs something. A comfortable patient allows for a successful procedure. Every attempt should be made to make the patient comfortable and able to tolerate the procedure.

If moderate sedation is required for cooperation with a longer or more painful procedure, all assessments, monitors, staff, equipment, medications, and capacity to rescue must be present prior to beginning sedation. Deep sedation, monitored anesthesia care, or general anesthesia should not be administered in the outpatient office setting without an anesthesia provider.

Monitoring for all patients should include blood pressure, heart rate and rhythm, respiratory rate, oxygen saturation, level of sedation, and pain at least every 15 minutes or as indicated by the patient's condition. End-tidal carbon dioxide monitoring is strongly advised when procedures are performed in a dark room and/or when patients are at risk for apnea.

Recovery and Discharge

Recovery

There should be a safe physical space for recovery from sedation under the direct supervision of a sedation-qualified RN. The recovery area should be calm and quiet. It must be appropriately equipped with standard monitors, oxygen, non-rebreather face masks, nasal cannulas, suction, and other airway management devices such as masks, oral and nasal airways, laryngeal mask airways and intubation equipment, bag-valve masks, a crash cart, emergency medications, reversal agents, and intravenous fluids. If anesthesia is administered in the outpatient office setting, a malignant hyperthermia kit must be immediately available.

The recovery nurse may care for at most two patients at a time – either two recovering patients or one recovering patient and one pre-procedural patient. The nurse who is administering sedation is focused solely on that one patient.; they may not recover a second patient. A nurse should never be alone in an isolated area with a potentially unstable patient.

Patients should be monitored for at least 60 minutes after the last transmucosal, intramuscular, or intravenous drug administration, or until they have returned to their baseline mental status. During recovery, the patient's status should be assessed and documented at least every 15 minutes until the patient reaches the defined discharge criteria. If a reversal agent (flumazenil or naloxone) has been administered, the patient should be monitored for at least 2 hours following the last dose of the reversal agent in order to assess for possible re-narcotization or re-sedation.

Discharge

When the patient is ready for discharge, the patient and another responsible adult should be given written discharge instructions. After sedation medications, a patient who seems entirely oriented at discharge may forget what was explained to them after leaving the facility. Discharge instructions should include diet, activity, special care of the procedural wound, and names of all medications received. This is to ensure that if the patient needs to seek emergency care, the emergency providers may consider the events/medications associated with the procedure and render care appropriately. The patient should have a reliable adult escort them home and remain with the patient for the rest of the day and possibly overnight to monitor for any adverse post-procedure events. Discharge instructions should include conditions for seeking emergency care and post-procedure follow-up instructions. This written paperwork should be signed by the patient and witnessed by either a physician or a nurse prior to departure.

Contingency Plan

There is no substitute for preparation. Even if the outpatient setting is adequately equipped and staffed, unexpected or adverse events do occur. Errors may be made or patients may react in unexpected ways. It is important to recognize a problem immediately and to know when a situation is beyond the capabilities of the team.

In a remote office location, it is important to call for emergency ambulance services as soon as rescue measures are initiated. Time is critical to avoid permanent harm to a patient who suffers an adverse event during sedation. Low- or high-fidelity simulation of rare but life-threatening situations can help the entire team function effectively during a true crisis situation.

Summary

A highly skilled and experienced team is essential to providing safe sedation in an outpatient office setting. Both the procedure and the patient should be carefully selected prior to developing a plan for sedation. Development of a contingency plan is critical in a location distant from immediate aid.

References

1. Gawande A. *The Checklist Manifesto: How to Get Things Right.* New York, NY: Metropolitan Books, 2009.

2. Joint Commission. Hospital: 2024 National Patient Safety Goals. www.jointcommission.org/standards/national-patient-safety-goals/hospital-national-patient-safety-goals

3. AORN. AORN position statement on a healthy perioperative practice environment. www.aorn.org

4. AORN. AORN position statements on perioperative registered nurse circulator dedicated to every patient undergoing an operative or other invasive procedure. www.aorn.org

5. American Society of Anesthesiologists Task Force on Preanesthesia Evaluation. Practice advisory for preanesthesia evaluation: an updated report by the American Society of Anesthesiologists Task Force on Preanesthesia Evaluation. *Anesthesiology* 2012;116:522–38.

6. American Society of Anesthesiologists Task Force on Preanesthesia Evaluation. Practice guidelines for moderate procedural sedation and analgesia 2018: a Report by the American Society of Anesthesiologists Task Force on Moderate Procedural Sedation and Analgesia, the American Association of Oral and Maxillofacial Surgeons, American College of Radiology, American Dental Association, American Society of Dentist Anesthesiologists, and Society of Interventional Radiology. *Anesthesiology* 2018; 128: 437–79.

Additional Reading

Catchpole K, Mishra A, Handa A, McCulloch P. Teamwork and error in the operating room: analysis of skills and roles. *Ann Surg.* 2008;247:699–706.

Jani SR, Shapiro FE, Gabriel RA, et al. A comparison between office and other ambulatory practices: analysis from the National Anesthesia Clinical Outcomes Registry. *J Healthc Risk Manag.* 2016; 35(4):38–47.

Nestel D, Kidd J. Nurses' perceptions and experiences of communication in the operating theatre: a focus group interview. *BMC Nurs.* 2006;5 1.

Ogg M, Burlingame B. Clinical issues: recommended practices for moderate sedation/analgesia. *AORN J.* 2008;88:275–7.

Reynolds A, Timmons S. The doctor–nurse relationship in the operating theatre. *Br J Perioper Nurs.* 2005;15:110–15.

Shapiro FE, Jani SR, Liu X, Dutton RP, Urman RD. Initial results from the National Anesthesia Clinical Outcomes Registry and overview of office-based anesthesia. *Anesthesiol Clin.* 2014; 32(2):431–44.

Shapiro FE, Punwani N, Rosenberg NM, et al. Office-based anesthesia: safety and outcomes. *Anesth Analg.* 2014;119(2):276–85.

Chapter 26

Sedation in Dentistry

Alan D. Kaye, Ghali. E. Ghali, Elyse M. Cornett, and Charles J. Fox III

Introduction

Modern dentistry has made much progress in pain control and in providing a patient-friendly service, which has expanded the dentist's ability to perform a wide range of treatments in a pain-free environment. Nevertheless, despite revolutionary new dental techniques, it is well recognized in the dental literature that substantial fear exists concerning seeking dental care. This fear can be so extensive that people from all races and socioeconomic categories can be affected by it in some form.

The literature shows that approximately 15% of the US population fears the dentist enough to avoid care completely. Among dental patients who regularly seek care, as many as 50% report some level of fear and anxiety toward their dental experiences and view many of the routine procedures in a dental office as *frightening* [1, 2]. These results are supported by the recent survey released by the American Association of Endodontists (AAE) [3]. Not surprisingly, the report from the AAE shows that fear of pain is the root cause, more so than previous experiences. For the purpose of definition, there is a difference between fear and anxiety. Fear refers to a response to an immediate event, whereas anxiety is a response to an anticipated event.

Levels of Anxiety/Phobia in Dentistry

The levels of anxiety in the typical dental patient can be classified into severe, moderate, or low to moderate.

Severe dental anxiety: These patients are rare, but create a dual problem for the dentist and the dental team. They delay treatment to the extreme. Now, instead of only treating the physiological concern (pain and/or infection), we must treat a psychological emergency as well. The dental pain is exacerbated by the patient's fear of pain, creating a vicious cycle. If the patient's fear is not addressed, treating the dental problem only creates more stress and increased frustration for the dentist and dental team while furthering the fear and distrust felt by the patient.

Moderate dental anxiety: These patients are the easiest to identify, as they will typically avoid routine care but usually will come to the office with problems before they become emergencies. Their signs of anxiety and/or fear will be somewhat obvious: rescheduling routine care and signs and symptoms of anxiety in the waiting room and dental chair. These patients may sit in the chair, but they will be hyperresponsive to tactile stimulation and the clinician may require permission to perform even a routine dental examination [4].

Low to moderate dental anxiety: Patients with low to moderate dental anxiety are the most common patients seen in the dental office [4]. These are patients who have no irrational fears of dentistry; however, they do feel some form of anxiety as the day approaches. This fear does not prevent them from coming in, because the desire to maintain oral hygiene and health, and/or to obtain relief from pain, overrides any fear of avoidance, because they know the consequences. However, while in the dental office, this patient has some signs of anxiety: sweaty palms, tachycardia – and admittedly would much rather be somewhere else.

The many techniques of behavioral modification, iatrosedation, and pharmacologic intervention can help control fear and anxiety in dental patients [5]. Although a number of behavioral techniques are available for the treatment of dental fear, minimal/moderate sedation and general anesthesia are the mainstay to provide dental treatment to phobic patients [1] (Figure 26.1).

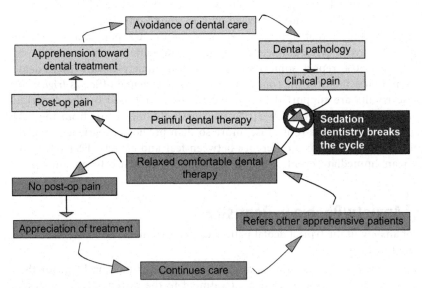

Figure 26.1 Breaking the vicious cycle: the role of sedation in dentistry.

Sedation in Dentistry: Aims and Indications

The following general goals can be achieved with the use of various sedation methods:

- reduced anxiety and fear
- analgesia
- amnesia
- control secretions
- monitor safely blood pressure, ventilation, oxygenation, ECG, and temperature
- counteract hyperactive gag reflex
- allow for lengthy and difficult dental procedures
- enable treatment of medically compromised patients (unable to tolerate the stress of the dental visit)
- enable treatment of special populations:
  - developmentally disabled patients
  - children

History of Sedation in Dentistry

Anxiety and pain control for medical and dental surgery began with two dentists in the nineteenth century. In 1844 Horace Wells discovered the use of nitrous oxide as an anesthetic, and in 1846 William T. G. Morton was the first to successfully demonstrate anesthesia to the medical establishment, using ether.

In the twentieth century, several dentists, including Allison, Hubbell, and Monheim, advanced the training and practice of general anesthesia in dentistry. Other dentists, including Jorgensen, Driscoll, and Trieger, recognized the potential of combining the ideal sedative and amnesic effects of general anesthetic drugs with the analgesic effects of local anesthetics. They became advocates of moderate (conscious) sedation, which produced an altered state of consciousness, analgesia, and amnesia without producing unconsciousness. By the end of the twentieth century, the dental profession had developed several different anxiety and pain control options, including local anesthesia alone; minimal, moderate, and deep sedation with local anesthesia; and general anesthesia [6].

Guidelines, Rules, and Regulations

According to the American Dental Association (ADA), the administration of local anesthesia, sedation, and general anesthesia is an integral part of dental practice [7]. A number of organizations – including the ADA, the American Association of Oral and Maxillofacial Surgeons (AAOMS), the American Academy of Pediatric Dentistry, the American Academy of Periodontology, and the American Dental Society of Anesthesiology – have developed strict guidelines for the use of anesthesia and sedation in the dental setting by appropriately educated and trained dentists. The goal of these guidelines is to assist dentists in the delivery of safe and effective sedation and anesthesia. The existing guidelines incorporate definitions, educational requirements, clinical guidelines for the dentist and auxiliary personnel, including patient evaluation, preoperative preparation, personnel and equipment requirements, monitoring and documentation, recovery and discharge, emergency management, and the management of children [7–12].

Dentists providing sedation and anesthesia should also be in compliance with their state rules and regulations. Most state dental boards require dentists to have additional training (postgraduate residency or continuing education) in order to be licensed to provide nitrous oxide sedation, minimal and moderate sedation via enteral (oral) or parenteral routes, and/or general anesthesia. The legislation by state board typically focuses on the *intent* of sedation by dentists, and also takes into consideration the route of administration. Minimal sedation (anxiolysis) and moderate sedation by the enteral route are the most commonly used methods, followed by moderate/deep sedation via the parenteral route, and then general anesthesia. The ADA has adopted the definitions of the American Society of Anesthesiologists [13], and the ADA's definitions of levels of sedation are as set out as follows [7].

Levels of Sedation

Minimal Sedation (Anxiolysis)

According to the American Society of Anesthesiologists (ASA) and the American Society of Dentist Anesthesiologists [14, 15], minimal sedation is "a minimally depressed level of consciousness, produced by a pharmacologic method, that retains the patient's ability to independently and continuously maintain an airway and respond normally to tactile stimulation and verbal command. Although cognitive function and coordination may be modestly impaired, ventilatory and cardiovascular functions are unaffected."

The drug(s) and/or techniques used should carry a margin of safety wide enough never to render unintended loss of consciousness and the appropriate initial dose of a single drug should never exceed the maximum recommended dose (MRD) prescribed for unmonitored home use [14, 15].

Typically, a patient can take a single dose of a drug at home the night before the appointment (optional), and a second dose of the same or a different drug can be administered by the dentist on the morning of the appointment [4]. This technique may be used in combination with nitrous oxide and still be considered minimal sedation, but it should be noted that this combination may be capable of producing higher levels of sedation including moderate, deep, or general anesthesia. Once a patient's only response is reflex withdrawal from repeated painful stimuli, this is no longer considered minimal sedation [7].

According to the ADA guidelines, "The use of preoperative sedatives for children (aged 12 and under) prior to arrival in the dental office, except in extraordinary situations, must be avoided due to the risk of unobserved respiratory obstruction during transport by untrained individuals" [7]. Oral sedation can be challenging to titrate in children, rendering it easier to obtain a moderate level of sedation though the intended level is minimal.

It is best practice to follow the guidelines for the use of sedation and general anesthesia by dentists set forth by the ADA [7].

Moderate Sedation

According to the ADA, moderate sedation is "a drug-induced depression of consciousness during which patients respond *purposefully* to verbal commands, either alone or accompanied by light tactile stimulation. No interventions are required to maintain a patent airway, and spontaneous ventilation is adequate. Cardiovascular function is usually maintained.

The drug(s) and/or techniques used should carry a margin of safety wide enough to render unintended loss of consciousness unlikely. If repeat dosing is considered, the practitioner must be careful that the effect of the previous dosing is fully recognized before considering additional administration of drugs. A patient whose only response is reflex withdrawal from a painful stimulus would not be considered to be in a state of moderate sedation" [7]. Monitoring of moderate sedation requires ECG, blood pressure, oxygenation with pulse oximetry, ventilation with quantitative end-tidal CO_2, and temperature based on standards set forth by the American Society of Anesthesiologists [16].

Deep Sedation

According to the ASA, deep sedation is "a drug-induced depression of consciousness during which patients cannot easily be aroused but respond purposefully following repeated or painful stimulation. The ability to independently maintain ventilatory function may be impaired. Patients may require assistance in maintaining a patent airway, and spontaneous ventilation may be inadequate. Cardiovascular function is usually maintained" [7]. As with moderate sedation, monitoring of deep sedation requires ECG, blood pressure, oxygenation with pulse oximetry, ventilation with quantitative end-tidal CO_2, and temperature based on standards set forth by the American Society of Anesthesiologists [16].

General Anesthesia

General anesthesia is "a drug-induced loss of consciousness during which patients are not arousable, even by painful stimulation. The ability to independently maintain ventilatory function is often impaired. Patients often require assistance in maintaining a patent airway, and positive pressure ventilation may be required because of depressed spontaneous ventilation or drug-induced depression of neuromuscular function. Cardiovascular function may be impaired" [7].

The levels of sedation and general anesthesia occur on a continuum. A practitioner must have the knowledge, skill set, and training to not only recognize a patient's level of anesthesia, but to manage the physiologic state of the patient and the possible complications associated with anesthesia. Monitoring of moderate sedation requires ECG, blood pressure, oxygenation with pulse oximetry, ventilation with quantitative end-tidal CO_2, and temperature based on standards set forth by the American Society of Anesthesiologists [17, 18].

Physical and Psychological Assessment

Dental care can have a profound effect on both the physical and psychological well-being of the patient, and it is extremely important for the person treating the patient to know beforehand the most likely problems to be encountered. Asking pertinent questions and uncovering answers until you are satisfied will help you prepare for any possible situations or emergencies. In developing a sedation plan, there are specific goals of the assessment. The clinician must remain diligent not only in the physical assessment but also in the psychological examination, because the sedative and hypnotic drugs that are typically used may have unpredictable effects on patients with poorly controlled psychological conditions. The considerations during the physical and psychological assessment are described as follows.

Goals of the Physical and Psychological Assessment

1. Determine the patient's ability to tolerate the physical and psychological stress associated with dental treatment.
2. Determine whether treatment modification is indicated to enable the patient to better tolerate the procedure.
3. Decide which sedation technique is most appropriate for the case.
4. Analyze whether contraindications exist to the dental procedure or sedation.

Physical and Psychological Evaluation

The physical and psychological evaluation for anesthesia in dentistry consists of the following three components:

- full medical, social, family, and anesthetic history
- physical examination
- dialogue to determine patient's current psychological state to include anxiety and/or fear of dental procedures

Patients should be classified according to their medical risk when undergoing a dental/surgical procedure. Depending on the classification, the sedation level and route of administration can best be determined to avoid complications or emergencies. The system most commonly used is the ASA physical status classification system, which has been in use continually since 1962. See Table 26.1.

A thorough physical examination is also a requirement for assessing a patient prior to sedation/anesthesia for a dental procedure. Of particular importance is the heart/lung examination, neck mobility and range of motion, jaw mobility and maximum incisal opening (MIO) measurement, thyromental distance, the general condition of the dentition and an airway examination. Most commonly, the Mallampati classification[8] is used to help determine the difficulty of intubation if necessary and assess the risk of upper airway obstruction during anesthesia [9].

Sedation Techniques for Dentistry

In this chapter we focus on enteral (oral) and parenteral (intravenous) sedation techniques for adults, although we recognize that inhalation (nitrous oxide) is one of the more commonly used techniques for sedation in outpatient dental clinics. The combination of nitrous oxide–oxygen administered safely with appropriate armamentarium provides a fast and effective means of sedation that is extremely safe because of its ease of titration and the limited side effects for patients. However, there are limitations to nitrous oxide–oxygen in a dental office, including issues concerning storage, cost, and side effects to dental personnel, and these have limited its use [4]. Many practitioners regularly use nitrous oxide–oxygen in conjunction with both oral and intravenous (IV) sedation in the dental office. For the remainder of this chapter, however, we focus on

Table 26.1 Current definitions and examples

ASA physical status classification*	Definition	Examples, including, but not limited to
ASA I	A normal healthy patient	Healthy, non-smoking, no or minimal alcohol use
ASA II	A patient with mild systemic disease	Mild diseases only without substantive functional limitations. Examples include (but not limited to): current smoker, social alcohol drinker, pregnancy, obesity (30 < BMI <40), well controlled diabetes mellitus or hypertension, mild lung disease
ASA III	A patient with severe systemic disease	Substantive functional limitations; One or more moderate to severe diseases. Examples include (but not limited to): poorly controlled diabetes mellitus or hypertension, chronic obstructive pulmonary disease, morbid obesity (BMI ≥ 40), active hepatitis, alcohol dependence or abuse, implanted pacemaker, moderate reduction of ejection fraction, end-stage renal disease undergoing regularly scheduled dialysis, premature infant post-conceptual age < 60 weeks, history (> 3 months) of myocardial infarction (MI), cerebrovascular accident (CVA), transient ischemic attack (TIA) or coronary artery disease (CAD)/stents.
ASA IV	A patient with severe systemic disease that is a constant threat to life	Examples include (but not limited to): recent (< 3 months) MI, CVA, TLA, or CAD/stents, ongoing cardiac ischemia or severe valve dysfunction, severe reduction of ejection fraction, sepsis, disseminated intravascular coagulation; acute respiratory distress syndrome; or end-stage renal disease not undergoing regularly scheduled dialysis
ASA V	A moribund patient who is not expected to survive without the operation	Examples include (but are not limited to): ruptured abdominal/thoracic aneurysm, massive trauma, intracranial bleed with mass effect, ischemic bowel in the face of significant cardiac pathology or multiple organ/system dysfunction
ASA VI	A declared brain-dead patient whose organs are being removed for donor purposes	

*The addition of "E" to the ASA class denotes Emergency: (An emergency is defined as existing when delay in treatment of the patient would lead to a significant increase in the threat to life or body part).

enteral and parenteral sedation techniques, in each case discussing the indications, advantages, and disadvantages.

Oral (Enteral) Sedation

Oral sedation dentistry (OSD) provides dentists with an almost ideal form of outpatient surgery sedation technique by allowing the practitioner to manage the patient's anxiety before the appointment. The goal with most oral sedation dentistry is that of *minimal sedation* or, in some cases, *moderate sedation* [7]. Oral sedation dentistry has significant advantages for the patient and the dentist, but also a number of disadvantages.

Particular advantages of OSD include the ability to manage anxiety before a dental appointment by prescribing an anxiolytic at home before the appointment. The typical drug/dose would be a long- or medium-acting benzodiazepine at or below the MRD for unmonitored home use. This can be given the night before and repeated in the dental office before the appointment. Other advantages include the almost universal acceptance (children and special-needs patients being exceptions), ease of administration, and relative safety of orally administered drugs [4]. Unwanted side effects may occur with any drug, but they are less likely and less intense with the oral than the parenteral route, so in general the routine medications used for OSD are safe when used in the correct manner. Another distinct advantage of OSD is that postoperative pain control is well managed, because of the long duration of action of orally administered drugs.

Oral sedation dentistry, however, does possess several significant disadvantages that must also be considered, as they may serve to limit the clinical use of the oral route in the management of pain and anxiety [4]. Some of these include a long latent period, unreliable drug absorption, an inability to easily achieve a desired drug effect (lack of titration), and the prolonged duration of action. If one understands the pharmacology of the chosen sedative, however, its properties can be used for greater success. Also, if the drug is given prior to arriving to the dentist's office, appropriate transportation should be confirmed for the patient and the patient should not sign consent for treatment while under the influence of these medications.

The pharmacology of orally administered drugs (absorption, metabolism, distribution, and excretion) presents unique problems in the case of oral sedatives, the clinical effect of which is usually not seen for up to 30 minutes, or longer, depending on a variety of factors. The greatest degree of clinical effectiveness is not seen until a peak plasma concentration is reached, and this is typically at around 60 minutes [4]. The rate-limiting step of OSD is the "time of clinical effect" that arises from this slow onset of action and the delay in reaching maximal effect. Because of this, titration to desired effect is not possible. The clinician must administer a predetermined dose, and many factors alter a patient's response and affect the desired outcome. It is up to the practitioners of oral sedation to properly plan and educate patients and staff, to eliminate the variables that can be controlled.

The duration of action for most orally administered pain-controlling and anxiolytic drugs is prolonged, approximately 3–4 hours. For OSD, this is a problem with the long-acting benzodiazepines and other anxiety-reducing drugs, as the patient will still be under influence after most appointments. The need for post-sedation instructions, postoperative monitoring, and escorts, and the inability to drive or operate machinery, is most critical for orally sedated patients. In this regard, it should be appreciated that many patients take opioids and sedatives that can result in additive and/or potentiated respiratory depressor effects with anesthetics during dental procedures.

Postoperative pain control is well managed by the longer duration of action, and many of the anxiety-reducing drugs help potentiate relief of postoperative discomfort. However, because of the disadvantages, *intraoperative control* of anxiety and pain (unplanned administration) is not highly recommended for an orally sedated patient [4].

A typical oral-sedation visit for a patient constitutes an at-home dosage of a chosen anxiolytic or sedative-hypnotic the night before (optional) and an hour before the dental appointment in the office. If one chooses to sedate the night before, a mild, long-acting anxiolytic is typically prescribed. In the dental office, a shorter-acting, more moderate sedative-hypnotic is chosen, and the dose is usually between 0.5 × and 1 × MRD.

Patients are then monitored for level of sedation by monitoring the levels of *oxygenation, ventilation*, and *cardiovascular function*, as required by state dental boards [7]. This usually includes pulse oximetry, non-invasive blood pressure, respiratory rate, and monitoring of central nervous system (CNS) depression by communication. It is ill-advised to "titrate" oral medications (continually administering doses until desired effect). However, many dentists will administer a second dose at half the initial dose, but not to exceed 1.5 × MRD. This is referred to as "supplemental dosing" by the ADA [7], and is only done after appropriate monitoring for effect of the first dose (one half-life).

Drugs for Oral Sedation Dentistry

For oral sedation dentistry, benzodiazepines represent the most popular class of drugs available today, ideal for the management of dental fear and anxiety. They are the most effective drugs currently available for the management of anxiety (both preoperatively and postoperatively), and they also possess skeletal-muscle-relaxant and anticonvulsant properties. The use of benzodiazepines continues to grow, due to their effectiveness, variation of effectiveness, and duration of action, combined with a wide margin of safety [4]. However, benzodiazepines do not have any analgesic properties.

Benzodiazepines provide a level of minimal to moderate sedation in most patients, and there are many drugs of this class currently available. Because there are significant differences in the onset of action and the duration of action among these medications, the choice of a specific drug should be made only after consideration of the needs of both the patient and the dentist during the consultation appointment. Diazepam, triazolam, lorazepam, and midazolam (typically for oral use in children) remain popular benzodiazepines for the reduction of dental anxiety, providing minimal to moderate sedation in most patients [4].

For *minimal sedation*, one drug should be used, with or without nitrous oxide–oxygen, to achieve the desired effect. If one chooses to use a combination of anxiolytics and sedative-hypnotics, the intent is *moderate sedation* and therefore appropriate education, training, preparation, equipment for monitoring, and emergency protocols should be established. Clinicians are advised to check with their state board of dentistry to verify requirements.

Anxiolytic drugs are used to manage mild to moderate daytime anxiety and tension. At therapeutic dosages they produce the level defined as minimal sedation without impairing the patient's mental alertness or psychomotor performance. Drugs categorized as anxiolytics that are commonly used in oral sedation dentistry include the benzodiazepines diazepam (Valium), oxazepam (Serax), and alprazolam (Xanax). In the past, benzodiazepines have been known by other names, such as minor tranquilizers, ataractics, anxiolytic sedatives, and psychosedatives. The term *antianxiety drugs* is also widely used for this group of drugs. *Sedative-hypnotics* are drugs that produce either sedation or hypnosis, depending on the dosage of the drug administered and the patient's response to it. Lower dosages of these drugs produce a calming effect (sedation), usually associated with a degree of drowsiness and ataxia, while higher dosages produce hypnosis (a state resembling physiologic sleep). The benefit of the use of benzodiazepines and non-benzodiazepines (vs. barbiturates) is a reduced "hangover" effect [4]. Drugs of this category typically used for oral sedation dentistry include the benzodiazepines midazolam (Dormicum, Versed, Hypnovel), triazolam (Halcion, Rilamir), and lorazepam (Ativan), and the non-benzodiazepines zolpidem (Ambien) and zaleplon (Sonata). A review of the pharmacology of benzodiazepines reveals why they are ideal for oral sedation dentistry. Typical benzodiazepines have sedative (relaxing) and hypnotic properties (inducing sleep and allowing for posthypnotic suggestion). Most benzodiazepines work on the gamma-aminobutyric acid (GABA) receptors in the brain's limbic system and thalamus, which is involved in emotions and behavior. Because of this interaction, they impair neuronal discharge in the amygdala and amygdala–hippocampus nerve transmission, and they depress the limbic system at smaller doses than those required to depress the reticular activating system and cerebral cortex. They therefore do not produce a generalized CNS depression as much as barbiturates [4]. Benzodiazepine receptors have been isolated in the spinal cord and brain. They parallel the GABA major inhibitory neurotransmitter for the brain and glycine (spinal cord). Benzodiazepines act by intensifying the physiologic inhibitory effects of GABA, increasing the affinity of GABA on the chloride channels and allowing more chloride ions to enter postsynaptic sites and further depolarizing the membrane, preventing conduction. Benzodiazepines are classified as short-, intermediate-, or long-acting, with the longer-acting benzodiazepines typically prescribed for treatment of anxiety, and those with short and intermediate duration of action used for insomnia. Dentists use short- and intermediate-acting benzodiazepines for the treatment of dental anxiety immediately before and during a dental appointment, with the occasional use of a long-acting drug the night before an appointment.

Benzodiazepines have a very wide margin of safety, which provides dentists some confidence to properly sedate to desired effect without negative side effects. With dental offices typically isolated from ambulatory surgery centers and/or hospitals, providing effective and safe sedation is paramount when choosing a drug. Some of the other benefits of benzodiazepines are a result of the interactions within the CNS: reduction of hostile and aggressive behavior; attenuation of the behavioral consequences of frustration and fear; skeletal-muscle relaxant; anticonvulsant (more effective when given intravenously); potential respiratory depression unlikely (but can occur when used in combination with other medications); and virtually no cardiovascular changes in ASA class I patients.

Metabolism of benzodiazepines occurs in the liver, and they may or may not have active metabolites; learning which ones do can assist in determining the best choice for a given procedure. Plasma half-life and time for peak plasma concentration vary significantly with class (short-, intermediate-, and long-acting), and because they interact with glycine they may also help potentiate local anesthesia. All benzodiazepines are excreted in the feces and urine, with the percentage of urinary excretion varying from 20% to 80% [4].

There is a potential for psychological and physiologic dependence on benzodiazepines to develop with long-term use; however, the incidence of physiologic dependence is considerably less than that of psychological dependence. For the *pretreatment* of dental anxiety, diazepam and oxazepam are indicated; however, diazepam is most often prescribed, as it can be given early and still have effects on the day of the appointment.

Contraindications to benzodiazepines include allergy to medication, psychoses, and acute narrow-angle glaucoma, but they may be administered to patients with open-angle glaucoma who are receiving appropriate therapy [4]. There are some precautions that must be observed when prescribing these anxiolytics and sedatives:

1. Patients must be advised against driving a motor vehicle or operating hazardous machinery.
2. Avoid other CNS depressants, such as alcohol, opioids, and barbiturates.
3. Avoid prescribing to pregnant patients as a precaution. There is some evidence of birth defects, and benzodiazepines will cross the placental barrier and be excreted in breast milk.
4. The use of oral diazepam tablets in children younger than 6 months of age is not recommended.

Drugs Commonly Used in Oral Sedation

Below we describe pharmacologic and clinical characteristics of the commonly used oral agents for sedation. The reader is also referred to Chapter 2 for an additional discussion of pharmacology.

Benzodiazepines

Diazepam

- Stimulates GABA receptors
- Produces mild sleep
- Onset approximately 1 hour
- Active metabolites
- Half-life about 50 hours (20–100 hours)
- Duration 6–8 hours
- Mild amnesia
- Supplied in 2 mg, 5 mg, 10 mg
- US Food and Drug Administration (FDA)-approved anxiolytic
- Indications
- Preoperative reduction of anxiety

Contraindications

- Pregnancy
- Known hypersensitivity
- Pediatric patients < 6 months
- Acute narrow-angle glaucoma

- Dental use
- 2.5–10 mg the night before and/or the morning of appointment

Triazolam

- Sedative-hypnotic, benzodiazepine
- Stimulates GABA receptors
- No long-term active metabolites
- Plasma half-life 2–3 hours
- Duration of action 1.5–5.5 hours
- Very little hangover effect
- Wide effective dose range (minimum effective concentration varies with patients)
- Peak plasma levels seen in little as 1.3 hours
- Anticonvulsant
- Respiratory depressant in high doses
- Relaxation adequate for pain control (difficult anesthesia patients)
- No nausea
- Lethal dose, 50% (LD50) is 5 g/kg in rats

Indications

- Preoperative sedation
- Nighttime sleep

Cautions

- Overdose may occur at 4 × MRD of 0.5 mg (2.0 mg, or eight 0.25 mg tablets)
- Hallucinations, paranoia, and depression (several reports with extended medication time)
- Anterograde amnesia
- Reduce dose in elderly or debilitated patients
- Dry mouth

Contraindications

- Acute narrow-angle glaucoma (can dry up eyes and increase ocular pressure)
- Known hypersensitivity
- Psychosis (absolute contraindication in schizophrenia)
- Pregnancy and breastfeeding: excreted in milk
- Concurrent use of alcohol can lead to severe respiratory depression

Dental Use

- 0.125–0.5 mg/day; 1 hour before dental appointment in office; MRD 0.5 mg
- Elderly: maximum 0.25 mg/day
- Always use lowest effective dose
- Typically given 1 hour before appointment (0.125–0.5 mg)
- Supplemental dose of half initial dose after one half-life has been observed, not to exceed 1.5 × MRD, is appropriate in some patients to achieve minimal sedation in a dental office setting

Lorazepam

- Works on GABA receptors
- Produces mild/moderate sleep
- Onset 1 hour
- No active metabolites
- Half-life 12–14 hours
- Duration 6–8 hours
- Moderate amnesia
- Dosage forms 0.5 mg, 1 mg, 2 mg tablets
- Metabolized by glucuronidation

Indications

- Preoperative sedation
- Nighttime sleep

Contraindications

- Known hypersensitivity
- Pregnancy
- Children less than 12 years old
- Acute narrow-angle glaucoma

Dental Use

- 1–5 mg adult (ASA I, II); ASA III or elderly: half the normal dose
- Taken 1 hour before appointment in the office
- Onset is slightly slower than other benzodiazepines, and possible to have patient take earlier
- Usually used in patients needing longer procedures (> 2 hours), patients with hepatic dysfunction, patients where triazolam was ineffective

Midazolam

- Oral dosage form in United States is 2mg/mL syrup
- Absorption and onset of clinical action faster than comparable benzodiazepines (mainly diazepam)
- Peak action within 30 minutes
- No active metabolites
- Half-life 1–3 hours
- Anterograde amnesia very good
- Mostly used for pediatric sedation; not as effective in adults

Non-benzodiazepine Sedative-Hypnotics

Zaleplon (a pyrazolopyrimidine) and zolpidem (an imidazopyridine) are used for the short-term management of insomnia. Although unrelated structurally to benzodiazepines, they interact with a GABA–benzodiazepine receptor complex and share some of the pharmacologic properties of benzodiazepines.

- They are strong sedatives with only mild anxiolytic, myorelaxant, and anticonvulsant properties. Both have been shown to be effective in inducing and maintaining sleep in adults. They are rapidly absorbed from the gastrointestinal tract and are metabolized in the liver. They are converted into inactive metabolites and eliminated primarily through renal clearance.
- Precautions include respiratory depression, but this is not usually seen in healthy patients receiving average doses. If they are used in patients with compromised respiratory function, however, the likelihood of depressed respiratory drive is increased.

Zaleplon (Sonata) and Zolpidem (Ambien)

- Used for short-term insomnia
- Work on benzodiazepine–GABA receptor sites
- Produce high sleep
- Onset 45 minutes (zaleplon); 30 minutes (zolpidem)
- Time to peak concentration 1 hour (zaleplon); 1.5 hours (zolpidem)
- No active metabolites
- Elimination half-life 1 hour (zaleplon); 2.5 hours (zolpidem)
- Duration of action 1–2 hours (zaleplon); 2–4 hours (zolpidem)
- Moderate amnesia
- Not an FDA-approved anxiolytic but similar to midazolam in efficacy
- Zaleplon is absorbed and eliminated more quickly, and is used for short appointments

Contraindications

- Children < 18 years
- Severely depressed patients

Warnings

- Cytochrome P450 inhibitors
- Aldehyde oxidase inhibitors (diphenhydramine)
- Elderly patients

Dental Use

- Dose 5–15 mg for zaleplon; 5–10 mg for zolpidem
- Administered 30 minutes to 1 hour before appointment and used in short appointments
- Onset of sedation is rapid and, because of short half-life, recovery is quick
- Histamine (H$_1$) blockers (antihistamines)
- CNS depression (sedation and hypnosis) is a known side effect of some drugs used primarily for other purposes. Such effects occur with many of the histamine blockers, drugs used primarily in the management of allergies, motion sickness, and parkinsonism.

Note, several histamine blockers demonstrate this property and are marketed primarily as sedative-hypnotics. These drugs include methapyrilene, pyrilamine, diphenhydramine, promethazine, and hydroxyzine. The two histamine blockers most frequently used for their sedative/anxiolytic properties are promethazine and hydroxyzine.

In dentistry, these drugs have proven to be quite useful, especially in pediatric dentistry. Hydroxyzine is the most common form used in oral sedation dentistry, used alone or most commonly in addition to a benzodiazepine or opioid. The sedative actions of hydroxyzine are not produced by cortical depression; it is thought to suppress some hypothalamic nuclei and extend its actions peripherally into the sympathetic portion of the autonomic nervous system.

The oral liquid form of hydroxyzine hydrochloride is more pleasant-tasting to most patients than the liquid form of hydroxyzine pamoate. This fact is of particular importance in pediatric dentistry.

When these drugs are administered in combination with benzodiazepines or opioids, their dosage should be decreased by 50%, because the depressant actions of opioids are potentiated by hydroxyzine. In dental practice, the use of hydroxyzine as a sole drug is almost always limited to the management of children with mild to moderate fear, and it is often used in combination with meperidine for the management of more fearful pediatric patients.

The incidence of side effects is quite low, with transient drowsiness observed most commonly. Fatal overdose with hydroxyzine is extremely uncommon, and withdrawal reactions after long-term therapy have never been reported.

Hydroxyzine

- Moderate sleep
- Anxiolytic, antihistaminic, and antiemetic actions
- Onset 1 hour
- Metabolized in liver/excreted via kidneys
- No active metabolites (cetirizine has minimal sedation activity)
- Half-life 3–7 hours
- Duration 3 hours
- No amnesia
- No specific antidote
- Helps those patients with increased nausea and vomiting, increased gag reflex, hypersalivation; useful in smokers

Indications
- Preoperative management of anxiety
- Potentiation of sedative effects of anxiolytics

Contraindications
- Early pregnancy
- Known hypersensitivity
- Nursing mothers
- Children < 1 year
- Acute narrow-angle glaucoma
- Dental use
- 10–50 mg dose for adults
- Typically, 1.1–2.2 mg/kg (reduced by 50% in combination) in children

- Taken at same time as other CNS depressants in the office
- Opioids ("narcotics")
- Opioids are classified as strong analgesics, and their primary indication is for the relief of moderate to severe pain. Mainly, opioids alter a patient's *psychological response* to pain and suppress anxiety and apprehension.

Note, in dentistry, many opioids are used *parenterally* as preanesthetic drugs because of their sedative, anxiolytic, and analgesic properties. Meperidine has lost favor with many because of its adverse side effects at the higher doses that are often required (because it is not as effective as newer opioid derivatives), and we only discuss it here because it is still occasionally used, especially in pediatric oral sedation.

In the absence of pain, opioids administered alone frequently produce dysphoria instead of sedation. To achieve anxiolytic and sedative effects, opioids should not be administered via the oral route in adults. Absorption following oral administration is not as consistent as it is with parenteral administration, and the incidence of unwanted side effects (postural hypotension, nausea, and vomiting) is considerably greater. For adults, it is recommended that opioids should generally be avoided for oral sedation dentistry, given their lack of effect and the increased risk of complications, especially in medically compromised patients. Opioids are included for the sake of completeness, and because they are used in pediatric dentistry in combination with histamine blockers and/or benzodiazepines.

Oral Sedation Protocols

As a guideline in the use of oral sedation in an outpatient setting, the following protocols are provided. Note, however, that they are only a guide, and that practitioners must be trained in advanced airway techniques and at a level of sedation above their intent for "rescue" purposes.

Minimal Sedation

The following sample protocols are typically used in dental offices where the intent is minimal to moderate sedation (depending on the response of the patient). The addition of diazepam the night before or the morning of the appointment is optional, and is not recommended on the first sedation visit.

Sample Protocol 1

- Approximately 45 minutes to 1 hour of treatment in adults (18 years and older)
- Diazepam 2.5–10 mg orally the night before the appointment
- Zaleplon 5–15 mg orally in the office 30–45 minutes before the appointment
- Nitrous oxide–oxygen during administration of local anesthesia, and at the end of the appointment if needed to extend the procedure

Sample Protocol 2

- Approximately 1–2 hours of treatment in adults (18 years and older)
- Diazepam 2.5–10 mg orally the night before the appointment
- Triazolam 0.125–0.5 mg orally in the office1 hour before the appointment. Typical protocol for ASA I or II minimally to moderately anxious patient:
  - 0.25 mg in office 1 hour before "doctor" time
  - 45 minutes later evaluate for signs of sedation and move to dental chair

- ◦ At 60–90 minutes, may administer a supplemental dose, no more than half initial dose and given only after clinical half-life has been exceeded. Should not exceed 1.5 × MRD
- Nitrous oxide–oxygen during administration of local anesthesia and at end of appointment if need to extend procedure
- This is a first-line attempt for minimal-sedation dentistry on a majority of dental patients using oral sedation dentistry. The reader should note the following:
- It is often used for a target appointment in patients where the desire is to perform examination, obtain radiographs, and attempt prophylaxis on moderate to severe dental-phobic patients
- In mild to moderate dental-phobic patients, one can get more profound anesthesia
- In special-needs or medically compromised patients, dosages are often decreased
- It is a great starting point for most new patients who are severely anxious and not sure if they want to proceed with deeper sedation

Sample Protocol 3
- Approximately 1–3 hours of treatment
- Diazepam 2.5–10 mg the night before the appointment
- Lorazepam 1–5 mg orally in the office 1–1.5 hours before the appointment
- Supplemental dosing is not recommended due to long the half-life and slow onset
- Nitrous oxide–oxygen during administration of local anesthesia and at the end of the appointment if needed to extend the procedure

Moderate Sedation
The following protocols are intended to provide a deeper level of sedation, where the patient's responses will be "purposeful" to verbal or light tactile stimulation and respiratory depression will be unlikely. Clinicians and patients should see more profound amnesia and more relaxation with the following protocols.

Sample Protocol 1
- Approximately 2 hours of treatment (varies)
- Diazepam 2.5–10 mg orally the night before the appointment
- Triazolam 0.125–0.5 mg (up to 0.75 mg) orally in the office 1 hour before the appointment
- Hydroxyzine 50–100 mg orally in the office 1 hour before the appointment
- Nitrous oxide–oxygen during administration of local anesthesia and at the end of the appointment, if there is a need to extend the procedure
- Hydroxyzine is great for "gaggers" and smokers
- Combination helps with more profound amnesia and deeper sedation, but patients will recover more quickly

Sample Protocol 2
- Approximately 3–4 hours of treatment, depending on the patient
- Diazepam 2.5–10 mg the night before or 1 hour before the appointment

- Lorazepam 1–5 mg orally in the office 1 hour before the appointment
- Hydroxyzine 10–50 mg orally in the office 1 hour before the appointment
- Nitrous oxide–oxygen during administration of local anesthesia and at the end of the appointment if needed to extend the procedure
- An alternative would be to substitute meperidine for hydroxyzine

Note, when learning oral sedation dentistry, it is advised that the clinician should learn two to three protocols and the drugs used. One should also remember that there are other benzodiazepines and non-benzodiazepines that vary in chemical structure and half-life, and that if a protocol is no longer working on a patient, the possible causes should be considered: the patient may be taking new medications that interfere with the metabolism of benzodiazepines, or the patient may have developed a tolerance. In either case, a different benzodiazepine may produce the desired effect. Learning to use appropriate drug reference resources will assist the clinician in making an informed decision.

Meperidine is still used by some clinicians for oral sedation dentistry, especially in the sedation of children and special-needs patients. Some practitioners occasionally use orally administered meperidine in conjunction with a benzodiazepine if there is a contraindication to hydroxyzine; they may use it with both drugs if the intent is moderate sedation in a patient who has not responded to normal protocols and IV sedation/general anesthesia is absolutely contraindicated. In these cases, it is wise to administer sedation in a setting with full advanced cardiovascular life support capabilities, advanced airway, and anesthesia support. If it is decided that meperidine is safe, it would replace hydroxyzine or the benzodiazepine in the above protocols at a dose of 50–100 mg by mouth.

Emerging Techniques

There has been some clinical use of clonidine as a premedication to supplement oral and IV sedation in dentistry. Especially in procedures that are expected to be longer in duration [19], or in patients who have not responded to the typical "recipe," there has been some evidence that preloading with 0.1–0.2 mg of clonidine has an additive effect for benzodiazepines, histamine blockers, and/or opioids without significant decrease in respiratory or cardiovascular function. This is not indicated in patients currently on clonidine or with low blood pressure, but it has proven effectiveness. Clonidine is an alpha-2-adrenergic agonist hypotensive medication that may decrease heart rate and vascular resistance, allowing smoother flow of blood. This is a direct counteraction of the effects that "fear" (which leads to catecholamine release) and epinephrine (injected with local anesthetic) have on the body, especially during a time of anxiety. Specifically, clonidine prevents the "fight or flight" response produced by stimulation of the sympathetic nervous system (tachycardia, hypertension), especially during high-anxiety events such as a dental visit. Clonidine has many uses as a pre-sedation adjunct prior to surgery [20–23].

The techniques described above will allow a clinician to achieve minimal or moderate sedation in a low to moderately anxious dental patient, and to do so with relative predictability. However, oral sedation still has its limitations, chief among which are the inability to titrate and the prolonged sedation time. Parenteral (IV) sedation techniques will eliminate those issues.

Intravenous (Parenteral) Sedation

The IV route of drug administration is a parenteral technique that represents the most effective method of ensuring predictable and adequate sedation at all levels (mild, moderate, and deep) in virtually all patients [4].

Armamentarium for Intravenous Sedation

The following supplies and monitoring equipment are generally necessary for the safe and effective administration of IV sedation. Additional equipment may be necessary:

- IV fluids
- delivery tubing and drug pump
- IV catheters
- drugs
- monitors
- electrocardiography
- blood pressure
- pulse oximetry
- respiration
- quantitative end tidal carbon dioxide (CO_2)
- temperature

Fluid Management and Intravenous Access

Most office-based IV sedation procedures are of short duration and involve minimal blood loss. The need for fluid resuscitation perioperatively is not a major concern in everyday practice. The intent of fluid management in office-based surgery is primarily to rehydrate a patient, as opposed to replacing intraoperative fluid losses. Normally patients who undergo sedation will be required to be nothing by mouth for at least 6 hours. An 8-hour fast will create a 750 mL fluid deficit in a 70 kg healthy patient.

For a short-duration dental IV procedure, the choice of fluids, between normal saline (0.9 NaCl), half normal saline (0.45 NaCl), lactated Ringer's, and 5% dextrose in water, depends on convenience. To administer drugs and fluids, constant IV access is required. The armamentarium, anatomy, and access techniques are discussed in greater detail in Chapter 5.

Pharmacology

Several different anesthetic drugs and techniques are used in IV sedation in dentistry to facilitate procedures and patient comfort. The ideal properties of IV sedation drugs in the dental setting include the following:

- amnesia
- analgesia
- suppression of stress response
- hemodynamic stability
- sedation/immobilization
- hypnosis
- rapid onset and short duration of action

The most commonly used drugs for IV sedation in the dental setting are benzodiazepines, opioids, ultra-short-acting anesthetic agents (e.g., propofol or methohexital), and ketamine. These drugs are administered in various combinations, and in combination with nitrous oxide–oxygen and local anesthetics, and are normally administered by incremental boluses [24]. The pharmacology of these drugs is extensively covered in Chapter 2; therefore, this chapter covers only the drugs most commonly used in IV sedation in the dental setting, and their relevant properties.

Benzodiazepines

Benzodiazepines are the most effective drugs in the management of anxiety. They have muscle-relaxant and anticonvulsant properties, and anterograde amnesic properties.

Midazolam (Versed) is water-soluble, and therefore causes no irritation or phlebitis when applied, and no second peak effect. Beta half-life: 1.7–2.4 hours; alpha half-life: 4–18 minutes. It has anterograde amnesic properties. It is more amnesic but less sedating than diazepam, and it is known to cause dizziness. It is contraindicated in acute pulmonary insufficiency, secondary to its respiratory-depressant properties, and in patients allergic to midazolam. Dosage: start with 1–2.5 mg, then titrate to effect. Titrate with 2 mg increments. Average sedative dose: 2.5–7.5 mg.

Diazepam (Valium) is lipid-soluble, creating local irritation of the vein, phlebitis, and even thrombosis when applied. It may have a rebound effect or a second peak effect. Peak blood level: 1–2 minutes. Beta half-life: 30 hours; alpha half-life: 45–60 minutes. It provides 45–60 minutes of sedation, and can cause respiratory depression, can elevate the seizure threshold, and has anterograde amnesic properties. It is contraindicated in patients with glaucoma and hypersensitivity to valium. Other adverse reactions include hyperactivity, confusion, nausea, changes in libido, decreased salivation, and emergence delirium. Dosage: 5–20 mg titrated slowly, usually in 5 mg increments.

Opioids

Opioids are administered primarily for their analgesic properties. Opioids may be classified as natural or synthetically derived. Reliable sedation cannot be achieved without producing some level of respiratory depression. Respiratory depression is worsened by the concomitant administration of benzodiazepines or ultra-short-acting anesthetics.

Fentanyl (Sublimaze) is a synthetic opioid. It is 100 times more potent than morphine. It has a rapid onset and is short-acting: onset in less than 1 minute with a blood and brain equilibration time of 6.4 minutes. Its effects are usually gone in about 30–60 minutes. It may cause muscular rigidity of thoracic and abdominal muscles, related to fast administration, and its respiratory-depressant effects outlast its analgesic effects. It is contraindicated in patients allergic to fentanyl, patients with chronic obstructive pulmonary disease (COPD), and patients with advanced respiratory disease. This drug has a very narrow therapeutic index and should be used with extreme caution. Dosage: start with 25–50 µg, then titrate to effect. Titrate in 25 µg increments. Average sedative dose: 100 µg.

Meperidine (Demerol) is a synthetic opioid. Historically, meperidine was the most commonly used opioid by dentists for IV sedation, falling out of favor because of side effects and cleaner alternatives such as fentanyl. It is one-tenth as potent as morphine. The onset of action is 2–4 minutes; duration of action is 30–45 minutes. It has vagolytic properties, increases heart rate, and decreases salivary secretions. It also triggers histamine release at the site of injection (resolves spontaneously), and it is known to cause seizures, secondary to its metabolite normeperidine. It is contraindicated in patients allergic to meperidine and patients with COPD and decreased respiratory reserve. Average sedative dose: 37.5–50 mg. Maximum single dose: 50 mg. Titrate to effect in doses of 25 mg.

Reversal Agents

Naloxone (Narcan) is an opioid antagonist. Its onset of action is 2 minutes and its duration is 30 minutes. It is contraindicated in patients allergic to naloxone and in patients with opioid dependency. Dosage: 0.1–0.2 mg every 2–3 minutes. Maximum dose: 1.2 mg.

Flumazenil (Romazicon) is a benzodiazepine antagonist. It has a short onset of action of 3–5 minutes and duration of approximately 60 minutes. It is contraindicated in patients allergic to flumazenil and in patients who have been given benzodiazepines for status epilepticus or increased intracranial pressure. Dosage: 0.2 mg every minute up to maximum dose of 1.0 mg.

It is important to note that patients who are reversed from sedation with any of these reversal agents will need to be monitored for approximately 2 hours. Reversal agents most of the time have a shorter duration of action than the sedative drugs, creating the risk of re-sedation.

Barbiturates

Barbiturates are sedative-hypnotic drugs, anticonvulsants (except for methohexital), and CNS and respiratory depressants. They have no analgesic properties. They are known to cause "hangover" effects, secondary to their redistribution to fat. Barbiturates are also known to cause idiosyncratic reactions such as excitement and lower pain threshold, and to increase rates of laryngospasm.

Propofol

Propofol (Diprivan) is a general anesthetic drug used for induction and maintenance of anesthesia as well as for sedation. It is not water-soluble, but is available in aqueous solution. The solution contains soybean oil, glycerol, and egg lecithin (egg yolks, not whites); therefore, it is recommended to be used within 6 hours of opening the bottle. It causes pain with IV administration that can be lessened by pretreatment with IV lidocaine. Propofol has high lipid solubility that results in a rapid onset of action and short duration. It is available in 10 mg/mL concentration. The typical recommended dose for sedation is 50–100 μg/kg per minute until the appropriate level of sedation is obtained, followed by a maintenance infusion of 25–75 μg/kg per minute. Its onset of action is 90–100 seconds and its duration of action is 2–8 minutes. However, prolonged administration can result in drug accumulation and a prolonged wake-up time.

Ketamine

Ketamine (Ketalar) is a dissociative anesthetic that dissociates the thalamus from the limbic cortex. The patient appears conscious (e.g., eye opening, swallowing, muscle contracture), but is unable to process or respond to sensory input. Ketamine can be administered through an IV or intramuscular (IM) route. It can increase blood pressure, heart rate, and cardiac output; therefore, it should be avoided in patients with coronary artery disease, congestive heart failure, arterial aneurysms, and uncontrolled hypertension. It is a potent bronchodilator, useful in patients with asthma, but it also increases salivation. Lithium may prolong the duration of action and diazepam attenuates its cardiostimulatory effects and prolongs its half-life. Ketamine is known to cause the so-called "emergence phenomenon," for which its use in combination with benzodiazepines is recommended. Maximum doses: 2mg/kg IV or 4mg/kg IM.

Anticholinergics

These drugs are competitive antagonists to acetylcholine in the parasympathetic nervous system, effective in dryness of the mouth and upper respiratory tract.

Glycopyrrolate (Robinul) does not cross lipid membranes (blood–brain barrier), with no CNS depression or delirium-type reactions. Its time of onset is 1 minute and its duration of action is 2–3 hours for its vagal effects and up to 7 hours as an anti-sialagogue. It is contraindicated in patients with glaucoma, adhesions between the iris and the lens, prostate disease, myasthenia gravis, contact lenses, and asthma. Its usual therapeutic dose is 0.1 mg, and it may be repeated every 2–3 minutes. Maximum dose: 0.3 mg.

Techniques of Administration

There are as many techniques for administering and combining drugs for IV sedation in the dental setting as there are practitioners administering IV sedation. In order to simplify the techniques, it may be helpful to classify the drugs in the following categories.

Premedication

- *Nitrous oxide–oxygen*: Widely available to the dental practitioner. It can be used to reduce anxiety, even before venipuncture, and as a support drug during IV sedation.
- *Steroids* (dexamethasone, methylprednisolone): Can be administered to decrease postoperative edema in traumatic procedures. Also can be given to decrease histamine release reactions created by some of the sedative drugs.
- *Antihistamines* (diphenhydramine): Used to decrease histamine release reactions created by some of the sedative drugs. Some antihistamines provide added sedative properties.
- *Anticholinergics* (glycopyrrolate, scopolamine, atropine): Used for control of secretions.

Anxiolysis/Analgesia

- *Nitrous oxide–oxygen.* Support drug during IV sedation to reduce amounts of sedative drugs used and to provide oxygen supplementation.
- *Benzodiazepines* (diazepam, midazolam): Most effective drugs in the management of anxiety. Most commonly used in combination with opioids in IV sedation.
- *Opioids* (fentanyl, meperidine): Administered primarily for analgesia.
  In combination with benzodiazepines accomplish ideal levels for moderate IV sedation.

Deep Sedation

- *Anesthetic drugs* (ketamine, propofol, barbiturates). Administered to increase the level of sedation during particularly painful or difficult portions of the procedure (e.g., local anesthesia injections), or when the ideal level of sedation cannot be accomplished with anxiolytic/analgesic drug combination.

Day of Procedure

On the day of the procedure, certain preoperative, documentation, and discharge planning requirements must be met. Below is a rough guide to help the practitioner improve patient comfort and safety, and to ensure proper documentation and monitoring during and after the procedure.

Preoperative Requirements
- Current medical history
- Pre-procedure diagnosis, appropriateness of procedure, rationale for sedation and sedation plan, i.e., medications to be administered
- Verify nothing by mouth status for at least 4 hours following oral intake of clear fluids and at least 6 hours following oral intake of nonclear fluids or food
- Physical examination, to include at least the patient's vital signs, airway, and blood oxygenation
- Signature on appropriate consent form for the procedure and for the administration of parenteral sedation/analgesia
- Verification of the presence of a patient escort, a responsible adult who will stay in the waiting area during the procedure and take the patient home upon completion of the procedure
- Loose-fitting garments
- Morning appointments
- Short waiting-room time
- Restroom (urine pregnancy test as needed)
- Monitors
- Oxygen–nitrous oxide
- IV line placement

Documentation
- Respiratory rate (documented every 5 minutes and preoperatively, intraoperatively, and postoperatively)
- Level of consciousness (documented every 5 minutes); can be assessed by different scales (e.g., AVPU [Alert, Voice, Pain, Unresponsive] scale)
- Heart rate (documented every 5 minutes and preoperatively, intraoperatively, and postoperatively)
- Blood pressure (documented every 5 minutes and preoperatively, intraoperatively, and postoperatively)
- Pulse oximetry with continuous auditory and visual display of oxygen saturation (documented every 5 minutes and preoperatively, intraoperatively, and postoperatively)
- Quantitative end-tidal CO_2 monitoring: continuous with documentation every 5 minutes

- ECG monitoring (three–five-lead ECG): constant, with printing capabilities (not required for oral sedation dentistry)

Recovery and Discharge
- Never leave patient unattended
- Adjust dental chair position slowly
- Vital signs must return close to normal
- Never discharge alone after sedation
- Written and verbal instructions to patient and escort
- Discharge on wheelchair and with escort
- Continue to document until patient is discharged

Discharge Criteria
- Patient has stable vital signs
- Patient easily arousable and with intact protective reflexes
- Adequately patent airway
- Adequately hydrated
- Patient can talk, and can sit unaided
- Patient can walk with minimal assistance
- Can use a scoring system to document adequacy of discharge (e.g., modified Aldrete or PADDS [Post Anesthesia Discharge Scoring System])

Complications Associated with Intravenous Sedation for Dental Treatment

The literature shows that the administration of IV sedation and general anesthesia during dental treatment is a safe and effective modality, and the overall complication rate is similar to or less than the rates reported in hospital-based anesthesia practices [25–30]. Boynes and colleagues showed that the overall complication rate for IV sedation during dental treatment is 24.7%, with *airway obstruction* (5.8%) and *nausea and vomiting* (4.7%) as the primary complications [27]. Airway obstruction is the complication reported more frequently in the dental setting when compared with hospital-based practices (2–4%). This could be explained by the nature of the procedures, in which the airway is shared by both the dentist and anesthesia provider working in the same area. Other complications were not reported to be very different than in the hospital-based practices, and these are discussed at length in Chapter 11. As noted earlier in this chapter, it takes 5.5 half-lives for medication regularly taken by patients to leave the body and, therefore, anesthetics in patients taking opioids, sedatives, and other medications that can cause dose-dependent respiratory depression must be carefully considered in ensure that hypoventilation or respiratory depression intraoperatively does not occur and underscores the critical importance of monitoring of ventilation with quantitative end-tidal CO_2 monitoring in addition to pulse oximetry.

Monitoring

The ASA has five basic standards for anesthetic monitoring that are required by all practicing anesthesia healthcare providers:

- temperature
- ECG
- blood pressure
- pulse oximetry
- Quantitative end-tidal CO_2

It should be noted that, in 2011, the ASA task force included end-tidal CO_2 which allows for real-time assessment of ventilation. Because procedures in dentistry involve the critical elements of the airway, the provider delivering sedation for modern dentistry procedures needs to include all five of these important monitors for any procedure.

Summary

Every dental visit must begin with the recognition that dental phobia exists, and clinicians will begin to "sedate" their patients the moment they enter the dental office. By relying solely on the use of drugs, in enteral or parenteral sedation, you invite the occasional failure and expose yourself to risk of oversedation and/or adverse drug reaction. Remember that regardless of the severity of the phobia and the level of sedation chosen, a clinician must always utilize iatrosedation as the foundation of every visit.

Minimal, moderate, and deep sedation are major modalities of pharmacologic intervention and behavior modification that assist the dental profession in providing dental treatment to patients with different levels of dental anxiety and fear, and they have become an integral part of dental practice.

There are many safe and effective medications available to the dental practitioner for sedation, all possessing slightly different clinical characteristics and various degrees of risk. Careful consideration needs to be given to the objectives of the sedation when deciding which pharmacologic agents and route of administration to use. The appropriateness of the procedure, the rationale for sedation, and the sedation plan should be reviewed to ensure that the sedation procedure is as safe as possible.

Careful attention also needs to be given to physical and psychological assessment of the patient, to determine his or her ability to tolerate (both physically and psychologically) the stresses involved with the planned dental treatment, and to determine whether treatment modifications, including modification of sedation protocols, are indicated to enable the patient to better tolerate these stresses.

The dental practitioner should have a complete understanding of, and should be in compliance with, the national and/or state regulations that define moderate and deep sedation, including the educational requirements, clinical guidelines, and licensure.

Finally, even though the administration of moderate and deep sedation during dental treatment is a safe and effective modality, basic preparation for all emergency situations is critical for the successful management of any unexpected sedation-related emergencies that may arise.

Acknowledgments

The authors wish to thank Jennifer E. Woerner and Melissa Wibowo for the contributions to the first edition of this chapter.

References

1. Slovin M, Falagario-Wasserman J. Special needs of anxious and phobic dental patients. *Dent Clin North Am.* 2009;53:207–19.

2. Gale E. Fears of the dental situation. *J Dent Res.* 1972;51:964–6.

3. American Association of Endodontists. Dealing with anxious patients. www.aae.org/specialty/dealing-with-anxious-patients

4. Malamed, SF. *Sedation: A Guide to Patient Management*, 5th ed. St Louis, MO: Mosby, 2009.

5. Rubin J, Slovin M, Kaplan A. Assessing patients' fears: recognizing and reacting to signs of anxiety. *Dent Clin North Am.* 1986;1:14–18.

6. Weaver JM. Two notable pioneers in conscious sedation pass their gifts of pain-free dentistry to another generation. *Anesth Prog.* 2000;47:27–8.

7. American Dental Association. Guidelines for the use of sedation and general anesthesia by dentists. www.ada.org/-/media/project/ada-organization/ada/ada-org/files/resources/research/ada_sedation_use_guidelines.pdf

8. Mallampati S, Gatt S, Gugino L, et al. A clinical sign to predict difficult tracheal intubation:a prospective study. *Can Anaesth Soc J.* 1985;32(4):429–34.

9. Karakoc O, Akcam T, Gerek M, Genc H, Ozgen F. The upper airway evaluation of habitual snorers and obstructive sleep apnea patients. *ORL J Otorhinolaryngol Relat Spec.* 2012;74(3):136–40.

10. Glassman P, Caputo A, Dougherty N, et al. Special Care Dentistry Association consensus statement on sedation, anesthesia, and alternative techniques for people with special needs. *Spec Care Dentist* 2009;29:2–8.

11. American Dental Association. Guidelines for teaching pain control and sedation to dentists and dental students. www.ada.org/-/media/project/ada-organization/ada/ada-org/files/resources/library/oral-health-topics/ada_sedation_teaching_guidelines.pdf

12. American Academy of Pediatrics, American Academy of Pediatric Dentistry, Coté CJ, Wilson S, Work Group on Sedation. Guidelines for monitoring and management of pediatric patients during and after sedation for diagnostic and therapeutic procedures: an update. *Pediatrics* 2006;118:2587–602.

13. American Association of Oral and Maxillofacial Surgeons. Statement by the American Association of Oral and Maxillofacial Surgeons concerning the management of selected clinical conditions and associated clinical procedures: the control of pain and anxiety. www.aaoms.org/docs/practice_resources/clinical_resources/control_of_pain_and_anxiety.pdf

14. American Association of Anesthesiologists. Statement on continuum of depth of sedation: definition of general anesthesia and levels of sedation/analgesia. www.asahq.org/standards-and-practice-parameters/statement-on-continuum-of-depth-of-sedation-definition-of-general-anesthesia-and-levels-of-sedation-analgesia

15. American Society of Dentist Anesthesiologists: Parameters of Care. *Anesth Prog.* 2018;65(3):197–203. doi:10.2344/anpr-65-03-19 .PMID:30235432

16. Weaver J. The latest ASA mandate: CO_2 monitoring for moderate and deep sedation. *Anesth Prog.* 2011;58(3):111–2. doi: 10.2344/0003-3006-58.3.111. PMID: 21882985

17. American Association of Anesthesiologists. Standards for basic anesthetic monitoring. www.asahq.org/standards-and-practice-parameters/standards-for-basic-anesthetic-monitoring

18. Eden N, Rajan S. ASA monitoring standards. In Abd-Elsayed A, ed., *Advanced Anesthesia Review*. Oxford: Oxford University Press, 2023, 19–C8.S13.

19. American Association of Oral and Maxillofacial Surgeons (AAOMS). Anesthesia in outpatient facilities.

In *AAOMS Parameters of Care: Clinical Practice Guidelines*, 5th ed. Rosemont, IL: AAOMS, 2012, e24–37.

20. American Society of Anesthesiologists. Continuum of depth of sedation: definition of general anesthesia and levels of sedation/analgesia. Committee of origin: Quality Management and Departmental Administration (approved by the ASA House of Delegates on October 13, 1999, and last amended on October 23, 2019). www.asahq.org/standards-and-practice-parameters/statement-on-continuum-of-depth-of-sedation-definition-of-general-anesthesia-and-levels-of-sedation-analgesia

21. Hall DL, Tatakis DN, Walters JD, Rezvan E. Oral clonidine pre-treatment and diazepam/meperidine sedation. *J Dent Res.* 2006;85:854–8.

22. Fazi L. A comparison of oral clonidine and oral midazolam as preanesthetic medications in the pediatric tonsillectomy patient. *Anesth Analg.* 2001;92:56–61.

23. Wright PMC, Carabine UA, McClune S, Orr DA, Moore J. Preanesthetic medication with clonidine. *Br J Anaesth.* 1990;65:628–32.

24. Carabine UA, Wright PMC, Moore J. Preanesthetic medication with clonidine. *Br J Anaesth.* 1991;67(1):79–83.

25. Segal IS, Jarvis DJ, Duncan SR, White PF, Maze M. Clinical efficacy of oral transdermal clonidine combinations during the perioperative period. *Anesthesiology.* 1991;74:220–5.

26. Treasure T, Bennett J. Office-based anesthesia. *Oral Maxillofac Surg Clin N Am.* 2007;19:45–57.

27. Boynes SG, Lewis CL, Moore PA, Zovko J, Close J. Complications associated with anesthesia administered for dental treatment. *Gen Dent.* 2010;58:e20–5.

28. D'Eramo EM. Mortality and morbidity with outpatient anesthesia: the Massachusetts experience. *J Oral Maxillofac Surg.* 1999;57:531–6.

29. Nkansah PJ, Haas DA, Saso MA. Mortality incidence in outpatient anesthesia for dentistry in Ontario. *Oral Surg Oral Med Oral Pathol Oral Radiol Endod* 1997;83:646–51.

30. Hines R, Barash PG, Watrous G, O'Connor T. Complications occurring in the postanesthesia care unit: a survey. *Anesth Analg* 1992;74:503–9.

Additional Reading

Green SA, Saxen MA, Urman RD. A review of scientific literature of interest to office-based anesthesiology practice. *Anesth Prog.* 2017;64(2):119–21.

Lunn JN, Hunter AR, Scott DB. Anaesthesia related surgical mortality. *Anaesthesia.* 1983;83:1090–6.

Tarrac SE. A description of intraoperative and post anesthesia complication rates. *J Perianesth Nurs* 2006;21:88–96.

Sedation for Assisted Reproductive Technologies

Vesela Kovacheva and Patricia M. Sequeira

Introduction

Assisted reproductive technologies (ART) refers to a set of techniques utilizing reproductive cells and/or embryos outside of the body to help patients conceive. These technologies have been made possible by advances in endocrine assays, controlled ovarian stimulation, cryopreservation, ultrasonography, and a range of procedures on oocytes, sperm, and embryos. An ART physician is a gynecologist specially trained in reproductive endocrinology. In vitro fertilization (IVF) is a term used to describe the process of obtaining an oocyte and uniting it with sperm outside of the body, and later transferring the developing embryo into the uterus. The most common method for obtaining oocytes is the transvaginal ultrasound-guided oocyte retrieval. This procedure is also the most painful part of an IVF cycle and therefore requires sedation and analgesia. This chapter focuses on sedation for oocyte retrieval and related ART procedures.

Infertility is defined as the inability to conceive after regular, unprotected intercourse for 1 year or more [1]. Infertility may be due to female factors like fallopian tube obstruction, ovulatory dysfunction, diminished ovarian reserve, endometriosis, abnormalities of the uterus; or male factors like very low sperm count, abnormal sperm motility, and/or unknown or idiopathic factors. Approximately one-third of infertility is attributed to female factors, one-third to male factors, and the remaining third is due to a mixture of both or unknown factors.

Assisted Reproductive Technologies Overview

Each IVF cycle consists of a series of treatments in several steps over a period of approximately 2 weeks. The cycle starts with the administration of hormonal drugs aimed to stimulate oocyte production, or with ovarian monitoring, with the intention of having embryos transferred. If the ovarian stimulation was successful, the mature oocytes are retrieved under ultrasound guidance. Next, the oocytes are fertilized with sperm and incubated under standardized protocols. Depending on the embryo development and the couple's wishes, the next step is to transfer one or more embryos to the uterus. Further monitoring and/or tests may be indicated until normal pregnancy is documented. The IVF cycle may require discontinuation due to inadequate oocyte production, ovarian hyperstimulation syndrome, other medical reasons, or patient wishes.

Controlled Ovarian Hyperstimulation

Controlled ovarian hyperstimulation is a process through which the ovaries are induced to develop more than one dominant follicle, utilizing a combination of hormones (Figure 27.1). This is the start of an IVF cycle. This process is used to promote the development of a relatively synchronous cohort of ovarian follicles and thus assists in the timing of oocyte retrieval. Multiple dominant follicles increase the number of oocytes retrieved and the likelihood of pregnancy. The controlled ovarian hyperstimulation process also helps with the development of the proper endometrial environment for embryo transfer. A typical protocol uses a combination of a gonadotropin-releasing-hormone agonist (GnRH-a), follicle-stimulating hormone (FSH), human menopausal gonadotropin (hMG), and human chorionic gonadotropin (hCG). Ovarian and pituitary suppression are achieved with GnRH-a. Both FSH and hMG induce the development of multiple synchronous ovarian follicles. Oocyte maturation is stimulated by hCG. Oocyte retrieval is usually scheduled 36 hours after the start of hCG. There is variation in the ovarian stimulation protocols based on provider preference and the patient's hormonal response. The response to controlled ovarian hyperstimulation is carefully monitored throughout with hormonal blood levels and serial ultrasound examination to document the follicle size and count.

Ovarian Hyperstimulation Syndrome

Controlled ovarian hyperstimulation can have adverse effects. Ovarian hyperstimulation syndrome (OHSS) is an iatrogenic consequence of controlled ovarian

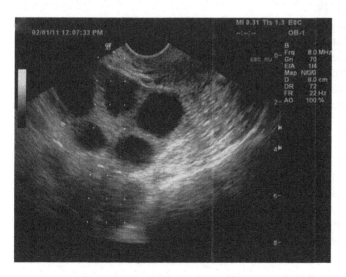

Figure 27.1 Ultrasound view of a hyperstimulated ovary with five follicles.

hyperstimulation, and at its most severe stage can have life-threatening complications. The patient with moderate to severe OHSS may have signs of rapid weight gain, oliguria, hemoconcentration, leukocytosis, hypovolemia, electrolyte imbalance, ascites, pleural, pericardial effusions, acute respiratory distress syndrome, hypercoagulability, thromboembolic events, and multiorgan failure. OHSS is usually self-limiting, and regression takes place as long as prompt and appropriate supportive medical care is provided. Exogenous and endogenous hCG will worsen OHSS. On rare occasions, the patients may need emergency laparoscopy/laparotomy for a ruptured ovarian cyst or ovarian torsion, paracentesis to drain ascites, or anticoagulants if there is thromboembolism.

Oocyte Retrieval

The reproductive gynecologist retrieves oocytes under direct ultrasound visualization from the individual ovarian follicles that have been stimulated via controlled ovarian hyperstimulation. The oocytes may be retrieved transvaginally, the most common approach, or transabdominally, in case of technical challenges, such as in morbidly obese patients. There is a window of time in which the oocytes can be retrieved; if that window is missed, spontaneous ovulation of multiple oocytes may occur. Thus, oocyte retrieval is a specially scheduled and timed procedure. Retrievals may be performed 7 days a week in a busy ART center.

Embryo Transfer

Fertilization is performed *in vitro,* and the embryos may be incubated for 3 to 5 days. Subsequently, the embryos may be transferred to the uterus or cryopreserved for future pregnancy. Embryo transfer is a very short ART procedure. The process consists of transferring embryos from the laboratory to the patient's uterus. This procedure is usually painless; however, patients with abnormal vaginal or uterine anatomy and those who are extremely anxious may require sedation.

Dilatation and Curettage

The ART patient is at a higher risk for miscarriage. The dilatation and curettage (D&C) procedure in a setting outside the operating room, such as an ART center, should be done only on carefully screened patients. These patients should be overall healthy and of normal weight, with normal coagulation, no risk of excessive bleeding, and with pregnancies less than 12 weeks. Patients with morbid obesity, full stomach, comorbidities, and pregnancies greater than 12 weeks should be scheduled for the operating room with an anesthesiologist.

Sperm Retrieval

In cases of male-factor infertility, several invasive techniques can be utilized to obtain sperm. Microscopic epididymal sperm aspiration (MESA), percutaneous epididymal sperm aspiration (PESA), and testicular sperm extraction (TESE) are sperm retrieval procedures that can be done at an ART center. They are performed by a urologist experienced in male infertility. The MESA technique consists of microsurgical techniques to obtain sperm from the epididymis. The TESE technique involves the removal of a small sample of testicular tissue followed by the extraction of the sperm. The PESA technique involves needle aspiration of sperm from the epididymis.

The patient is in the supine position with the scrotum sterilely prepped and draped. The urologist administers local anesthesia and may use an operating microscope for the sperm retrieval. The procedure usually lasts less than 1 hour and is typically done under sedation.

Patient Demographics

The patients are usually healthy adult women and men. Overweight and obese patients are occasionally encountered. Patients with mild, well-controlled comorbidities like asthma and hypertension can be scheduled as well. Anxiety, depression, and stress due to infertility status may arise. In recent years, there has been an increase in older patients and those with complex comorbidities like congenital heart disease and cancer. These patients may need to be evaluated and cared for by an anesthesiologist. The age range for the ART patient is the late twenties to mid-forties.

Procedural Risks

Procedural risks for transvaginal ultrasound-guided oocyte retrieval include bleeding, infection, and injury to pelvic or abdominal organs. These complications may require hospitalization and possibly surgery. Oskowitz et al. reported on a series of 6,776 procedures performed in a freestanding surgical facility dedicated to ART [2]. Following 4,199 vaginal oocyte retrieval procedures, seven patients required hospital admission during the first 24 hours after surgery. Two patients had serious morbidity, defined as requiring major intervention such as surgery. Nausea and vomiting, syncope, hemoperitoneum, and ovarian hematoma were included in the admitting diagnoses.

Assisted Reproductive Technologies Facilities and Personnel

According to a postal questionnaire conducted in 2004, 69% of ART centers in the United Kingdom perform oocyte retrieval outside of the general operating room environment [3]. A typical ART procedure room may be located within a university-based or free-standing fertility clinic. The embryology and andrology laboratories are adjacent to the procedure room, for immediate processing of the oocytes and sperm.

Another postal questionnaire of ART centers in the UK revealed significant variations in personnel present during oocyte retrievals, the use of drugs, degree of monitoring, and the availability of emergency drugs [4]. Eighty-four percent of the ART centers used intravenous (IV) sedation and 16% used general anesthesia for transvaginal oocyte retrieval.

Results from a telephone survey of 278 ART programs in the United States revealed that 91 private (68%) and 41 academic (56%) programs used personnel from the department of anesthesiology [5]. A large number of ART programs used their own trained personnel to provide sedation. Ninety-five percent of the transvaginal oocyte retrieval and transcervical embryo transfer were performed under sedation. For the remaining 5%, general, regional, or local anesthesia was used. The majority of the ART personnel typically used meperidine and midazolam, while 90% of the anesthesiology personnel used midazolam and/or propofol with fentanyl.

Sedation for ART Procedures

The procedure that most commonly requires sedation during an IVF cycle is oocyte retrieval. Occasionally, an embryo transfer procedure can be scheduled with sedation. The D&C procedure is infrequently encountered. On very rare occasions, the urologist incorporates MESA and TESE procedures in the ART sedation schedule.

Sedation Goals

The sedation goals for oocyte retrieval and related procedures are effective pain relief and anxiolysis with minimal postoperative nausea and vomiting. The procedure should be executed in a safe manner, and the goals also include ease of administering IV medications and patient monitoring. The medications should be short-acting and easily reversible. The drugs should minimally affect the oocytes, embryos, and the endocrine and immune systems. The procedures in ART are costly, and economic factors should be considered.

Sedation Considerations

The principal consideration for the ART patient in the pre-procedural period is the management of patient anxiety. The patients may have stress, anxiety, and depression due to their infertile status. They may arrive with anxiety from the expectant wait for the oocyte count. Empathy from all those involved in their care, including the nursing staff, the procedure-room staff, the embryologist, the reproductive medicine physician, and the sedation provider, is invaluable.

Pre-procedural sedation concerns are typically minor, because of the overall healthy ART patient population. Airway issues can arise from patients who have a history of loud snoring, sleep apnea, or obesity. Patients with mild, well-controlled comorbidities like asthma or hypertension are usually good candidates for sedation. The hyperstimulated patient may feel bloated and nauseated prior to the ART procedure. A history of postoperative nausea and vomiting (PONV), or motion sickness, should be obtained, and a reduction of baseline risks initiated. Pain management should be discussed with the patient. The nothing by mouth (nil per os [NPO]) status merits special consideration. Since this is not an elective procedure, even patients who have not been compliant with NPO guidelines will need to proceed with the oocyte retrieval. In such cases, full aspiration precautions need to be implemented, and possibly the assistance of an anesthesiologist should be considered.

Airway issues should be communicated to the ART physician, since the sedation level may be different than the usual. Care should be taken in the placement of the patient in the dorsal lithotomy position. Positioning while awake and not sedated ensures proper padding and avoidance of nerve compression injury. Adequate sedation should ensure a cooperative patient and help avoid injury to the pelvic vessels or organs due to inadvertent patient movement.

Sedation Risks

Hypoventilation or apnea are risks associated with the administration of IV sedation agents, especially when using two or more different medications. Reducing or stopping the sedation and providing greater stimulus (chin lift or jaw thrust) may help overcome the loss of ventilatory drive. Control of the airway with a bag-valve mask may be necessary. Opioid or benzodiazepine reversal should be available, but not routinely used. The desired sedation level should be achieved by careful titration of the IV agents.

Patients at risk for aspiration should be identified. Suctioning equipment should be readily available. Laryngospasm is a risk in the oversedated and obtunded patient. Successful laryngospasm management includes early recognition followed by positive-pressure ventilation and waking up the patient. Hypotension from sedation agents is treated with generous fluid hydration and reduction of sedation. Vasopressors are rarely needed. This patient population may have PONV, and those at risk should be identified and treated prophylactically. Patients who are not good candidates for sedation, for example, due to high body mass index or concern for the airway may need to be referred to large academic centers and anesthetized by an anesthesiologist; in those cases, there are many choices for anesthesia, including general and spinal anesthesia [6].

Selection of Sedation and Analgesia
The selection of medications for sedation and analgesia will depend on the ART center and the physician's preference. The sedation provider should be familiar with the ART procedures, the fertility center's choice of sedation/analgesia, the individual physician's needs, and those of the ART patient. Most ART centers usually have established sedation protocols.

Sedation for Oocyte Retrieval
Transvaginal ultrasound-guided oocyte retrieval can be performed under a paracervical block, moderate sedation, deep sedation, or general anesthesia. The literature concerning effective sedation and analgesia should be interpreted with caution. There are insufficient data to support any one method as superior to others in terms of pregnancy outcomes, pain relief, and patient satisfaction [7]. Specific anesthetic drugs and techniques should be evaluated for their compatibility. Animal data may not reflect the human experience. In general, short-acting opioids like fentanyl, alfentanil, and remifentanil and benzodiazepines like midazolam are considered safe and have no adverse effect on the fertilization rate and quality of the embryos [8–11].

Moderate IV sedation for transvaginal ultrasound-guided oocyte retrieval is the most commonly used anesthetic strategy. Multimodal analgesia with acetaminophen may be considered. The personnel may include nursing staff and/or an ART physician trained and experienced in sedation for ART procedures. A paracervical block can be used in combination with sedation [7].

The patient's chart is reviewed; medications and allergies, height and weight, as well as baseline vital signs are noted. The patient interview includes the NPO status, medical, surgical, and sedation/anesthesia history, as well as a history of PONV or motion sickness. The discussion of the sedation plan and the expectations of the peri-procedure period are explained to the patient. This explanation helps alleviate some of the anxiety associated with the procedure. The discussion should include the information that the patient will be sleepy yet responsive to touch or voice for the evaluation of pain or discomfort. The patient should be reassured that comfort and pain control are the goals of sedation.

The readiness of the ART procedure team is checked so that the patient can be brought into the procedure room. This is necessary because the embryology laboratory also participates in this procedure by accepting the collected oocytes and reporting the oocyte count. Once in the procedure room, the ART staff together with the embryologist will identify the patient, and perform a safety checklist.

The patient is positioned supine on the operating-room table. The routine monitors that are placed include a continuous electrocardiogram, pulse oximetry, and non-invasive blood pressure. Capnography is necessary, especially for deep sedation. An IV catheter is placed. Oxygen is usually provided via a nasal cannula or face mask. The patient is repositioned in the dorsal lithotomy position with the perineum at the edge of the table, just as for a vaginal examination.

The opioid is usually the first agent given since the primary goal of sedation is pain management during oocyte retrieval. The most frequently used opioid is fentanyl. The usual dose of fentanyl is in the range of 50–100 μg, intravenously. Once fentanyl titration is begun, the anxiolytic is administered. The most common agent is a benzodiazepine, such as midazolam or diazepam. Usually, 2–4 mg of midazolam IV is given, titrated, so the patient is relaxed yet responsive to light touch and voice.

When the desired sedation level is achieved, the surgeon places the vaginal ultrasound into the vagina. Both ovaries are examined, and the physician reports to the sedation provider an approximate estimate of the oocyte number expected to be retrieved. This helps gauge the length of time that the procedure is expected to take. Generally, younger patients have more oocytes than older patients. The placement of the vaginal probe can be very stimulating when the ovaries are difficult to visualize, and maximal pressure may need to be applied into the posterior vaginal wall. The next stimulus is the puncture through the vaginal wall into the ovary. A 16-gauge needle is used alongside the vaginal ultrasound probe. The follicles are aspirated under direct visualization. This process is then repeated on the contralateral ovary. Once the retrieval is complete, the probe is used to evaluate the ovaries for possible bleeding or tissue injury. The probe is withdrawn, and a vaginal speculum is then placed to evaluate for bleeding or vaginal wall injury. Pressure is typically held at the vaginal wall puncture sites. Additional medication is not needed at this point because the inspection of the vagina is usually not too painful. If the physician needs to place a suture or hold extensive vaginal pressure, additional opioids may be needed as well as further verbal reassurance. Once this part is complete, the patient is transferred to the recovery area. Box 27.1 summarizes the steps involved in sedation for oocyte retrieval.

Sedation for Embryo Transfer

Embryo transfer usually does not require sedation. The ART center will administer an oral benzodiazepine for those with mild to moderate anxiety. On occasion, the extremely anxious patient will request sedation for the embryo transfer. The main reason is to alleviate the procedural anxiety and discomfort of the vaginal speculum and cervical stimulation. The reproductive medicine physician may also request moderate sedation for a patient with abnormal cervical or uterine anatomy. Having the patient under moderate sedation will facilitate maneuvering the small plastic catheter containing the embryos into the uterus.

The patient chart is reviewed, and the history and physical examination are obtained. The goal of the procedure is discussed with the patient. Patient safety, comfort, and anxiolysis are emphasized. Describing the sedation/ART procedure helps ease any pre-procedural anxiety.

> **Box 27.1 Sedation for transvaginal ultrasound-guided oocyte retrieval: a summary**
>
> - Preparation in the procedure room
> - Check availability of emergency equipment
> - Pre-procedure interview and documentation
> - Confirm patient identification in the room
> - Place routine monitors
> - Peripheral IV
> - Give oxygen via nasal cannula
> - Position patient in dorsal lithotomy position
> - Start sedation with fentanyl 50 µg IV
> - Give midazolam 2 mg IV
> - Titrate IV fentanyl and midazolam
> - Keep communicating with the patient
> - Give reassurance throughout the retrieval
> - Treat pain with fentanyl
> - Follow the progression by talking to the ART physician

In the procedure room, the patient identification is verified by the ART staff and again by the embryologist. The patient is positioned supine on the table. The routine monitors and an IV catheter are placed. Then the patient is repositioned into the dorsal lithotomy position. Pressure points are padded and checked. The sedation is started during the surgical preparation, which also includes the placement of a vaginal speculum by the procedure technician. Moderate sedation can be accomplished with a combination of fentanyl and midazolam. Approximately 50 µg of fentanyl is titrated along with 2–4 mg of midazolam. Verbal reassurance is also very important when administering moderate sedation.

Sedation for Dilatation and Curettage

The sedation provider will occasionally be scheduled to administer moderate to deep sedation for a missed abortion. This is not unusual since this patient population is at higher risk of missed abortion. The patients scheduled for a D&C in the ART center should be healthy, NPO, and at minimal risk for complications. The reproductive physicians who elect to do the D&C in the ART facility may facilitate moderate sedation with a paracervical block.

The patient's chart is reviewed, and the gestational age is noted. The laboratory work is reviewed for the hematocrit, platelet count, and blood type. When a rhesus-negative woman carries a rhesus-positive pregnancy, RhoGAM is given to prevent the woman's immune system from reacting to rhesus-positive blood in any subsequent pregnancy.

The goals of ART sedation are reviewed with the patient. Safety and comfort are emphasized. Empathy and reassurance help with pre-procedural anxiety.

The procedural risks include uterine bleeding and perforation. The reproductive medicine physician will request a dose of antibiotic to prevent pelvic infection. The most stimulating part of the D&C is the serial dilatation of the cervical os and canal.

In the procedure room, the nursing staff verifies the patient and performs a procedure check. The patient is positioned supine on the operating-room table. The routine monitors are placed. An IV catheter (minimum 20-gauge) is placed. The patient is then repositioned in the dorsal lithotomy position, with the perineum at the lateral edge of the table. Pressure points are padded. Oxygen is administered via a nasal cannula or face mask. Midazolam 2–4 mg is given for anxiolysis and amnesia. A few minutes later, fentanyl is titrated in doses of 25 μg. The usual required doses of fentanyl range from 50 μg to 100 μg, with the most common total being a 100 μg dose. Titrating the sedation agents carefully will ensure that the patient breathes spontaneously with minimal airway assistance.

Post-sedation Considerations

Patient care is transferred to the recovery-room nurse. The patient care transfer begins with proper patient identification, followed by a description of the procedure, the sedation agents used, drug allergies, antiemetics, antibiotics, and fluids administered. Sedation or procedure complications encountered are communicated. Pertinent patient details such as a history of PONV, extreme pre-procedural anxiety, large amounts of sedation medications given, retrieval of few or no oocytes, or many oocytes should be communicated. A young patient or egg donor with many oocytes retrieved will probably require additional analgesics in the recovery period.

Upon arrival to the recovery area, attention is focused on oxygenation, ventilation, and circulation by monitoring pulse oximetry, breathing frequency, airway patency, systemic blood pressure, and heart rate. Supplemental oxygen and suction should be readily available. The vital signs are recorded every 15 minutes. On occasion, care may be directed toward the need for airway support for the sedated patient, who is usually treated by verbal stimulation and a chin lift. Hypotension is usually secondary to sedation and is typically self-limiting. Continuing the IV fluids and waking the patient usually resolves the hypotension. Moderate to severe pain on admission should be immediately treated with IV fentanyl 25–50 μg. Proactively addressing pain management should aid in the prompt discharge of the patient, and avoidance of PONV.

The patients undergoing ART usually stay in the recovery area for 90–120 minutes. Typical causes for a delay in the discharge from the recovery room are abdominal cramping or pain, PONV, a vasovagal event, or a delay in urination.

Moderate to severe pelvic pain is treated with IV opioids, whereas mild pain is treated with non-opioids such as acetaminophen. In most centers, non-steroidal anti-inflammatory medications are avoided due to concern for adverse effects on the subsequent embryo implantation; however, a recent study of ketorolac showed that it is likely safe and efficient [12]. In addition, as many patients may not be planning pregnancy immediately following the retrieval cycle, non-steroidal anti-inflammatory medications may be considered provided that there are no concerns about bleeding. Verbal reassurance also helps with pain control. The reproductive medicine physician should evaluate unrelenting pain. A full bladder may also be responsible for ongoing abdominal pain. The patient is encouraged to urinate. Rarely, catheterization of the bladder is needed.

The considerations for PONV should start during the pre-procedure period, recognizing that the ART population is at high risk. According to Apfel and colleagues, the four primary risk factors for PONV are female gender, non-smoking status, a history of PONV, and opioid use [13]. The typical ART patient has at least three of the four risk factors. A history of PONV and motion sickness can be specifically determined during the patient interview. Strategies to reduce baseline PONV risk factors should be deployed. These include reduction in pre-procedural anxiety, aggressive IV hydration, supplemental oxygen, and minimizing opioids. These strategies coupled with an antiemetic prophylaxis form a multimodal approach to PONV.

When PONV occurs in the recovery area, and the patient has not received prophylaxis, a 5-hydroxytryptamine (serotonin) receptor 3 (5-HT$_3$) antagonist such as ondansetron should be administered. In the event that PONV prophylaxis with a 5-HT$_3$ antagonist is inadequate, an additional dose of 5-HT$_3$ antagonist should not be used as a rescue agent since it does not give additional benefit when used within the first 6 hours after surgery [14]. The use of antiemetics like compazine, droperidol, and metoclopramide is controversial due to the transient hyperprolactinemia, which can adversely affect the procedure's outcome [15, 16].

On occasion, a patient may experience lightheadedness and nausea as a result of a vasovagal event. This event may be accompanied by nausea, bradycardia, and hypotension. The patient should be placed in the supine position, and a bolus of crystalloid fluid should be administered. Symptoms usually resolve quickly. If bradycardia and hypotension persist, a dose of vasopressor, like ephedrine 5–10 mg or anticholinergic medications like glycopyrrolate 0.2 mg or atropine 0.4 mg IV should be administered. Crampy pain may be responsible for the vasovagal event, and this should be treated.

Very rarely, brisk vaginal bleeding is observed in the recovery area. The reproductive medicine physician should evaluate the patient. The patient may be brought back to the procedure room for a thorough vaginal/pelvic examination.

The ART nursing staff documents the patient recovery course. Once the criteria for discharge are met, the patient and the adult escort are given written discharge instructions. A post-procedure follow-up telephone call is made the following morning by the ART staff.

Summary

Oocyte retrieval is a very important part of the IVF cycle. Transvaginal ultrasound-guided oocyte retrieval remains the most painful part of an IVF cycle. Moderate/deep sedation is commonly used for oocyte retrieval and related procedures in the United States and the United Kingdom. There is a large variability in personnel and medications used. A significant number of ART centers are providing their own sedation teams. The best sedation and anesthetic practice for ART procedures should be tailored to the individual patient and provider needs.

References

1. Zegers-Hochschild F, Adamson GD, de Mouzon J, et al. International Committee for Monitoring Assisted Reproductive Technology (IMART) and the World Health Organization (WHO) revised glossary of ART terminology, 2009. *Fertil Steril*. 2009;92:1520–4.

2. Oskowitz SP, Berger MJ, Mullen L, et al. Safety of a freestanding surgical unit for the assisted reproductive technologies. *Fertil Steril*. 1995;63:874–9.

3. Yasmin E, Dresner M, Balen A. Sedation and anaesthesia for transvaginal oocyte collection: an evaluation of practice in the UK. *Hum Reprod* 2004;19:2942–5.

4. Elkington NM, Kehoe J, Acharya U. Intravenous sedation in assisted conception units: a UK survey. *Hum Fertil (Camb)*. 2003;6:74–6.

5. Ditkoff EC, Plumb J, Selick A, Sauer MV. Anesthesia practices in the United States common to in vitro fertilization (ART) centers. *J Assist Reprod Genet*. 1997;14:145–7.

6. Guasch E, Gómez R, Brogly N, Gilsanz F. Anesthesia and analgesia for transvaginal oocyte retrieval. Should we recommend or avoid any anesthetic drug or technique? *Curr Opin Anaesthesiol.* 2019;32(3):285–90.

7. Kwan I, Wang R, Pearce E, Bhattacharya S. Pain relief for women undergoing oocyte retrieval for assisted reproduction. *Cochrane Database Syst Rev.* 2018;5(5): CD004829.

8. Gejervall AL, Lundin K, Stener-Victorin E, et al. Effect of alfentanil dosage during oocyte retrieval on fertilization and embryo quality. *Eur J Obstet Gynecol Reprod Biol.* 2010;150:66–71.

9. Bruce DL, Hinkley R, Norman PF. Fentanyl does not inhibit fertilization or early development of sea urchin eggs. *Anesth Analg.* 1985;64:498–500.

10. Casati A, Valentini G, Zangrillo A, et al. Anaesthesia for ultrasound guided oocyte retrieval: midazolam/remifentanil versus propofol/fentanyl regimens. *Eur J Anaesthesiol.* 1999;16:773–8.

11. Swanson RJ, Leavitt MG: Fertilization and mouse embryo development in the presence of midazolam. *Anesth Analg.* 1992;75:549–54.

12. Mesen TB, Kacemi-Bourhim L, Marshburn PB, et al. The effect of ketorolac on pregnancy rates when used immediately after oocyte retrieval. *Fertil Steril.* 2013;100:725–8.

13. Apfel CC, Läärä E, Koivuranta M, Greim CA, Roewer N. A simplified risk score for predicting postoperative nausea and vomiting: conclusions from cross-validations between two centers. *Anesthesiology.* 1999;91:693–700.

14. Kovac AL, O'Connor TA, Pearman MH, et al. Efficacy of repeat intravenous dosing of ondansetron in controlling postoperative nausea and vomiting: a randomized, double-blind, placebo-controlled multicenter trial. *J Clin Anesth.* 1999;11:453–9.

15. Kauppila A, Isotalo H, Kirkinen P, et al. Metoclopramide-induced hyperprolactinaemia: effects on corpus luteum function, endometrial steroid receptor concentrations and 17 beta-hydroxysteroid dehydrogenase activity. *Clin Endocrinol (Oxf).* 1987;26:145–54.

16. Forman R, Fishel SB, Edwards RG, et al. The influence of transient hyperprolactinemia on in vitro fertilization in humans. *J Clin Endocrinol Metab.* 1985;60:517–22.

Additional Reading

Bokhari A, Pollard BJ. Anaesthesia for assisted conception. *Eur J Anaesthesiol.* 1998;15:391–6.

Elkington M, Kehoe J, Acharya U. Policy and Practice Committee of the British Fertility Society. Recommendations for good practice for sedation in assisted conception. *Hum Fertil (Camb).* 2003;6:77–80.

Gan TJ, Meyer T, Apfel CC, et al. Consensus guidelines for managing postoperative nausea and vomiting. *Anesth Analg.* 2003;97:62–71.

Kwan I, Bhattacharya S, Knox F, McNeil A. Conscious sedation and analgesia for oocyte retrieval procedures: a Cochrane review. *Hum Reprod* 2006;21:1672–9.

Kwan I, Wang R, Pearce E, Bhattacharya S. Pain relief for women undergoing oocyte retrieval for assisted reproduction. *Cochrane Database Syst Rev.* 2018;5: CD004829.

Schenker JG, Ezra Y. Complications of assisted reproductive techniques. *Fertil Steril.* 1994;61:411–22.

Toledano RD, Kodali BS, Camann WR. Anesthesia drugs in the obstetric and gynecologic practice. *Rev Obstet Gynecol.* 2009;2:93–100.

Trout SW, Vallerand AH, Kemmann E. Conscious sedation for in vitro fertilization. *Fertil Steril.* 1998;69:799–808.

Tsen LC. From Darwin to desflurane? Anesthesia for assisted reproductive technologies. *Anesth Analg.* 2002;94 (Suppl):109–14.

Wallach EE, Zacur HA. *Reproductive Medicine and Surgery.* St Louis, MO: Mosby, 1995:849.

Chapter 28

Interventional Pain Management Procedures

Alan D. Kaye and Laxmaiah Manchikanti

Introduction

The administration of anesthetics for sedation during pain management procedures is a challenge to any provider. While minor and interventional procedures are routinely performed in operating theaters, it is increasingly common for these same procedures to be performed in a variety of other settings and even without sedation at all. These sites include remote locations within the hospital, outpatient pain management centers, diagnostic centers, and physician offices.

Practitioners must be aware of the specific characteristics of their location to ensure patient safety. This includes, for example, logistics for contacting medical assistance or obtaining equipment for medical emergencies. It is equally prudent to realize that standards of care are unchanged regardless of practice setting. Multiple guidelines by various organizations, such as The Joint Commission (TJC), the American Society of Anesthesiologists (ASA), and the Occupational Safety and Health Administration (OSHA), describe the requirements for intravenous sedation in any given location that should be utilized. All practitioners and assisting personnel must survey the site prior to the commencement of a procedure to ensure that adequate care is delivered in a controlled and routine manner.

Established Standards of Care

The ASA has established several guidelines including the requirements for anesthesia delivery in an office-based setting and for interventional pain procedures. The concept of anesthesia delivery in the office, referred to as office-based anesthesia, is considered a subset of ambulatory anesthesia. Policies of accreditation and licensure bodies require that a licensed physician be in attendance at the facility and at least available by telephone in the event of overnight patient care until discharge criteria are met. Resuscitation equipment and emergency transfer should be immediately available to the facility. Additionally, minimal care standards such as appropriate written consent, patient education regarding follow-up, and discharge instructions apply to all patients undergoing procedures. Office-based anesthesia is unique in that, unlike a hospital or licensed ambulatory surgical facility, physician offices have minimal regulatory control or oversight by government agencies. However, this underscores the importance of meeting requirements for delivering sedation for pain procedures. The practitioner must be confident that all issues are addressed in order to reduce risk and liability.

The ASA's statement on anesthesia delivered for interventional pain procedures outlines that, unless unique circumstances are present, patients should only need local anesthesia. This is also consistent with sedation guidelines published in 2019 from the American Society of Interventional Pain Physicians (ASIPP) and both societies specifically do not recommend propofol for sedation for routine interventional pain procedures, such as epidurals, facet injections, sacroiliac injections, and other relatively quick and straightforward pain procedures. Any procedures that are prolonged and/or painful should follow the guidelines for sedation or monitored anesthesia care (MAC) discussed in this chapter. Procedures performed with sedation, MAC, or local anesthesia must balance the risk of possible harm to the patient, especially those undergoing elective cervical spine procedures. Patients must be alert enough during a pain procedure to be able to communicate with the pain practitioner if they are experiencing pain when a needle is misplaced intraneurally, within the spine itself, or in another aberrant location.

Specific standards are also set by OSHA for the care of patients in settings outside of the operating suite. Their guidelines cover safety items such as radiation exposure, high sound levels, and heavy mechanical equipment, which can all be applicable to the practice of pain management.

Accreditation agencies including TJC, and licensure agencies, outline several standards for the anesthetic care of patients, from environmental guidelines and emergency management to leadership structure and infection control. There are aspects of office-based surgery outlined in accreditation handbooks for office-based surgery specific to the delivery of sedation and anesthesia. In this regard, permission given to a practitioner to administer sedation stipulates that he or she must be able to rescue the patient from any depth of anesthesia (e.g., "when the patient slips from moderate into deep sedation or from deep sedation into full anesthesia"). It is further clarified that the availability of a cardiorespiratory rescue team is not acceptable in lieu of a practitioner who is qualified to administer sedation, and thus also qualified to rescue a patient from any depth of anesthesia.

Facilities and Equipment

There are basic characteristics of non-operating-room sites that need to be met for adequate delivery of anesthesia care to patients. The ASA, OSHA, TJC, other accreditation agencies, and licensure agencies outline the standards that each remote location should fulfill prior to administration of sedation for pain management procedures. At the conclusion of procedures, travel distances to recovery areas vary, and therefore it is vital to have an adequate supply of supplemental oxygen with fully functional backup, monitoring equipment, and immediate access with keys to elevators or corridors. In the event of an emergency, there should be efficient access to oxygen, suction, emergency drugs, monitors, and defibrillator. The crash cart should be stocked and within reasonable distance from the patient area, along with instruments for intravenous access (gloves, tourniquets, alcohol wipes, catheters, tubing, syringes). Furthermore, reliable transfer to an outside facility should also be in place for emergent situations requiring a higher level of care. Additionally, the practitioner and staff should be familiar with the exact location of the nearest defibrillator, fire extinguisher, and exit. Pain management procedures often require fluoroscopy, and radiation safety is therefore of the utmost importance. Advanced preparation should be made for proper storage and handling of machines, lead aprons or glass shields, and thyroid shields. Dosimetry data should comply with state and federal regulations. The remote locations where pain procedures are performed should also have adequate illumination, power outlets, and fault circuit breakers. There should be ample provision of physical space for equipment and all participating personnel.

Personnel and Staffing

An anesthesiologist is not always involved in the care of the patient, and sedation/analgesia is frequently administered by non-anesthesiologists or other non-anesthesia professionals. Delivery of anesthesia requires the understanding that sedation and general anesthesia are on a continuum. But not all those who are administering medications may be able to appreciate the importance of this concept, based on their background and training. The ASA has established standards for granting privileges for administering moderate sedation to practitioners who are not anesthesia professionals. Only physicians, dentists, or podiatrists who are qualified by education, training, and licensure should supervise the administration of moderate sedation. The non-anesthesiologist should not only be able to pre-assess patient comorbidities and be competent in the use of routine sedation medications, but also be trained and skilled in the use of airway equipment and emergency resuscitative care (e.g., oral airway, laryngoscope, endotracheal tubes, and resuscitation bag-mask). These qualifications are needed in order to provide complete care for patients undergoing routine pain procedures in remote locations where emergent situations may arise.

There are numerous people involved in the care of a patient before, during, and after the procedure, including nurses, radiology technicians, and surgical technicians. Open communication between parties is essential for adequate anesthetic delivery to the patient in an environment where staff members are skilled in different areas. This is extremely important in a situation where skilled anesthesia care may not be in the immediate vicinity. It may also be prudent to ensure that staff members are able to assist in patient resuscitation, if needed (basic life support, advanced cardiac life support).

Patient Evaluation

Appropriate pre-procedural evaluation of each patient is recommended. The pre-assessment allows for reduction in risk of adverse outcomes and in turn leads to improved patient outcomes. Qualified practitioners should familiarize themselves with and document major organ-system abnormalities, previous exposure to sedation anesthesia, and noted complications, current medical history and medications, allergies, and social history including tobacco, alcohol, and substance abuse. The subpopulation of patients undergoing interventional pain management procedures requires that the provider have a detailed understanding not only of routine medications, but additionally of various analgesics, muscle relaxants, sedatives, and other adjunct medications, to avoid oversedation and other adverse events perioperatively. This includes knowing how many of these drugs were taken in recent days, including on the day of the pain procedure, and a good understanding of the baseline level of sedation. Complete physical examination assessing the heart, lungs, and airway should be completed. Many pain procedures are performed with the patient in the prone position, and a thorough evaluation for airway limitations is prudent for a successful outcome. Extra precautions should be taken for patients with increased body habitus, short neck, limited range of motion of head and neck, dysmorphic features of the head and neck, small mouth, trismus, or history of sleep apnea, because these factors increase the likelihood of airway obstruction during spontaneous ventilation and difficult airway management. Additional laboratory workup is indicated for underlying medical conditions that have the potential to affect the delivery of anesthetic care.

Obtaining consent for anesthetic care is required in most situations. Since many of these procedures are performed with mild or moderate sedation only, it is important that patients have a good understanding that they may feel a portion of the procedure, in particular a local anesthesia wheal at the surface of the injection site. They need to understand that it is against local, regional, and national standards to render a pain patient unconscious for typical interventional pain procedures and that deep sedation or general anesthesia can increase the risk of catastrophic consequences including injection into the wrong area such as the spinal cord, causing neurologic injury and hypoventilation resulting cardiopulmonary collapse and even death. In this regard, if the injection is placed directly into the spine, the patient will not be able to communicate effectively that the injectable is being placed into the wrong area. Further, the patient must be informed that routine measures are taken to ensure safe delivery of medical care, but more invasive techniques may need to be employed if sedation fails to provide adequate analgesia and the patient and surgeon wishes to proceed with the procedure. Additionally, there is always a rare chance for an unanticipated procedural complication or an acute reaction to medications, which can include the potential for catastrophic allergic response with loss of the airway, cardiovascular instability, and even death. The risks and benefits of all types of anesthetic care should be explained and questions answered, to ensure that the patient clearly understands the plan of action. It is recommended that procedures not be performed if a responsible adult is not available to accompany the patient home after the procedure.

Monitoring

Since a primary cause of morbidity associated with sedation is drug-induced respiratory depression, adequate monitoring of ventilatory function beyond observation of chest rise and auscultation is recommended by the ASA with moderate or deep sedation to avoid adverse outcomes. Additional monitors should be employed to ensure proper oxygenation and circulation with pulse oximetry and ECG and this is a national standard. Blood pressure, quantitative end-tidal carbon dioxide (CO_2), and temperature monitoring should be employed and are also a national standard for patients undergoing moderate or deep sedation. The healthcare practitioner providing sedation for pain procedures will be ill-equipped to ascertain the cause of symptoms such as sudden onset of

Table 28.1 The Ramsay scale for monitoring of sedation level

Sedation level	Description
1	Anxious and agitated
2	Cooperative, tranquil, oriented
3	Responds only to verbal commands
4	Asleep with brisk response to light stimulation
5	Asleep without response to light stimulation
6	Nonresponsive

Modified from: Ramsay MAE, Savege TM, Simpson BRJ, Goodwin R. Controlled sedation with alphaxalone–alphadolone. *Br Med J.* 1974;2:656–9.

lightheadedness, shortness of breath, oversedation, nausea, or changes in mental status, without appropriate monitors.

As cited earlier, the depth of anesthesia, from sedation to general anesthesia, is a continuum (see Table 1.1). The adequate delivery of anesthesia requires the practitioner to understand the difference between conscious sedation and MAC, because the level of care can change from moment to moment based on the titration of a given drug. The essential component of MAC is the assessment and management of anticipated physiologic changes during the case, with the provider of the anesthetic prepared and qualified to convert to general anesthesia if necessary. For practitioners administering moderate or deep sedation, there should not be such an expectation, meaning that the integrity of the patient's physiologic status and airway should remain intact for the entirety of the procedure. The patient should also respond purposefully to verbal command and to tactile stimulation. In this regard, the degree of postoperative care required for patients after MAC is higher (e.g., assessment for return to baseline mental status, relief of pain).

In addition to physiologic monitoring, assessment of the level of sedation and pain is vital for adequate sedation for pain procedures. Some facilities use brain-wave monitors such as the bispectral index (BIS) and Sedline to help the clinician assess the depth of anesthesia of pain patients under sedation. Common additional tools include the Ramsay Sedation Scale (RSS; Table 28.1) and the Richmond Agitation–Sedation Scale (RASS; see Tables 4.1 and 22.1). While RSS is scaled 1 (anxious and agitated) to 6 (non-responsive), the RASS is from +4 (combative) to −5 (unarousable). The Visual Analog Scale and the Faces Pain Scale (see Figure 3.1) are most commonly used to assess and document a patient's comfort level.

Drugs

Various sedatives, opioids, and dissociative agents are used in the management of patients undergoing pain procedures. As referenced from the ASA and ASIPP, propofol is *not* recommended for common pain procedures that are relatively quick and straightforward. Here we present a brief review of the effects of other sedative drugs; see Chapter 2 for fuller details of the pharmacology of sedative agents. Obviously, it is imperative for the practitioner to have immediate access to airway equipment when administering any of these medications.

Midazolam (Versed), diazepam (Valium), and remimazolam (Byfavo) are common benzodiazepines used in the premedication of pain patients prior to their pain procedure. These drugs interact with discrete benzodiazepine receptors in the cerebral cortex, and while they have no direct analgesic properties they do have anxiolytic, amnesic, sedative, and muscle-relaxant properties. Benzodiazepines cause minimal cardiovascular depression, which can be seen as a decrease in blood pressure or decreased heart rate mediated via decreased vagal tone. These medicines also cause respiratory depression from a decreased response to CO_2, especially when administered intravenously. The relatively high potency of midazolam necessitates careful titration to avoid overdose and resulting apnea. The use of opioids with benzodiazepines has a synergistic effect on cardiovascular depression, which can be especially pronounced in patients with ischemic heart disease. Careful review of a patient's chart is also warranted, to avoid drug interactions. Cimetidine reduces the metabolism of diazepam, erythromycin inhibits metabolism of midazolam, and heparin increases the free drug concentration of diazepam in blood twofold.

The commonly used opioids fentanyl and alfentanil are used for pain control. These drugs inhibit postsynaptic responses to noxious stimulus in nociceptive neurons. The high lipid solubility of these two drugs is reflected in the rapid onset of action, but the duration of action is considerably shorter. If multiple doses are administered, plasma concentrations do not decrease rapidly, and this may prolong the duration of analgesia and suppression of ventilation. Alfentanil is one-fifth to one-tenth as potent as fentanyl and has about one-third the duration of action, which provides many clinical advantages over fentanyl for analgesia. Side effects are similar to those of morphine (e.g., reduced peristalsis leading to constipation) without the accompanying histamine release and hypotension. Opioids do not depress cardiac function, but high doses may cause vagus-mediated bradycardia. However, opioid-mediated respiratory depression is subject to close titration. In addition to blunting a patient's response to CO_2, these drugs also induce chest wall rigidity, which may impair adequate ventilation.

Propofol is an induction agent used for general anesthesia that can also be used for deep sedation in a variety of settings. Combined with active hypnotic and antiemetic properties, its short duration of action makes it an ideal anesthetic adjuvant for deep sedation for certain complex and lengthy interventional pain procedures, as well as resulting in a prompt recovery. Physiologic changes result in decreased arterial blood pressure, in which large changes occur with large intravenous doses, rapid injection, and advanced age. Careful titration and adequate monitoring of patient vital signs during administration is critical, because profound respiratory depression can be seen, which may lead to apnea with multiple or larger doses. Furthermore, patients under deep sedation are unable to communicate effective with the pain practitioner, including when a needle is placed in the wrong place and cause nerve injury.

Ketamine is a highly lipid-soluble dissociative anesthetic that renders patients unable to process sensory information while appearing to be conscious. Uniquely, the cardiovascular effects are increased blood pressure and heart rate, which typically needs to be avoided in patients with coronary artery disease. Respiratory drive is minimally affected and, in fact, it is a bronchodilator, which is an advantage for asthmatic patients (although the drug also increases secretions in a dose-dependent manner). Although this drug is not considered a first-line sedation drug for interventional pain procedures, it can be a useful agent for difficult patients and/or challenging pain procedures. Patients should be educated about the undesirable psychotomimetic effects (e.g., illusions, disturbing dreams, delirium). Drug interaction with diazepam prolongs ketamine's elimination half-life.

Dexmedetomidine is a selective alpha-2 agonist with sedative properties and some analgesic effects. There is no significant depression of respiratory drive, but excessive sedation may cause airway obstruction. Other side effects include bradycardia, heart block, hypotension, and nausea. Therefore, dexmedetomidine should be used with caution in patients taking vasodilators, beta-blockers, or drugs that decrease heart rate.

Competitive antagonists (reversal agents) should also be available to the practitioner, such as naloxone and flumazenil. Naloxone is an opioid reversal agent that can rescue patients from the effects of opioid overdose. But reversal of opioid overdose (e.g., respiratory depression) can also reverse opioid analgesia and result in sympathetic stimulation from sudden increased perception of pain. Flumazenil is a benzodiazepine reversal agent that antagonizes the hypnotic effects more effectively than the amnesic properties. Side effects include anxiety reactions and nausea and vomiting. Both reversal agents can also cause withdrawal symptoms if patients are tolerant or have long-standing treatment with the given opioid or benzodiazepine.

Emergency rescue drugs, including epinephrine, diphenhydramine (Benadryl), and dexamethasone (Decadron), should always be available in a crash cart that is easily accessible to the site of procedure. The practitioner and staff should be prepared for situations such as sudden loss of consciousness, seizure, allergic reaction, and adverse procedural outcomes.

Procedures

Typical procedures in pain management are varied, and the clinician providing sedation should have an understanding so that appropriate sedation can be delivered effectively and efficiently (Box 28.1). It is critical to perform a time-out before the interventional pain physician starts the procedure, to ensure that the correct procedure on the correct side is being performed. Many busy pain practitioners perform 10–20 procedures in a day, and confusion must be minimized. Fairly straightforward interventional pain procedures, which are typically between 10 and 60 minutes in duration and can be managed effectively with moderate sedation, include diagnostic and therapeutic procedures, epidural injections, transforaminal injections, caudal injections, sacroiliac joint injections, hip and knee injections, radiofrequency neurotomy, discograms, epidurolysis, and most sympathetic blocks. There are many other types of injections and most of them can be performed successfully with local or mild to moderate sedation. In most cases, experience with the pain practitioner, appropriate monitoring (in particular quantitative end-tidal CO_2 for ventilation assessment), careful titration of drugs, and effective communication will ensure success for these patients. Key anesthetic considerations are outlined in Box 28.2.

Patient Recovery

Immediately following a pain procedure, the patient should be transported with the practitioner providing the sedation to a recovery area. Supplemental oxygen and

---

Box 28.1 Overview of pain procedures for the non-anesthesiologist

Short-duration procedures (15–30 minutes)

- Diagnostic blocks and infusions
- Trigger-point/myofascial injections (e.g., injections directly into muscle beds)
- Cryoablation injections
- Facet joint injections
- Epidural steroid injections, including cervical, thoracic, and lumbar
- Transforaminal nerve root injections
- Caudal injections
- Sacroiliac joint injections
- Hip injections
- Radiofrequency thermocoagulation
- Pulsed electromagnet field injections
- Knee injections
- Most sympathetic/ganglion blocks, including sphenopalatine ganglion, stellate ganglion, dorsal root ganglion, splanchnic nerve, celiac plexus block, thoracic and lumbar sympathetic, hypogastric plexus, and ganglion of Impar
- Intercostal nerve blocks
- Suprascapular nerve blocks

Longer-duration procedures (30–60 minutes)

- Discograms: cervical, thoracic, lumbar
- Epidurolysis/epiduroscopy
- Augmentation techniques, including spinal cord stimulation (dorsal column stimulation testing and permanent implantation) of the occipital nerve, cervical, thoracic, lumbar, or sacral spinal cord
- Intrathecal implantation
- Neurolytic and neurolysis blocks, including ethyl alcohol, phenol, hypotonic, hypertonic, and glycerol injections
- Decompressive neuroplasty (Racz procedure)
- Vertebroplasty
- Sacroiliac joint fusion

Box 28.2 Key anesthetic considerations for the non-anesthesiologist

- Ensure supplemental oxygen supply
- Ensure that tools for intravenous access and airway equipment are functional and available
- Develop skills for early recognition in oversedation
- Document vital signs before, during, and after procedure
- Ensure personnel are on standby for emergency
- Be vigilant!

---

monitors for transport may be required if a long distance to recovery care is expected. Upon arrival, vital signs, level of sedation, and degree of pain should be immediately reassessed. The patient's general condition should be noted, and staff should be available to accept the transfer of care. Because stimulation from the procedure is no longer present, prolonged effects of the sedatives or decreased metabolism may contribute to cardiorespiratory suppression. Prior to release from the facility, appropriate discharge criteria should be met such as return to baseline mental status, stable vital signs, and a sufficient time elapsed since last documented dose of medication. Discharge from the facility should only be done when the patient is accompanied by a responsible adult. Finally, it is imperative that discharge instructions are provided to the patient, indicating appropriate diet, medications, acceptable activities, and contact information in case of emergency.

Summary

Providing safe and effective sedation for pain patients can be challenging and rewarding. Even for longtime anesthesia providers, interventional pain procedures require careful planning and prudent decision making. Many interventional pain practitioners perform procedures without sedation, which can be both terrifying and painful for the patient in need of these treatments. Regardless of the location, whether in an office, a radiology suite, an ambulatory facility, or a hospital operating room, sedation can be a critical component of an interventional pain procedure. However, in ill-equipped hands, pain patients can potentially have morbidity and mortality when sedation is utilized. Competence and defined standards of experience and expertise are not only warranted but essential for successful sedation of the pain patient. Monitoring of these pain patients, many of whom are in the prone position and not intubated, should include standard ASA monitors, including quantitative end-tidal CO_2 for ventilation in the setting of moderate or deep sedation and general anesthesia.

Acknowledgments

The authors wish to thank Dr. Ron Banister and Dr. Rahul Mishra for the contributions to the first edition of this chapter.

Additional Reading

Kaye AD, Jones MR, Kaye AM, et al. Prescription opioid abuse in chronic pain: an updated review of opioid abuse predictors and strategies to curb opioid abuse: Part 1. *Pain Physician.* 2017;20(2S): S93–109.

Kaye AD, Jones MR, Kaye AM, et al. Prescription opioid abuse in chronic pain: an updated review of opioid abuse predictors and strategies to curb opioid abuse: Part 2. *Pain Physician.* 2017;20(2S): S111–33.

Kaye AD, Jones MR, Viswanath O, et al. ASIPP guidelines for sedation and fasting status of patients undergoing interventional pain management procedures. *Pain Physician.* 2019;22(3):201–7.

Manzi JE, Jones MR, Cornett EM, Kaye AD. Moderate and deep procedural sedation-the role of proper monitoring and safe techniques in clinical practice. *Curr Opin Anaesthesiol.* 2021;34(4):497–501.

Practice guidelines for sedation and analgesia by non-anesthesiologists. *Anesthesiology.* 2002;96:1004–17.

Miller RD, ed. *Anesthesia*, 7th ed. Philadelphia, PA: Churchill Livingstone, 2009.

Raj PP, Lou L, Erdine S, et al. *Interventional Pain Management: Image-Guided Procedures*, 2nd ed. Philadelphia, PA: Elsevier, 2008.

Ramsay MAE, Savege TM, Simpson BRJ, Goodwin R. Controlled sedation with alphaxalone–alphadolone. *Br Med J.* 1974;2:656–9.

Sessler CN, Gosnell MS, Grap MJ, et al. The Richmond Agitation–Sedation Scale: validity and reliability in adult intensive care patients. *Am J Respir Crit Care Med.* 2002;166:1338–44.

Stoelting RK, Miller RD. *Basics of Anesthesia,* 5th ed. Philadelphia, PA: Churchill Livingstone, 2007.

The Joint Commission. Office-based surgery accreditation fact sheet.

www.jointcommission.org/resources/news-and-multimedia/fact-sheets/facts-about-office-based-surgery-accreditation

ASA Guidelines

Statement on continuum of depth of sedation: definition of general anesthesia and levels of sedation/analgesia. Committee of origin: Committee on Quality Management and Departmental Administration (original approval on October 13, 1999 and last amended on October 23, 2019)

Distinguishing monitored anesthesia care ("MAC") from moderate sedation/analgesia (conscious sedation). Committee of origin: Economics (approved by the ASA House of Delegates on October 27, 2004 and last amended on October 21, 2009).

Guidelines for ambulatory anesthesia and surgery. Committee of origin: Ambulatory Surgical Care (approved by the ASA House of Delegates on October 15, 2003, and last amended on October 22, 2008).

Guidelines for office-based anesthesia. Committee of origin: Ambulatory Surgical Care (approved by the ASA House of Delegates on October 13, 1999, and last affirmed on October 21, 2009).

ASA Statements

Statement on anesthetic care during interventional pain procedures for adults. Committee of origin: Pain Medicine (approved by the ASA House of Delegates on October 22, 2005 and last amended on October 20, 2010).

Statement on granting privileges for administration of moderate sedation to practitioners who are not anesthesia professionals. Committee of origin: Ad Hoc Committee on Credentialing (approved by the ASA House of Delegates on October 25, 2005, and amended on October 18, 2006).

Statement on nonoperating room anesthetizing locations. Committee of origin: Standards and Practice Parameters (approved by the ASA House of Delegates on October 15, 2003 and amended on October 22, 2008).

Statement on qualifications of anesthesia providers in the office-based setting. Committee of origin: Ambulatory Surgical Care (approved by the ASA House of Delegates on October 13, 1999, and last amended on October 21, 2009).

Chapter 29

Emergency Resuscitation Algorithms: Adults

Jue Teresa Wang

Introduction

Moderate and deep sedation occurs in numerous settings, and healthcare providers may unexpectedly find themselves in situations where emergency resuscitation of patients will be required. A discussion of key concepts found in the latest American Heart Association (AHA) guidelines follows, to prepare the provider for these potential emergencies. For more detailed information, the reader is referred to the 2020 AHA guidelines for cardiopulmonary resuscitation and emergency cardiovascular care [1].

Basic Life Support

Basic life support (BLS) skills for the healthcare provider include immediate recognition of sudden cardiac arrest (SCA), early cardiopulmonary resuscitation (CPR), and rapid defibrillation with an automated external defibrillator (AED) [1] (Figure 29.1).

The first step is to check for the patient's responsiveness. The healthcare provider can check for the absence of breathing or normal breathing, as well as try to appreciate a response to stimulus (e.g., voice and touch). Immediate activation of the emergency response system should follow if the patient is unresponsive, and an AED should be obtained if it is nearby and easily accessible.

It is important to note the provider should take no longer than 10 seconds to check for a pulse, and if no pulse is appreciated in that time, chest compressions should be initiated without further delay. However, if the patient suddenly collapses or is not breathing, pulse checks should not even be attempted and the provider should assume that SCA has occurred and begin chest compressions [2].

As in the previous update, chest compressions should be initiated before ventilation (compression–airway–breathing [CAB] rather than airway–breathing– compression [ABC]), and this priority shift is a result of growing evidence on the importance of chest compressions to ensure oxygen delivery to the heart and brain.

However, if a definite pulse is palpable, the healthcare provider should not initiate chest compressions, but give one rescue breath every 5–6 seconds and recheck the patient's pulse every 2 minutes. The patient should also be placed in a recovery position on his/her side with the lower arm in front of the body.

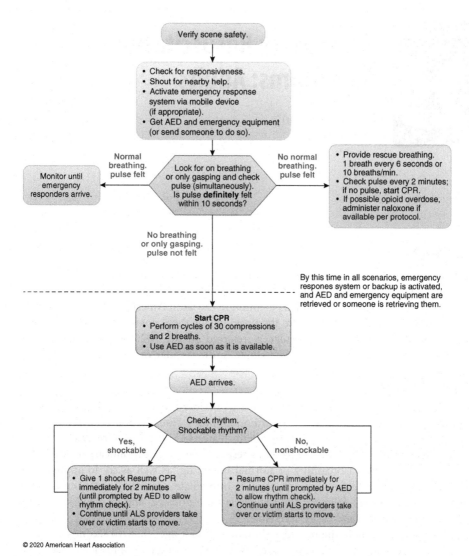

Verify scene safety.

- Check for responsiveness.
- Shout for nearby help.
- Activate emergency response system via mobile device (if appropriate).
- Get AED and emergency equipment (or send someone to do so).

Look for on breathing or only gasping and check pulse (simultaneously). Is pulse **definitely** felt within 10 seconds?

Normal breathing. pulse felt → Monitor until emergency responders arrive.

No normal breathing. pulse felt →
- Provide rescue breathing. 1 breath every 6 seconds or 10 breaths/min.
- Check pulse every 2 minutes; if no pulse, start CPR.
- If possible opioid overdose, administer naloxone if available per protocol.

No breathing or only gasping. pulse not felt

By this time in all scenarios, emergency respones system or backup is activated, and AED and emergency equipment are retrieved or someone is retrieving them.

Start CPR
- Perform cycles of 30 compressions and 2 breaths.
- Use AED as soon as it is available.

AED arrives.

Check rhythm. Shockable rhythm?

Yes, shockable
- Give 1 shock Resume CPR immediately for 2 minutes (until prompted by AED to allow rhythm check).
- Continue until ALS providers take over or victim starts to move.

No, nonshockable
- Resume CPR immediately for 2 minutes (until prompted by AED to allow rhythm check).
- Continue until ALS providers take over or victim starts to move.

© 2020 American Heart Association

Figure 29.1 Adult basic life support healthcare provider cardiac arrest algorithm – 2020 update.

To start chest compressions, the patient should be placed on a firm surface, or a backboard should be placed under the patient if he/she is in a hospital bed. The heel of one hand should be placed on the center of the patient's chest, with the heel of the other hand on top of the first. The chest wall should be allowed to completely recoil after each compression to prevent higher intrathoracic pressure and allow the heart to refill, in order to improve hemodynamic outcomes. The new 2020 AHA guidelines recommend chest compression rates should be 100–120 compressions per minute, and the sternum should be depressed 2 inches (5 cm) ("push hard and fast"). If two or more providers are present, they should alternate every 2 minutes to prevent fatigue and poor compression quality. It is also important to note that chest compressions should be minimally interrupted to check for a pulse, analyze rhythm, or other activities. If an interruption occurs, it should be limited to less than 10 seconds. CPR should continue until an AED arrives, the patient wakes up, or advanced life support personnel arrive.

After the initiation of chest compressions, ventilation should be attempted. The compression/ventilation ratio is 30:2 if there is no advanced airway, such as an endotracheal tube. Ventilation can be performed using the head-tilt/chin-lift maneuver if there is no evidence of head or neck trauma. A tight seal should be obtained between the face and mask, and the bag should be squeezed just enough to produce visible chest rise. In all of the ventilation methods, the compression/ventilation ratio is still 30:2. Once an advanced airway (endotracheal tube, or laryngeal mask airway [LMA]) is placed, one breath should be delivered every 6–8 seconds, or 8–10 breaths per minute, with no interruption of chest compressions. These recommendations are given to prevent excessive ventilation, which can lead to gastric inflation and complications such as regurgitation and aspiration.

Early defibrillation with an AED is the next key step in the adult BLS sequence and is the treatment of choice for ventricular fibrillation (VF) of short duration. Defibrillation is performed after a 2-minute cycle of CPR in the BLS sequence. Early defibrillation is key, and should not be delayed until a cycle of CPR has been done. For in-hospital settings where an AED is available, the defibrillator should be used as soon as possible. If more than one healthcare provider is present, one provider should initiate compressions while the other activates the emergency response system and obtains an AED. Once the AED has been obtained, the defibrillation sequence is as follows: power AED on, follow AED prompts to check rhythm and give one shock if the rhythm is "shockable," and resume CPR immediately after shocking. If the rhythm is "not shockable," CPR should resume immediately, and the rhythm should be checked every 2 minutes. CPR should be continued while the AED is being turned on and pads are being applied to minimize disruptions in chest compressions.

Lastly, there are special situations that warrant discussion, especially because the healthcare provider can have a significant impact on patient outcome if they are properly recognized. Two of those situations are discussed here.

Acute coronary syndrome is commonly manifested by chest pain, radiation of pain to the upper body, shortness of breath, sweating, nausea, and lightheadedness. Immediate activation of the emergency medical service (EMS) system should follow when these symptoms are present. When appropriate, EMS providers are trained to administer chewable, non-enteric aspirin 160–325 mg, obtain a 12-lead ECG, administer oxygen to keep oxygen saturation $\geq$ 94%, administer nitroglycerin in select patients, and administer analgesics such as morphine. Additionally, if an ECG demonstrates ST-segment elevation myocardial infarction (STEMI), the patient must then be rapidly transported to a percutaneous coronary intervention (PCI) facility. Prompt PCI has been associated with improved outcomes in STEMI [2].

Acute ischemic stroke is another situation in which proper recognition and immediate activation of the EMS system can have a significant impact on the patient's outcome. Commonly manifested symptoms of stroke are acute in onset and can include the following: numbness and weakness of the face, upper or lower extremities, confusion, difficulty speaking or understanding, difficulty walking, dizziness, loss of balance or coordination, and severe headache. If fibrinolytic therapy is given within the first 3 hours of symptom onset, neurologic injury is reduced and patients can have improved outcomes. Patients should be transported directly to a stroke center when possible.

As with any other situation, if the patient is unresponsive, the BLS sequence, as well as the following advanced cardiac life support (ACLS) components, are critical and should not be delayed, regardless of whether or not the root cause is acute coronary syndrome or acute ischemic stroke.

Advanced Cardiac Life Support

Advanced cardiac life support (ACLS) builds on the BLS sequence and includes airway management and ventilation support, management of cardiac arrest, and treatment of bradyarrhythmias and tachyarrhythmias [1].

Advanced airway placement and ventilation support allow for oxygenation and elimination of carbon dioxide (CO_2). There are not sufficient data to recommend when to place an advanced airway in relation to other interventions during resuscitation. However, airway placement should not delay initial CPR and defibrillation, and it is important to note that airway placement can be achieved without interruption of chest compressions. Additionally, only those healthcare providers who have been trained in airway placement should do this, and the guidelines suggest frequent training for skill maintenance. If advanced airway placement cannot be achieved, bag-valve-mask ventilation can be used as a backup. Oropharyngeal airways and nasopharyngeal airways can all be used as adjuncts until an advanced airway is placed.

Once an endotracheal tube or supraglottic airway (e.g. LMA) is placed, an immediate assessment for proper placement should follow. Physical examination should reveal bilateral chest rise, bilateral breath sounds, no breath sounds over the epigastrum, and exhaled CO_2 detectors should also be used to confirm correct placement. Additionally, continuous waveform capnography is now recommended, as it is the most reliable method to confirm and monitor for correct placement of an endotracheal tube. Continuous waveform capnography also has the advantage of reflecting poor-quality CPR if partial-pressure end-tidal CO_2 ($PETCO_2$) decreases below 10 mmHg, and reflecting the return of spontaneous circulation (ROSC) if there is an abrupt and sustained increase in $PETCO_2$ (> 40 mmHg) [3].

After successful placement of an advanced airway, chest compressions should immediately resume with the 2020 AHA guideline rate of 100–120 compressions per minute with no interruptions for ventilation. Ventilation should be given as one breath every 6–8 seconds, or 8–10 breaths per minute. Providers should switch roles every 2 minutes to prevent fatigue. There are not sufficient data to suggest the goal tidal volume, respiratory rate, and inspired oxygen concentration, but 100% inspired oxygen is often empirically used.

In addition to CPR and ventilation support, management of cardiac arrest involves rhythm-based management with an AED and early defibrillation when appropriate [4]. The adhesive pads or paddles of an AED should be placed in an anterior-lateral position. Other positions are anterior-posterior, anterior-left infrascapular, and anterior-right infrascapular. VF, pulseless ventricular tachycardia (VT), pulseless electrical activity (PEA), and asystole are heart rhythms that can lead to cardiac arrest. p VT and VF are "shockable" rhythms, whereas PEA and asystole are "not shockable" rhythms. If a rhythm check with an AED reveals VF or pulseless VT, the initial shock should be delivered at 120–200 J for a biphasic defibrillator and 360 J for a monophasic defibrillator (Figure 29.2). After shocking, CPR should resume immediately for 2 minutes, followed by another rhythm check. If VF or pulseless VT is revealed again, another shock is delivered, immediately followed by CPR. Additionally, during this 2-minute cycle of CPR, epinephrine 1 mg intravenous/intraosseous (IV/IO) can be given and repeated every 3–5 minutes. Again, if in 2 minutes VF or VT is revealed at the rhythm check, another shock is delivered, immediately followed by CPR. During this cycle of CPR, a bolus dose of amiodarone 300 mg IV/IO can be given. Subsequent to this initial round of cycles, medications given should alternate between epinephrine 1 mg IV/IO and amiodarone 150 mg IV/IO. The new 2020 AHA guidelines also suggest the use of lidocaine at 1–1.5 mg/kg IV/IO with a possible second dose at 0.5–0.75 mg/kg. If a rhythm check at any time reveals PEA or asystole, which are not shockable rhythms, the sequence outlined as follows is initiated.

For PEA or asystole, CPR (and not defibrillation) should continue for 2 minutes, followed by another rhythm check. Epinephrine 1 mg IV/IO every 3–5 minutes can be given during this cycle of CPR. If PEA or asystole is revealed again, CPR resumes for 2 minutes. If a rhythm check at any time reveals VF or VT, the preceding sequence for shockable rhythms is initiated. For the treatment of PEA or asystole, atropine is no longer recommended for routine use, because of a lack of supporting evidence.

Medications given during cardiac arrest have the primary goal of facilitating ROSC. Epinephrine hydrochloride is a vasopressor with alpha-adrenergic agonist properties including increasing coronary perfusion pressure and cerebral perfusion pressure. The benefits of epinephrine's beta-adrenergic agonist properties are less clear, and it may increase myocardial work and reduce subendocardial perfusion. There is evidence that vasopressors may be associated with an increased rate of ROSC, although not necessarily an increase in the rate of neurologically intact survival to hospital discharge. Amiodarone is an antiarrhythmic drug and is preferred for treatment of VF and pulseless VT. It acts at sodium, potassium, and calcium channels, as well as alpha- and beta-adrenergic receptors as an antagonist. There is evidence that amiodarone increases short-term survival to hospital admission compared to lidocaine or placebo, but there has been no evidence suggesting increased survival to discharge.

It is important to note that other ACLS interventions, such as obtaining vascular access, administering drugs, placing an advanced airway, and monitoring continuous waveform capnography, are recommendations in the AHA guidelines and should not interrupt CPR or defibrillation. Additionally, timely identification and treatment of the underlying cause of cardiac arrest is essential. The "Hs and Ts" are identified in the guidelines as potentially reversible causes of cardiac arrest and are as follows: hypovolemia, hypoxia, hydrogen ion excess (acidosis), hypoglycemia, hypo-/hyperkalemia, hypothermia, tension pneumothorax, tamponade (cardiac), toxins, thrombosis (pulmonary), and thrombosis (coronary). Examples of interventions that may be critical for effective resuscitation include crystalloid administration for hypovolemia due to sepsis, empiric fibrinolytic therapy for suspected pulmonary embolism, and needle decompression for tension pneumothorax.

Another integral component of ACLS is the timely identification and treatment of unstable bradyarrhythmias and tachyarrhythmias. "Unstable" is defined by the AHA guidelines as "a condition in which vital organ function is acutely impaired or cardiac arrest is ongoing or imminent," and it can be manifested as acute mental status changes,

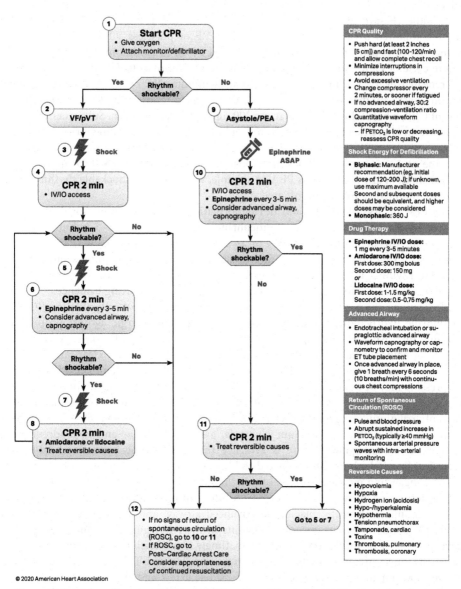

Figure 29.2 Adult cardiac arrest algorithm – 2020 update. pVT, pulseless VT; ET tube, endotracheal tube.

chest pain, acute heart failure, shock, and hypotension. Hypoxemia is a common cause of unstable bradycardia and tachycardia, and as a result each ACLS treatment algorithm begins with an evaluation of the patient's breathing by physical examination and monitors such as pulse oximetry. Patients often require supplemental oxygen and assistance with breathing.

Bradycardia is a heart rate less than 60 beats per minute and should be immediately treated if it is the cause of the patient's instability. The first-line treatment is atropine 0.5 mg IV, which can be repeated every 3–5 minutes up to a maximum dose of 3 mg. If the patient is unresponsive to atropine, a dopamine infusion at 2–10 μg/kg per minute, epinephrine at 2–10 μg per minute, or temporary transcutaneous pacing may be utilized. Expert consultation and/or transvenous pacing may also be required.

There are many types of tachycardia, and they can be classified according to whether they are narrow-complex or wide-complex, or regular or irregular. Additionally, they may or may not require treatment. However, for an unstable tachyarrhythmia, immediate synchronized cardioversion should follow. IV access and patient sedation should be established prior to cardioversion when possible, but should not delay cardioversion if the patient is too unstable.

Cardioversion is synchronized with the QRS complex, and the energy dose is adjusted depending on the nature of the rhythm. For unstable atrial fibrillation, the initial biphasic energy dose is 120–200 J. For unstable atrial flutter, the initial energy dose is 50–100 J. For unstable monomorphic/regular VT, the initial energy dose is 100 J. If synchronization is not possible, if the QRS complex has a polymorphic appearance, or if the appearance of the QRS complex cannot be determined, the energy dose should be set as high-energy unsynchronized shocks (i.e., energy doses used for defibrillation). It is important to note that with a heart rate less than 150 beats per minute and the absence of ventricular dysfunction, the tachyarrhythmia is more likely a secondary manifestation of the underlying condition, rather than the root cause of the patient's instability. If the patient is not hypotensive, the AHA guidelines suggest a trial of adenosine 6 mg IV with a 12 mg second dose if needed. In a stable patient with a tachyarrhythmia, further evaluation and intervention can be considered depending upon the nature of the QRS complex. If the QRS complex is wide ($\geq$ 0.12 seconds), the following can be considered: IV access, 12-lead ECG, adenosine if monomorphic, antiarrhythmic infusion, and cardiology consultation. The following antiarrhythmic infusions can be given: procainamide, amiodarone, or sotalol. If heart failure or QT prolongation is absent, procainamide should be administered at 20–50 mg per minute until arrhythmia resolves, hypotension occurs, or QRS increases to greater than 0.18 seconds (50% increase). After this initial dose, the maintenance dose of procainamide is 1–4 mg per minute. Alternatively, amiodarone can be given as 300 mg over 10 minutes and repeated at 150mg as necessary, followed by a maintenance dose of 1 mg/min for the first 6 hours. If QT prolongation is absent, sotalol can also be considered and given as 100 mg (1.5 mg/kg) over 5 minutes.

If the QRS complex is narrow ($\leq$ 0.12 seconds) in a stable patient with a tachyarrhythmia, the following can be considered: IV access, 12-lead ECG, vagal maneuvers (i.e., Valsalva maneuver, carotid sinus massage), adenosine if monomorphic, beta-blocker or calcium channel blocker, and cardiology consultation.

There are many pharmacologic treatment options for the various types of tachyarrhythmias, and a discussion of each is beyond the scope of this book. However, the current AHA guidelines provide drug tables that explain indications for use, dosing, common side effects, and contraindications for use.

Once ROSC has been achieved, the guidelines emphasize the need for prompt transition to post-cardiac-arrest care. For patients in an outpatient setting, transport to a hospital that can provide coronary intervention, neurologic care, critical care, and

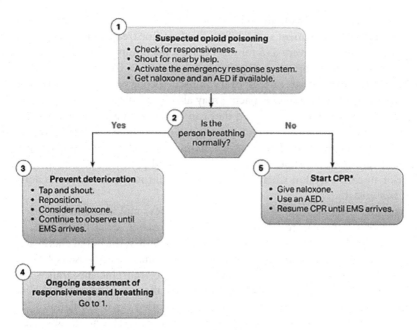

Figure 29.3 Adult opioid overdose management algorithm from 2020 AHA Guideline.

hypothermia is the first step. For inpatients who are in a hospital setting, transfer to a critical care unit is the next step. What the best care is for patients after an SCA is an ongoing area of research, but a timely initiation of a multidisciplinary, multisystem approach to patient care is vital, as most deaths occur in the first 24 hours.

Initial management of resuscitation for an opioid overdose should focus on the patient's airway and breathing (Figure 29.3). Begin by opening the airway followed by initiation of rescue breaths, ideally with the use of a bag-mask or barrier device and subsequent escalation of care to CPR if return of spontaneous breathing does not occur. Early activation of the emergency response system is critical as rescuers cannot be certain opioids alone are responsible for the person's status. Naloxone can be administered along with standard advanced cardiovascular life support care if it does not delay components of high-quality CPR [3]. Recurrent central nervous system and/ or respiratory depression may recur once the effect of naloxone has worn off. Thus, patients may require longer periods of observation or an infusion of naloxone before safe discharge.

Summary

The most recent AHA guidelines re-emphasize the role for early compressions (CAB). High-quality chest compressions (100–120 compressions a minute with enough force to depress the sternum approximately 5 cm and adequate time for complete recoil between compressions) are required to provide adequate blood flow to vital organs and achieve return of spontaneous circulation.

Early defibrillation for shockable rhythms should not be delayed in order to optimize resuscitation outcomes.

Two rescue breaths should be given after 30 compressions with immediate application of defibrillator pads. In a patient with an advanced airway in place, a breath should be given every 6–8 seconds (or 8–10 breaths per minute).

Minimizing disruptions to CPR is paramount, with no more than 10 seconds for any disruption.

Due to the extent of the opioid epidemic, if the cause of respiratory depression is suspected to be from an acute opioid overdose, resuscitation should begin with initiation of rescue breaths with escalation of care to CPR if no response is noted. Naloxone should be given to reverse opioid-induced respiratory depression, but should not delay CPR or activation of the emergency response system.

References

1. Panchal AR, Bartos JA, Cabañas JG, et al. Part 3: Adult basic and advanced life support: 2020 American Heart Association Guidelines for Cardiopulmonary Resuscitation and Emergency Cardiovascular Care. *Circulation.* 2020;142(16_Suppl_2): S366–468. doi:10.1161/ CIR.0000000000000916: PMID:33081529

2. Marsch S, Tschan F, Semmer NK, et al. ABC versus CAB for cardiopulmonary resuscitation: a prospective, randomized simulator-based trial. *Swiss Med Wkly.* 2013;143:w13856. doi:10.4414/ smw.2013.13856

3. Dezfulian C, Orkin AM, Maron BA, et al. Opioid-associated out-of-hospital cardiac arrest: distinctive clinical features and implications for health care and public responses: a scientific statement from the American Heart Association. *Circulation.* 2021;143(16):e836–70. doi:10.1161/CIR.0000000000000958; PMID:33682423

4. Swor RA, Jackson RE, Cynar M, et al. Bystander CPR, ventricular fibrillation, and survival in witnessed, unmonitored out-of-hospital cardiac arrest. *Ann Emerg Med.* 1995;25:780–4. doi: 10.1016/s0196-0644(95)70207-5

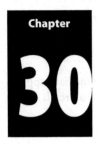

Emergency Resuscitation Algorithms: Infants and Children

Jue Teresa Wang

Introduction

Healthcare practitioners must always be prepared for an emergency situation in which they are responsible for the initial resuscitation of their patient. While the principles behind the emergency resuscitation of adults can be broadly applied to pediatric patients, there are many important differences to be noted. In infants and children, cardiac arrest most commonly occurs as the end result of progressive respiratory failure – hypoxemia, hypercapnia, and acidosis leading to bradycardia and hypotension, and, ultimately, cardiac arrest. This is in contrast to adults, in whom cardiac arrest is most often due to a primary cardiac cause. Pulseless ventricular tachycardia (VT) and ventricular fibrillation (VF) are found as the initial cardiac rhythm in approximately 7–10% of pediatric patients, with their incidence increasing with age. This chapter outlines an approach toward the resuscitation of pediatric patients adapted from the 2020 American Heart Association (AHA) guidelines for cardiopulmonary resuscitation and emergency cardiovascular care [1].

Pediatric Basic Life Support

Pediatric basic life support (BLS) encompasses prevention, early cardiopulmonary resuscitation (CPR), and prompt access to the emergency response system (Figure 30.1). As was the case in the 2015 AHA guidelines, in the 2020 AHA guidelines there continues to be a stronger emphasis on early chest compressions (compression–airway–breathing [CAB]).

Even stronger emphasis is placed on minimizing interruptions to chest compressions, such as during pulse and rhythm checks, with the time limited to less than 10 seconds as evidence shows worse resuscitation outcomes with increasing disruptions in CPR.

If a child is found unresponsive and not breathing (or only gasping), the healthcare provider should immediately send someone to activate the emergency response system and obtain an automated external defibrillator (AED) or other defibrillator. The healthcare provider should begin CPR (with chest compressions) after spending no longer than 10 seconds searching for a pulse. Any prolonged search for a pulse may be unreliable and time-consuming, delaying the onset of CPR. In infants, one should check for a brachial

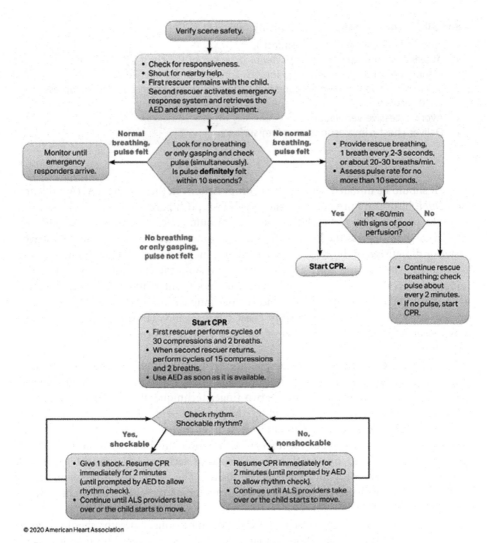

Figure 30.1 Pediatric basic life support algorithm for healthcare providers – two or more rescuers.

pulse, and in children, a femoral or carotid pulse. In the event that there is a lone rescuer, CPR should begin immediately with chest compressions and rescue breathing with a ratio of 30 compressions to 2 breaths for 2 minutes prior to activating the emergency response system and obtaining a defibrillator (if not already done). If 2 providers are present the ratio of compressions to rescue breaths should be 15:2.

If a child is found with a palpable pulse of 60 beats per minute or more but inadequate breathing, a rescue breath should be given every 2–3 seconds, or 20–30 breaths per minute, with pulse checks (lasting up to 10 seconds) every 2 minutes. If the pulse is less than 60 beats per minute and there are signs of poor perfusion despite support via oxygenation and ventilation, chest compressions should be initiated, as cardiac output in children is heavily dependent on the heart rate (HR).

> **Box 30.1** Characteristics of high-quality CPR
> - Rate 100–120 per minute ("push fast")
> - At least one-third the anterior-posterior diameter of the chest ("push hard") compressed: 1.5 inches (4 cm) in infants, 2 inches (5 cm) in children
> - Complete recoil between compressions Minimize interruption between compressions < 10 seconds
> - Avoid excessive ventilation
> - Deliver chest compressions on a firm surface

CPR should be initiated with 30 chest compressions. In the new 2020 AHA guidelines for a *child*, healthcare providers should "push fast, push hard," using the heel of 1 or 2 hands to provide 100–120 compressions per minute. Chest compression should have enough force to depress the lower half of the sternum at least one-third of the anterior-posterior dimension of the chest (approximately 2 inches, or 5 cm). One should take care to avoid the xiphoid and ribs. After each compression, the chest should be allowed to completely recoil so that the heart can refill with blood. Interruptions between compressions should be minimized, but to avoid rescuer fatigue, the compressor role should be rotated every 2 minutes. High-quality chest compressions (Box 30.1) are required to provide adequate blood flow to vital organs and achieve return of spontaneous circulation (ROSC).

In *infants*, the two-finger chest compression technique should be used when there is a lone healthcare provider, and the two-thumb-encircling hands technique should be used when there are two rescuers [2]. In the two-finger technique, the two fingers are placed below the intermammary line, avoiding the xiphoid and ribs. In the two-thumb–encircling hands technique, the infant's chest is encircled with both hands – fingers around the thorax and thumbs together over the lower third of the sternum – and the sternum is compressed by the thumbs. This latter technique is thought to provide improved coronary artery and systemic perfusion. The depth of compression should be at least one-third the anterior-posterior diameter of the chest (approximately 1.5 inches, or 4 cm).

In a scenario with a single rescuer, after 30 compressions, 2 breaths should be given with a jaw-thrust or head-tilt/chin-lift maneuver. For two-rescuer CPR, one provider is responsible for chest compressions and the other provider maintains an open airway and delivers ventilations at a 15:2 ratio. Ventilation is by bag-valve-mask ventilation. The patient's airway should be opened with a chin lift and a tight seal must be maintained between the mask and the patient's face [3].

When additional healthcare practitioners are present, a two-person bag-valve-mask technique may provide for more efficient ventilation. A small self-inflating bag with a volume of at least 450–500 mL should be used for infants and small children and an adult-sized bag (1,000 mL) should be used for older children.

Pediatric Advanced Life Support

Pediatric advanced life support (PALS) builds upon BLS and relies on a team of organized healthcare providers working effectively, rapidly, and simultaneously to resuscitate a patient [1]. While chest compressions begin, other providers must provide ventilation, obtain a defibrillator, connect monitors, establish vascular access (peripheral intravenous [IV] or intraosseous [IO] access), and determine which medications are to be administered. Also, extracorporeal life support should always be considered early, if available, when cardiac arrest is refractory to standard resuscitation and there is a potentially reversible cause (Figure 30.2). Emergency drugs can be administered IV or IO. Given the general difficulty in obtaining central venous access, this should be deferred until the patient has been stabilized. Initial resuscitation medications should be dosed based on actual body weight (not exceeding the standard adult dose) or determined with the use of a body-length tape with precalculated doses.

Beyond standard monitoring (electrocardiography, pulse oximetry, non-invasive blood pressure measurement), arterial catheterization and end-tidal carbon dioxide (CO_2) monitoring can be helpful in PALS resuscitation. An arterial waveform can be used to provide important information on adequacy of hand position and depth during chest compressions, as well as to indicate ROSC. In addition to confirmation of endotracheal tube position, capnography is essential to assess quality of compressions during CPR. With partial-pressure end-tidal CO_2 ($PETCO_2$) < 10–15 mmHg, one must be aware of the possibility of excessive ventilation or inefficient chest compressions. On the other hand, an abrupt and sustained increase in $PETCO_2$ may herald ROSC and may be able to prevent stopping compressions for an additional pulse check.

The PALS cardiac arrest algorithm organizes care around 2-minute periods of uninterrupted CPR. Based on a trained healthcare provider's interpretation of the ECG, or by AED analysis, the rhythm will either be "shockable" (e.g., VF or rapid pulseless VT) or "not shockable" (e.g., pulseless electrical activity [PEA] or asystole). For shockable rhythms defibrillation should be delivered early as it could be curative. Ideally, there should be minimal time between the last compression and shock delivery, after which compressions should immediately begin again. Compressions can continue while the defibrillator is charging, and, as described earlier, the initial shock can be given at a dose of 2 J/kg. If the rhythm is still shockable after 2 minutes of CPR, a shock should be given at 4 J/kg. And subsequent shocks should be given at 4 J/kg. This is in contrast to the 2015 guidelines to escalate the shock dose up to 10 J/kg. During CPR, epinephrine 0.1 mg/kg IV (maximum of 1 mg) should be administered every 3–5 minutes with chest compressions [2]. If epinephrine has been dosed, amiodarone (5 mg/kg IV bolus) can also be given repeated up to 2 times. In the absence of amiodarone, lidocaine 1 mg/kg IV loading dose with 20–50 µg/kg per minute infusion can be given. Attempts should be made to treat reversible causes of cardiac arrest. (These include analysis of events leading to the arrest as well as checking for the "H's and T's" that can lead to or cause PEA; see Figure 30.2.)

If defibrillation is successful, a pulse must be verified and, if present, post-cardiac-arrest care should commence. If VF or pulseless VT recurs, CPR should be restarted, amiodarone should be administered, and a shock should be delivered at a dose at least equal to the previous successful dose. If at any time the rhythm becomes "non-shockable," management switches to the PEA/asystole algorithm. In non-shockable rhythms, CPR is the mainstay of therapy. Epinephrine should be administered as described previously, and the rhythm should be rechecked every 2 minutes for either an organized or shockable rhythm. Reversible causes should be explored and treated.

Since ventilation is key, various airway devices may aid in ventilating the patient. Oropharyngeal and nasopharyngeal airways may help to maintain a patent airway. It is important to select an appropriate size in order to maintain an open airway but avoid

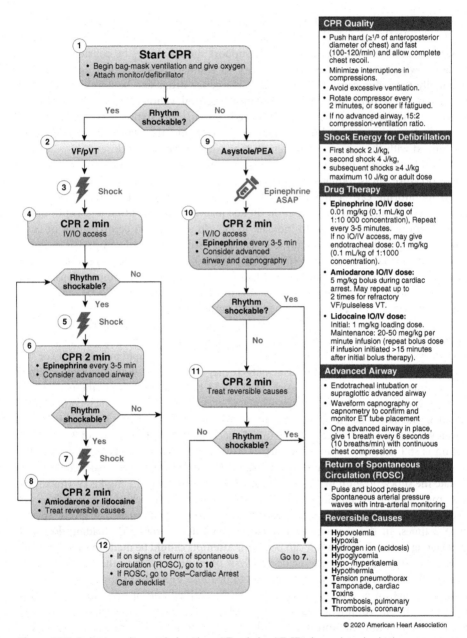

Figure 30.2 Pediatric cardiac arrest algorithm. pVT, pulseless VT; ET tube, endotracheal tube.

obstruction. A laryngeal mask airway can be considered when ventilation is unsuccessful and endotracheal intubation is not possible. Endotracheal intubation requires a trained provider, as the pediatric airway poses challenges given the different airway anatomy in children. When appropriate, endotracheal intubation should be facilitated with rapid sequence induction and confirmed with condensation on endotracheal tube, bilateral chest rise and equal breath sounds, exhaled CO_2 on capnometry or capnography, and chest X-ray. When an advanced airway is in place, a breath is given every 6–8 seconds (or 8–10 breaths per minute). If a patient's condition worsens, consider dislocation or obstruction of the tube, pneumothorax, or equipment errors.

When circulation has been restored and arterial oxyhemoglobin saturation monitoring is possible, begin titrating down the inspired oxygen concentration (if appropriate equipment is available). Given the risk of harm from hyperoxemia, there is a recommendation to titrate down inspired oxygen to maintain an arterial oxyhemoglobin concentration $< 100\%$ and $\geq 94\%$. Note that adequate oxygen delivery to end organs is determined by arterial oxyhemoglobin saturation, as well as cardiac output and hemoglobin concentration.

In a child with bradycardia (HR $<$ 60 beats per minute), supplemental oxygen should be provided, IV access should be obtained, and an ECG monitor/defibrillator should be attached. No further action needs to be taken if ventilation and perfusion are adequate. However, if there are signs of cardiorespiratory symptoms such as poor perfusion in a patient with bradycardia, CPR should be initiated and the patient should be reevaluated after 2 minutes. Epinephrine 0.01 mg/kg IV should be given for persistent bradycardia. Atropine 0.02 mg/kg IV should be given for bradycardia due to increased vagal tone or atrioventricular block. Transcutaneous pacing should be used for complete heart block or sinus node dysfunction.

In a child with tachycardia, one should first check for pulses and assess perfusion. If the patient has poor perfusion or is pulseless, immediately begin the PALS algorithm as described earlier. Otherwise, place monitors, provide supplemental oxygen, obtain vascular access and a 12-lead ECG. Once the ECG is available, determine the QRS duration. A narrow-complex tachycardia (QRS $\leq$ 0.09 s) may be either sinus tachycardia (for which reversible causes should be explored and treated) or a supraventricular tachycardia. In a hemodynamically stable patient, begin with vagal stimulation by carotid sinus massage, Valsalva maneuver, or, in infants and young children, apply ice to the face. If this is unsuccessful, chemical cardioversion with adenosine 0.1 mg/kg IV given rapidly followed by an immediate saline flush should be attempted. Verapamil 0.1–0.3 mg/kg IV can also be used in older children. If this is ineffective, electric synchronized cardioversion is recommended, preferably with sedation, starting at a dose of 0.5–1 J/kg. If unsuccessful, the dose should be increased to 2 J/kg. Prior to a third shock, amiodarone 5 mg/kg IV (infused over 20–60 minutes) or procainamide 15 mg/kg IV (infused over 30–60 minutes) should be given. Expert consultation should be obtained prior to this if the patient is hemodynamically stable.

In a stable child with wide-complex tachycardia (QRS $>$ 0.09 s), expert consultation is strongly recommended, because all treatments have serious potential adverse effects. Pharmacologic and electric cardioversion are both part of treatment that should be guided by an expert in pediatric arrhythmias. Drugs used in the treatment of wide-complex tachycardias are amiodarone IV/IO 5 mg/kg over 20–60 minutes or procainamide IV/IO 15mg/ kg over 30–60 minutes. In hemodynamically unstable patients, electric cardioversion with 0.5–1 J/kg is recommended, and, if unsuccessful, the dose should be increased to 2 J/kg.

The resuscitation of infants and children with congenital heart disease is not described in this chapter. However, the 2020 AHA guidelines for CPR and ECC do contain recommendations for the emergency management of these patients and should be reviewed as necessary.

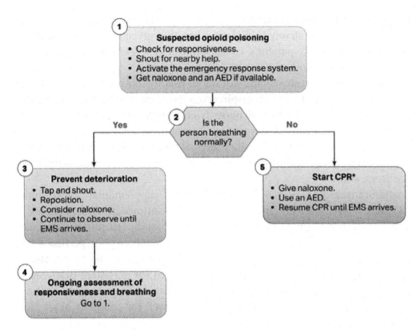

Figure 30.3 2020 AHA guideline for opioid-related emergency response.

Despite improvement in CPR outcomes, the majority of children with cardiac arrest either do not survive or survive but with significant impairment. Studies have shown that the inclusion of family members during resuscitation has helped family members cope with long-term grief and trauma following such an event.

Initial management of resuscitation for an opioid overdose should focus on the patient's airway and breathing. Begin by opening the airway followed by initiation of rescue breaths, ideally with the use of a bag-mask or barrier device and subsequent escalation of care to CPR if return of spontaneous breathing does not occur. Early activation of the emergency response system is critical as rescuers cannot be certain opioids alone are responsible for the person's status. Naloxone can be administered along with standard advanced cardiovascular life support care if it does not delay components of high-quality CPR. Recurrent central nervous system and/or respiratory depression may recur once the effect of naloxone has worn off thus patients may require longer periods of observation before safe discharge. There were no pediatric data supporting these recommendations; however, due to the urgency of the opioid crisis, the adult recommendations should be applied to children (Figure 30.3).

Summary

Most recent AHA guidelines re-emphasize the role for early compressions (CAB). High-quality chest compressions (100–120 compressions a minute with enough force to depress the sternum approximately 5 cm and adequate time for complete recoil between compressions) are required to provide adequate blood flow to vital organs and achieve return of spontaneous circulation.

Two rescue breaths should be given after 30 compressions if there is a single rescuer or after 15 compressions if there are two rescuers. In a patient with an advanced airway in place, a breath should be given every 6–8 seconds (or 8–10 breaths per minute).

In a child who is unresponsive or not breathing, the healthcare provider should delegate someone to activate the emergency response system and obtain a defibrillator, while the healthcare provider starts CPR with chest compressions. If there is a lone rescuer, 2 minutes of chest compressions with rescue breaths should be initiated prior to activating the emergency response system and obtaining a defibrillator.

The PALS cardiac arrest algorithm organizes care around 2-minute periods of uninterrupted CPR. If a patient's ECG rhythm is "shockable," defibrillation should occur immediately after the last compression and CPR should begin again with chest compressions immediately following delivery of the shock.

Due to the extent of the opioid epidemic, if a child is suspected of having respiratory depression from an acute opioid overdose resuscitation should begin with initiation of rescue breaths with escalation of care to CPR if no response is noted. Naloxone should be given to reverse opioid-induced respiratory depression, but should not delay CPR or activation of the emergency response system.

References

1. Topjian AA, Raymond TT, Atkins D, et al. Part 4: Pediatric basic and advanced life support: 2020 American Heart Association Guidelines for cardiopulmonary resuscitation and emergency cardiovascular care. *Circulation*. 2020;142(16_Suppl_2):S469–523. doi:10.1161/CIR.0000000000000901; PMID:33081526

2. Andersen LW, Berg KM, Saindon BZ, et al. Time to epinephrine and survival after pediatric in-hospital cardiac arrest. *JAMA*. 2015;314:802–10. doi:10.1001/jama.2015.9678

3. Hansen ML, Lin A, Eriksson C, et al. A comparison of pediatric airway management techniques during out-of-hospital cardiac arrest using the CARES database. *Resuscitation*. 2017;120:51–6. doi:10.1016/j.resuscitation.2017.08.015

Guidelines and Standards

Chelsi J. Flanagan, Paul B. Hankey, Jennifer S. Xiong, Alan D. Kaye, Richard D. Urman, and Elyse M. Cornett

American Academy of Pediatrics (AAP) and American Academy of Pediatric Dentistry (AAPD)

AAP: Guidelines for monitoring and management of pediatric patients before, during, and after sedation for diagnostic and therapeutic procedures: update 2019. Available at https://publications.aap.org/pediatrics/article/143/6/e20191000/37173/Guidelines-for-Monitoring-and-Management-of AADP 2019

Guideline for monitoring and management of pediatric patients during and after sedation for diagnostic and therapeutic procedures. Available at www.aapd.org/globalassets/media/policies_guidelines/bp_monitoringsedation.pdf?v=newAADP 2012

Policy on the use of deep sedation and general anesthesia in the pediatric dental office. Available at www.aapd.org/assets/1/7/P_Sedation1.PDF

American Association of Critical-Care Nurses (AACN)

Position statement on the role of the RN in the management of patients receiving IV moderate sedation for short-term therapeutic, diagnostic, or surgical procedures (2002). Available at www.aacn.org/policy-and-advocacy/position-statements

American Association of Nurse Anesthetists (AANA)

Standards for nurse anesthesia practice. Available at https://issuu.com/aanapublishing/docs/standards_for_nurse_anesthesia_practice_2.23

Position statement on the qualified providers of sedation and analgesia: considerations for policy guidelines for registered nurses engaged in the administration of sedation and analgesia (2003). Available at www.aana.com

Latex allergy protocol. Available at www.aana.com/practice-manual/aana-practice-manual-latex-allergy-management

Non-anesthesia provider procedural sedation and analgesia. Available at www.aana.com

American Association of Oral and Maxillofacial Surgeons (AAOMS)

Parameters of care: clinical practice guidelines for oral and maxillofacial surgery (AAOMS ParCare 2017). Available at www.aaoms.org/images/uploads/pdfs/parcare_assessment.pdf

Statement by the American Association of Oral and Maxillofacial Surgeons concerning the management of selected clinical conditions and associated clinical procedures: the control of pain and anxiety (2017). Available at –www.aaoms.org/docs/practice_resources/

clinical_resources/control_of_pain_
and_anxiety.pdf

Anesthesia in outpatient facilities
(AAOMS ParCare 2017). Available at
www.aaoms.org/images/uploads/pdfs/
parcare_anesthesia_1.pdf

American College of Cardiology (ACC) and American Heart Association (AHA)

ACC/AHA guidelines on perioperative
cardiovascular evaluation and care for
noncardiac surgery (2014). *J Am Coll
Cardiol.* 2007;130:e278–333. Available
at www.jacc.org/doi/abs/10.1016/j.jacc
.2007.09.003

2014 ACC/AHA guideline on
perioperative cardiovascular evaluation
and management of patients
undergoing noncardiac surgery: a
report of the American College of
Cardiology/American Heart
Association Task Force on Practice
Guidelines. Available at http://content
.onlinejacc.org/article.aspx?
articleid=1893784

Interventional cardiology: procedural
sedation for interventional cardiology
procedures 2013. *Int Anesthesiol Clin.*
2013; 51(2): 112–26

American College of Emergency Physicians (ACEP)

Procedural sedation and analgesia.
Available at www.acep.org/patient-care/
clinical-policies/procedural-sedation-
and-analgesia

ACEP policy statement: sedation in the
emergency department (2017 revision).
Available at www.acep.org/patient-care/
policy-statements/procedural-sedation-
in-the-emergency-department/

Clinical policy: procedural sedation and
analgesia in the emergency department.
AnnEmerg Med. 2014;63(2):247–58.e18.
Available at https://pubmed.ncbi.nlm
.nih.gov/24438649/

Policy statement: delivery of agents for
procedural sedation and analgesia by
emergency nurses (2022). Available at
www.acep.org

American College of Radiology (ACR) and Society of Interventional Radiology (SIR)

ACR–SIR practice guideline for
sedation and analgesia. Revised 2020.
Available at www.acr.org/-/media/acr/
files/practice-parameters/sed-analgesia
.pdf

American Dental Association (ADA) and American Dental Society of Anesthesiology (ADSA)

Guidelines for the use of sedation and
general anesthesia by dentists. Available
at www.ada.org/-/media/project/ada-
organization/ada/ada-org/files/
publications/cdt/anesthesia_guidelines
.pdf

American Nurses Association (ANA)

Procedural sedation consensus
statement (2008). Available at www
.nursingworld.org/practice-policy/
nursing-excellence/official-position-
statements/id/procedural-sedation-
consensus-statement

American Society for Gastrointestinal Endoscopy (ASGE)

Standards of practice guidelines.
Available at www.asge.org/publications/
publications

Position statement: nonanesthesiologist
administration of propofol for GI
endoscopy (2009). *Gastrointest Endosc.*
2009;70:1053–9

Sedation and anesthesia in GI
endoscopy (2008). *Gastrointest Endosc.*
2018;87(2):327–37.

Guidelines for conscious sedation and
monitoring during gastrointestinal

endoscopy (2003). *Gastrointest Endosc.* 2003;58:317–22

American Society of Anesthesiologists (ASA)

Standards for basic anesthetic monitoring (2020). Available at www.asahq.org/standards-and-guidelines/standards-for-basic-anesthetic-monitoring

Statement on anesthetic care during interventional pain procedures for adults. Available at www.asahq.org/standards-and-practice-parameters/statement-on-anesthetic-care-during-interventional-pain-procedures-for-adults

Statement on granting privileges for deep sedation to non-anesthesiologist sedation practitioners (2021). Available at www.asahq.org/standards-and-guidelines/statement-of-granting-privileges-for-administration-of-moderate-sedation-to-practitioners)

Continuum of depth of sedation: definition of general anesthesia and levels of sedation/analgesia. Available at www.asahq.org/standards-and-practice-parameters/statement-on-continuum-of-depth-of-sedation-definition-of-general-anesthesia-and-levels-of-sedation-analgesia

Distinguishing monitored anesthesia care ("MAC") from moderate sedation/analgesia (conscious sedation). Available at www.asahq.org/standards-and-practice-parameters/statement-on-distinguishing-monitored-anesthesia-care-from-moderate-sedation-analgesia

Guidelines for office-based anesthesia. Available at www.asahq.org/standards-and-guidelines/guidelines-for-office-based-anesthesia

Standards for postanesthesia care. Available at www.asahq.org/standards-and-practice-parameters/standards-for-postanesthesia-care

Statement on qualifications of anesthesia providers in the office-based setting. Available at www.asahq.org/standards-and-practice-parameters/statement-on-qualifications-of-anesthesia-providers-in-the-office-based-setting

Statement on safe use of propofol. Available at www.asahq.org/standards-and-practice-parameters/statement-on-safe-use-of-propofol

Statement on nonoperating room anesthetizing locations. Available at www.asahq.org/standards-and-guidelines/statement-on-nonoperating-room-anesthetizing-locations

Guidelines for ambulatory anesthesia and surgery. Available at www.asahq.org/standards-and-guidelines/guidelines-for-ambulatory-anesthesia-and-surgery

Statement on granting privileges for administration of moderate sedation to practitioners who are not anesthesia professionals. Available at www.asahq.org/standards-and-guidelines/statement-of-granting-privileges-for-administration-of-moderate-sedation-to-practitioners

Statement on granting privileges to non anesthesiologist practitioners for personally administering deep sedation or supervising deep sedation by individuals who are not anesthesia professionals (2022). Available at www.asahq.org/standards-and-practice-parameters/statement-on-granting-privileges-for-deep-sedation-to-non-anesthesiologist-physicians

Practice guidelines for sedation and analgesia by non-anesthesiologists (2002). *Anesthesiology.* 2002;96:1004–17. Available at https://pubs.asahq.org/anesthesiology/article/96/4/1004/39315/Practice-Guidelines-for-Sedation-and-Analgesia-by

Practice advisory for preanesthesia evaluation. *Anesthesiology* 2012: 116:522–38.

American Society of Interventional Pain Physicians (ASIPP)

Interventional techniques in the management of chronic pain: Part 2.0, *Pain Physician.* 2001;4(1):24–96. Available at https://pubmed.ncbi.nlm .nih.gov/16906171

ASIPP guidelines for sedation and fasting status of patients undergoing interventional pain management procedures. *Pain Physician.* 2019;22 (3):201–7. Available at https://pubmed .ncbi.nlm.nih.gov/31151329

Association of Perioperative Registered Nurses (AORN)

Guideline implementation: moderate sedation/analgesia. Available at https:// aornjournal.onlinelibrary.wiley.com/ doi/abs/10.1016/j.aorn.2016.03.001

Position statement on allied health care providers and support personnel in the perioperative practice setting. Available at www.aorn.org/guidelines-resources/ clinical-resources/position-statements

Position statement on creating a practice environment of safety. Available at www.aorn.org/guidelines-resources/clinical-resources/position-statements

Perioperative standards and recommended practices. Available at www.aornbookstore.org

Position statement on one perioperative registered nurse circulator dedicated to every patient undergoing a surgical or other invasive procedure. Available at www.aorn.org/guidelines-resources/ clinical-resources/position-statements

Recommended practices for managing the patient receiving moderate sedation/analgesia. Available at https://

health.ucdavis.edu/cppn/documents/ classes/sedation/AORN%20Guidelines_ 2011.pdf

AORN position statement on delegation in perioperative practice setting. Available at www.aorn.org/ guidelines/clinical-resources/position-statements

Centers for Medicare and Medicaid Services (CMS)

CMS interpretive guidelines for anesthesia and sedation (summary). Available at www.cms.gov/Regulations-and-Guidance/Guidance/Transmittals/ downloads/R59SOMA.pdf

Emergency medicine and CMS interpretive guidelines. Available at www.cms.gov/Regulations-and-Guidance/Guidance/transmittals/ downloads/R46SOMA.pdf

CMS revised hospital anesthesia services interpretive guidelines. Available at www.cms.gov/Medicare/ Provider-Enrollment-and-Certification/ SurveyCertificationGenInfo/ downloads/SCLetter10_09.pdf

CMS emergency preparedness interpretive guidelines. Available at www.cms.gov/medicare/provider-enrollment-and-certification/ surveycertificationgeninfo/downloads/ survey-and-cert-letter-17-29.pdf

The Joint Commission

Sedation under the JCI Standard 2011. Available at www.ncbi.nlm.nih.gov/ pmc/articles/PMC3198177

Comprehensive Accreditation Manual for Hospitals (CAMH): The Official Handbook (2023 update). Available at www.jcrinc.com

The Joint Commission office-based surgery accreditation. Available at www .jointcommission.org/resources/news-and-multimedia/fact-sheets/facts-about-office-based-surgery-accreditation/

Society of Critical Care Medicine (SCCM)

Clinical practice guidelines for the management of pain, agitation, and delirium in adult patients in the intensive care unit *Crit Care Med.* 2013;41(1):263–306. Available at journals.lww.com/ccmjournal/Fulltext/2013/01000/Clinical_Practice_Guidelines_for_the_Management_of.29.aspx

Index

Page numbers: **bold**=box or table, *italics*=figure